Llewellyn- nes

Fundamentals of **Obstetrics** and **Gynaecology**

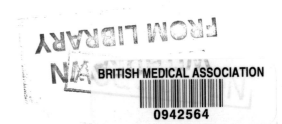

For Elsevier:

Commissioning Editor: Pauline Graham
Development Editor: Ailsa Laing
Project Manager: Kerrie-Anne McKinlay
Designer: Kirsteen Wright
Illustration Manager: Merlyn Harvey
Illustrators: Jennifer Rose, Amanda Williams, Debra Woodward and AntBits

Llewellyn-Jones
Fundamentals of Obstetrics and Gynaecology

9th
EDITION

Edited by

Jeremy Oats MBBS DM FRCOG FRANZCOG

Chair Victorian, Consultative Council on Obstetric and Paediatric Mortality and Mobility; Professional Fellow, Department of Obstetrics and Gynaecology, University of Melbourne; Adjunct Professor, School of Public Health, La Trobe University, Melbourne, Australia

Suzanne Abraham MSc PhD (Med) MAPS

Associate Professor, Department of Obstetrics and Gynaecology, Sydney Medical School, Royal North Shore Hospital, University of Sydney; Director, Eating Disorder Unit, Northside Clinic, University of Sydney, Australia

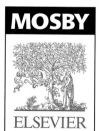

Edinburgh   London   New York   Oxford   Philadelphia   St Louis   Sydney   Toronto   2010

MOSBY
ELSEVIER

Ninth Edition © 2010, Elsevier Limited. All rights reserved.
Eighth Edition © Elsevier Limited 2005
Seventh Edition © Elsevier Limited 1999
Sixth Edition © Mosby Professional Ltd 1994

ISBN 978 0 7234 3509 9
International Edition ISBN 978 0 7234 3508 2

British Library Cataloguing in Publication Data
A catalogue record for this book is available from the British Library

Library of Congress Cataloging in Publication Data
A catalog record for this book is available from the Library of Congress

Notice

Knowledge and best practice in this field are constantly changing. As new research and experience broaden our knowledge, changes in practice, treatment and drug therapy may become necessary or appropriate. Readers are advised to check the most current information provided (i) on procedures featured or (ii) by the manufacturer of each product to be administered, to verify the recommended dose or formula, the method and duration of administration, and contraindications. It is the responsibility of the practitioner, relying on their own experience and knowledge of the patient, to make diagnoses, to determine dosages and the best treatment for each individual patient, and to take all approprate safety precautions. To the fullest extent of the law, neither the Publisher nor the Authors assume any liability for any injury and/or damage to persons or property arising out of or related to any use of the material contained in this book.

The Publisher

ELSEVIER your source for books,
journals and multimedia
in the health sciences
www.elsevierhealth.com

Working together to grow
libraries in developing countries

www.elsevier.com | www.bookaid.org | www.sabre.org

ELSEVIER BOOK AID International Sabre Foundation

The
publisher's
policy is to use
**paper manufactured
from sustainable forests**

Printed in China

Contents

Preface
to the ninth edition

Publication of this ninth edition of *Fundamentals of Obstetrics and Gynaecology* comes some 40 years later than the first edition, published by Derek Llewellyn-Jones in 1969. In his introduction to the first edition, Derek Llewellyn-Jones quoted from the World Health Organization Technical Report Series 1952, no. 51:

> *The object of maternity care is to ensure that every expectant and nursing mother maintains good health, learns the art of child care, has a normal delivery, and bears healthy children.*

In 2010 these objectives remain as salutary as they were in 1952. Intervention rates continue to climb and many women are embarking on pregnancy later in life and with more complex medical disorders; the need for those caring for women and their children to apply the best available standards of care is even more critical. In this ninth edition we have endeavoured to continue the tradition established by Derek Llewellyn-Jones and added where relevant a synthesis from the recommendations from high quality evidence-based guidelines and practice reports.

As with previous editions we have not included a bibliography of references as they are quickly rendered out-of-date. Our hope is that medical, midwifery and nursing students reading this book will use it as the basis on which to establish their 'fundamental' understanding of women's health and then pursue more detailed knowledge through the readily accessible electronic databases and their own experience.

We remain indebted to our colleagues and our readers for their many helpful suggestions and criticisms and corrections.

So, in the words of Derek Llewellyn-Jones, it is our hope 'that *Fundamentals of Obstetrics and Gynaecology* will continue to meet the needs of today's medical students and students of nursing and midwifery, and will encourage self-learning skills while providing essential information in a readable manner'.

Jeremy Oats and Suzanne Abraham

Acknowledgements

We particularly wish to thank the following for their substantial contribution to this ninth edition.

Dr Neil Roy for his meticulous revision of Chapters 26 and 27; Dr Helen Savoia for updating the section on haematological disorders in Chapter 15; Dr Amanda Sampson for her generous provision of all the ultrasound images; Associate Professor Suzanne Garland for her detailed review of Chapters 17 and 33, and for permission to use her photographs reproduced in Figs 34.1, 34.2 and 34.3; the Educational Resource Centre at the Royal Women's Hospital, Melbourne for allowing us to reproduce their illustrations on the management of shoulder dystocia (Fig. 22.5); Dr Aldo Vacca for the photograph of the Vacuum Extractor Omnicup (Fig. 24.16); Essure for the photograph of the Essure device (Fig. 31.9); Organon for the photograph of the Implanon device (Fig. 31.5).

Also: Dr John Bell, John Gocking, Dr Jenny King, Gwen Moody, Dr Diane Payton, Susan Hart and Down Syndrome Association for generously providing pathology and clinical photographs.

Figures 26.3 and 41.2 are reproduced from Lissauer T, Clayden G. *Illustrated Textbook of Paediatrics*, Second Edition, Mosby; 2001, with permission.

Figure credits

Fig. 3.3 redrawn from Patten. *Tend Act Gynecol et Obstet* 1959, Montreal: Beachemin

Fig. 3.5 redrawn from Hertig AJ and Rock. *J Contrib Embry Carnegie Inst* 1941, 29:127

Fig. 3.7 redrawn from Hamilton, Boyd and Mossman. *Human Embryology*, Cambridge: Heffer; 1962

Fig. 7.8 redrawn from Danforth DN and Ivy AC. *Amer J Obstet Gynecol* 1949, 57:831

Figs 7.16, 7.17, 7.18, 22.1, 22.2, 22.3 redrawn from Caldeyro-Barcia R and Poseiro JJ. *Trans Cong Int Gynecol et Obstet* 1958. Montreal: Libairie Beauchemin; 1959

Fig. 8.2 redrawn from J Studd

Fig. 8.3 redrawn from Greenhill. *Obstetrics*, 13th edn. Saunders; 1965

Fig. 42.3 reproduced with permission from Sambrook PN, Dequeker J and Rasp HH, Metabolic bone diseases. In: Klippel JH, Dieppe PA eds. Rheumatology, 2nd edn. London: Mosby; 1998: 8.36.1

Data

Fig. 2.2 data from Aptar D et al. *Acta Paediatr Scand* 1978, 67: 417

Fig. 3.11 data from Dawes GS. *Am J Obstet Gynecol* 1962, 84: 1643

Fig. 5.5 data from Hytten and Leitch, *The Physiology of Human Pregnancy*, 2nd edn. Oxford: Blackwell; 1971

Fig. 26.5 data from Cuckle et al. *Br Med J* 1987, 94: 387–402

Table 22.1 data from Cardozo LD et al. *BJ Obstet Gynaecol* 1982, 89: 33–38

Chapter | **1** |

Gynaecological and obstetric history and examination

THE WOMAN PRESENTING WITH GYNAECOLOGICAL PROBLEMS

It is generally accepted that most gynaecological problems are medical or psychological, rather than surgical. For this reason it is crucial that a careful history of the woman's complaints is obtained.

History

Doctors must be sensitive to the woman's beliefs and feelings, tactful, communicative, courteous, gentle and unhurried. The history of the patient's complaints should be recorded sequentially.

The manner in which the woman answers questions may give a clue to the origin of the complaint. This is important, as studies in the UK and Australia show that 14–17% of women have psychiatric morbidity. Other studies have noted a significant relationship between gynaecological symptoms, adverse life events and psychiatric morbidity. The doctor should exclude depression by inquiring about sadness, irritability, fatigue and so on. The questions should seek information about the woman's:

- **Menstrual history.** Age at menarche; duration of the menstrual cycle; menstrual pain; and the duration and severity of menstruation. This may cause some confusion. For example, if the woman says that she bleeds for 5 days every 20 days, the doctor may believe that her periods are occurring too frequently. The doctor may need to explain that the menstrual cycle starts on day 1 of bleeding and includes the menstrual phase as well as the interval between menstrual bleeds. The woman in the example given in this designation would bleed for 5 days every 25 days, which is normal. This designation is conveniently recorded as 5/25.
- **Obstetric history** (if any). The number of pregnancies and the outcome, that is, spontaneous miscarriages or induced abortions; ectopic gestation; children born, their birthweights and the year of the birth of each; complications occurring during pregnancy, labour or the puerperium (the end of the third stage of labour until involution of the uterus is complete, i.e. approximately 6 weeks).
- **Previous medical history (past illnesses and operations) and family history**
- **Psychological and psychiatric history and family history**
- **Current medications**
- **Sexual history.** This needs to be obtained with sensitivity, and matters such as physical and sexual abuse should be left until later in the interview. An explanation of why such questions are being asked will help communication.

- Details of contraceptive use, including any side-effects
- History of the main complaint.

In an older woman more emphasis should be placed on the menopausal history rather than menarche and menstruation.

Examination

Unless the patient has been seen recently, a general examination should be carried out as the gynaecological complaint may only be a local manifestation of a general disorder. This examination, which can be performed quite quickly, should include inspection of the head and neck, palpation of the supraclavicular areas for enlarged lymph nodes, auscultation of the heart and lungs, and determination of the pulse rate and blood pressure.

The gynaecological portion of the examination should include:

- A breast examination
- An abdominal examination
- An inspection of the external genitalia
- A pelvic examination, by speculum, and then digitally as a bimanual vaginoabdominal examination
- A rectal examination in certain instances.

Breast examination

With the patient sitting facing the examiner, the breasts are inspected, first with the patient's arms at her sides and then with her arms raised above her head (Fig. 1.1). The shape, contour and size of the breasts, their height on the chest wall, and the position of the nipples are compared, any nipple retraction being noted. The supraclavicular regions and axillae are next palpated. The latter can only be palpated satisfactorily if the pectoral muscles are relaxed. This relaxation can be obtained if the physician supports the patient's arms while palpating the axillae. Palpation is then performed with the patient lying supine, her shoulders elevated on a small pillow. Palpation should be gentle and orderly, using the flat of the fingers of one hand. Each portion of the breast should be palpated systematically, beginning at the upper, inner quadrant, followed by palpation of each portion sequentially until the upper, outer quadrant is finally examined.

The breast self-examination that many doctors recommend to women is similar to the breast examination made by the doctor, except that the woman usually does not palpate the axillary area. Figure 1.1 demonstrates how a woman should examine her breasts. The technique can easily be taught to her by her doctor.

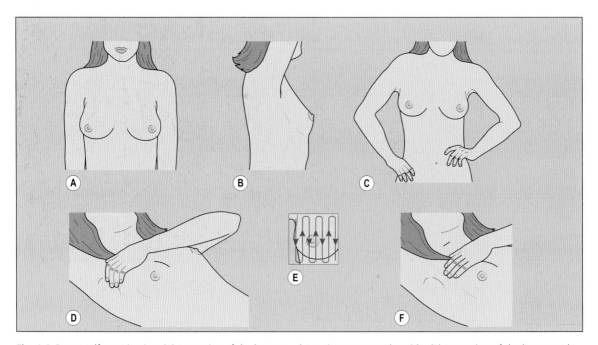

Fig. 1.1 Breast self-examination. (A) Inspection of the breasts – the patient's arms at her side. (B) Inspection of the breasts – the patient's arms raised above her head. During the inspection, the contour of the breasts, the size and shape of the areolae and the condition of the nipples are examined. An indentation or a bulge in the contour may indicate a lesion. (C) Placing hand on hip tenses the pectoralis major, accentuating any tethering from an infiltrating neoplasm. (D) Axillary palpation. (E) Systematic examination of four quadrants of the breast. (F) Palpation of the upper outer quadrant of the breast.

Abdominal examination

The examination is conducted with the patient lying comfortably on her back, having emptied her bladder immediately beforehand. Inspection of the abdomen will show its contour, and the presence of striae and scars or of dilated veins. If the patient raises her head and coughs, hernias and divarication of the recti abdominis muscles will be evident. Palpation of the viscera is performed systematically, the liver, the gallbladder, the spleen and the kidneys being palpated in turn. The caecum and colon are next palpated, the hand pressing down gently as the patient breathes out. Percussion may be required if the presence of free fluid is suspected.

Pelvic examination

The pelvic examination should follow the abdominal examination and should never be omitted unless the patient is a virgin. The external genitalia are first inspected under a good light with the patient in the dorsal position, the hips flexed and abducted, and knees flexed. If she or the doctor prefers, she may lie in the left lateral position. Some women are more comfortable and feel less exposed in the latter position. The patient must have voided just before the examination (unless she is complaining of stress incontinence), and should preferably have defacated that morning. If urinary infection is suspected, a midstream specimen of urine may be obtained at this time.

The patient is asked to strain down, to enable detection of any evidence of prolapse, after which a bivalve speculum is inserted and the cervix visualized. For the woman's comfort the speculum should be warmed and the doctor's approach sensitive and communicative. If the physician intends to take a cervical smear to examine the exfoliated cells, no lubricant apart from water should be used on the speculum. The vagina and cervix are inspected by opening the bivalve speculum (Fig. 1.2). If the patient has a prolapse, the degree of the vaginal wall or uterine descent can best be assessed if a Sims speculum is used, with the patient in the left lateral position (Fig. 1.3).

Digital examination follows, one or two fingers of the gloved hand being introduced. For the right-handed person it is usual to use the right hand as the fingers of this hand are more 'educated', and vice versa for the left-handed person. After the labia minora have been separated with the left hand to expose the vestibule, the fingers are introduced, passing upwards and backwards to palpate the cervix. The left hand simultaneously palpates the pelvis through the abdominal wall, so that the uterus and ovaries may be palpated. Normal Fallopian tubes (oviducts) are never palpable. As the intravaginal fingers push the cervix backwards, the abdominally located hand is placed just below the umbilicus and the fingers reach down into the pelvis, slowly and smoothly, until the fundus is caught between them and the fingers of the right hand in the anterior vaginal fornix (Fig. 1.4).

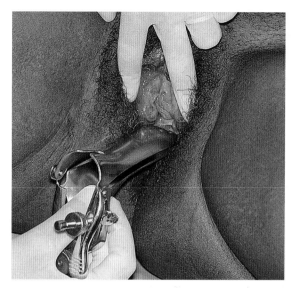

Fig. 1.2 Introducing the bivalve speculum. Care should be taken to avoid applying painful pressure on the urethra by inserting the speculum initially obliquely.

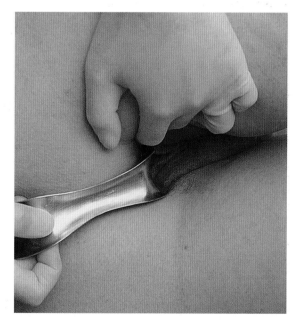

Fig. 1.3 The patient in the left lateral position; a Sims speculum has been inserted into the vagina.

The information obtained by bimanual examination includes:

- **By palpation of the uterus.** Position, size, shape, consistency, mobility, tenderness, attachments. The normal uterus is positioned either anteriorly or posteriorly and is about 9 cm long. It is pear-shaped

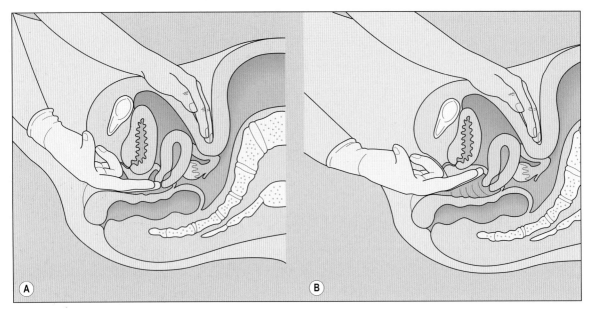

Fig. 1.4 Bimanual examination of the uterus. Note that the bladder is empty, the patient having voided just before the examination. (A) The vaginal fingers push the cervix back and upwards so that the fundus can be reached by the abdominally located fingers. (B) The vaginally located fingers now palpate the anterior surface of the uterus, which is held in position by the abdominally located fingers.

and firm in consistency, and can be moved in all directions. It is normally tender when squeezed between the two hands.

- **By palpation of the ovaries and Fallopian tubes.** The tips of the vaginally located fingers are placed in each lateral fornix in turn and then pushed backwards and upwards as far as possible without causing pain. The abdominally located fingers simultaneously press backwards about 5 cm medial and parallel to the superior iliac spine (Fig. 1.5). The normal oviduct cannot be palpated, and the normal ovary may or may not be felt. If the latter is palpable, it is extremely tender on bimanual pressure.

Rectal examination

A rectal examination, or a rectoabdominal bimanual examination, may replace a vaginal examination in children and in virgin adults, but the examination is less efficient and more painful than the vaginal examination. A rectal examination is a useful adjunct to a vaginal examination when either the outer parts of the broad ligaments or the uterosacral ligaments require to be palpated. On occasion, a rectovaginal examination, with the index finger in the vagina and the middle finger in the rectum, may help to determine if a lesion is in the bowel or between the rectum and the vagina. Box 1.1 describes the skills required in performing a gynaecological examination.

Tests

Appropriate tests may be required. For example, if the woman complains of a vaginal discharge, swabs should be taken to determine the cause (see p. 293). Urinary symptoms may require a midstream specimen of urine to assist in reaching a diagnosis.

Medical practitioners have a crucial role in encouraging sexually active women to have a cervical smear (Pap smear) taken at regular intervals, to detect abnormal cells. At present only half of women over the age of 40, who are at greatest risk of developing cervical carcinoma, have regular Pap smears.

Investigations

Pelvic ultrasound

The development of pelvic ultrasound scanning enables doctors to identify many disorders in the genital tract with greater accuracy than with clinical examination. Ultrasound is particularly helpful in establishing patency of the Fallopian tubes and in defining cystic, benign and malignant tumours of the internal genital organs. The examination may be made transabdominally through a full bladder, or transvaginally when the bladder is empty.

Colposcopy

The colposcope is a low-powered microscope for inspecting the cervix and vagina in cases where abnormal cells

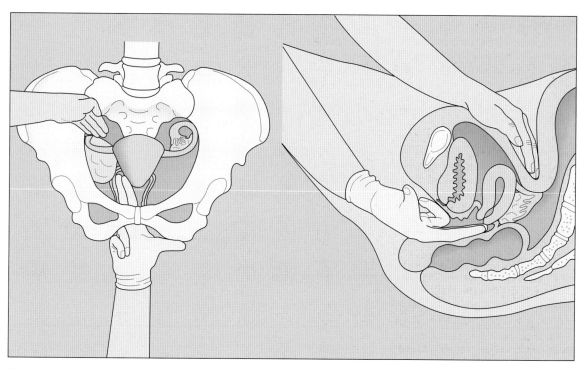

Fig. 1.5 Bimanual palpation of the adnexal area. Note the position of the fingers; normally the ovary cannot be felt. In this case a cystic mass lying in the position of the ovary can be identified.

Box 1.1 Patient–doctor skills needed during conduct of a gynaecological examination

- Ensure your patient understands what is involved and why the examination is being conducted
- Explain what you are about to do as you are conducting the examination
- When appropriate, make eye contact with your patient: do not always talk to the vulva
- Be efficient but not rushed
- Observe your patient's physical appearance and behaviour; be sensitive to anxiety, tension, withdrawal, signs of abuse, and inappropriate or unusual behaviour
- Be sensitive to her needs and preferences: having a third person present, using a sheet to cover herself
- Ask your patient to let you know if she is uncomfortable at any time during the examination
- Be reassuring and give feedback about what you are observing and feeling during the examination
- After the examination, allow the woman to dress and sit down with her to discuss your findings
- Use simple English and be prepared to draw diagrams: women are not always able to conceptualize their reproductive organs
- Give your patient the opportunity to ask you questions

---

have been detected by a Pap smear. The cervix and vagina are exposed by introducing a bivalve vaginal speculum. The colposcope is placed in front of the vagina and its focal length is adjusted to examine the suspect part of the lower genital tract (see p. 293).

Computed tomography and magnetic resonance imaging

These technologies have a role in assessing the nature and spread of malignant disease of the genital organs, but due to their costs should only be used when they are likely to provide information that would confer a real benefit.

Laparoscopy

Inspection of the pelvic organs with a laparoscope inserted into the peritoneal cavity through a small subumbilical incision may give valuable information about the state of the pelvic organs, particularly in cases of infertility, chronic pelvic pain and probable ectopic gestation. Techniques have been developed which enable operations to be conducted through a laparoscope, potentially reducing the postoperative analgesia requirements and the length of hospital inpatient stay.

Hysterosalpingography

The injection through the cervix of a radio-opaque substance and following its progress on a screen as it fills the uterus and Fallopian tubes provides information in cases of infertility.

Hysteroscopy

A small fibreoptic telescope is inserted through the cervix into the uterine cavity, which is inspected. The procedure may help the doctor to reach a diagnosis in cases of menstrual disorders. Endometrial polyps, submucous fibroids and intrauterine adhesions and septae can be removed and the endometrium ablated (see p. 225) using this technique.

Endometrial biopsy

This technique is used to obtain a sample of endometrium for histological examination, by introducing a small curette through the cervix without anaesthesia. Endometrial biopsy has a role in the investigation of infertility and in helping to reach a diagnosis in cases of postmenopausal bleeding.

THE MATERNITY PATIENT

Most women consulting a medical practitioner have a good idea that they are pregnant. The woman may have:

- Missed a menstrual period (has amenorrhoea)
- Noticed that her breasts are fuller and may be tender
- Nausea and perhaps may have vomited
- Frequency of micturition
- Purchased a 'home pregnancy test' or have had the test taken by her pharmacist.

The woman visits the doctor to confirm that she is pregnant and either to seek antenatal care from the doctor or to be referred to an obstetrician or to a hospital clinic.

History

At this first visit the doctor should take a history in the manner described earlier. The information includes more than that described for gynaecological examination. The history of previous pregnancies should be detailed and include information about:

- Spontaneous and induced abortions
- Complications during pregnancy
- The gestation period at delivery
- The method of delivery (spontaneous vaginal birth, forceps, ventouse delivery, caesarean section)
- Complications in the puerperium
- Birthweight of the baby, neonatal complications and long-term outcome

- Maternal physical and mental health during and after each pregnancy
- Breastfeeding history.

Once the pregnancy has been confirmed the medical practitioner should enquire about matters that may be associated with complications or a poor outcome:

- Whether the pregnancy was wanted
- Any problems, e.g. nausea or vomiting, bleeding, abdominal–pelvic pain
- Cigarette smoking, caffeine intake, alcohol and other prescribed and social drug use
- Prepregnancy body weight, recent and past history of weight loss or weight gain, and eating behaviour
- Family and community support
- Current and past history of depression and anxiety, and eating and weight disorders
- Current and past history of physical and sexual abuse
- Family history of hypertension, diabetes mellitus, and congenital and familial disorders
- Whether the woman has any concerns or worries about this pregnancy.

The medical practitioner should enquire about these matters again during the pregnancy.

Examination

Having taken a history the doctor should examine the woman as described earlier, although a vaginal examination does not need to be performed. Indications for conducting a vaginal examination include a vaginal discharge, active bleeding and to take a Pap smear if it has not been done in the previous 12 months. If the doctor performs a vaginal examination between 6 and 10 weeks after the woman's last menstrual period (LMP) the uterus may feel as if it is separate from the cervix. This is because the cervix has softened, and the examiner's fingers seem to meet below the ball-shaped uterus (Hegar's sign), as shown in Figure 1.6.

In most cases the doctor will confirm the pregnancy either clinically or by an immunological pregnancy test. The test depends on the fact that human chorionic gonadotrophin (hCG) is secreted into the circulation within 10 days of conception. Using a sensitive monoclonal antibody test, small amounts of the β fraction of hCG can be detected if the woman is pregnant.

A question invariably asked by the woman when the pregnancy has been confirmed is 'When can I expect my baby to be born?' This can be determined by asking the woman if the length of her menstrual cycle falls into the normal range (22–35 days). The calculation is to add 1 year and 10 days to the first day of her LMP and then to subtract 3 months. This gives the estimated date of confinement (EDC). Thus if her LMP began on 14 November 2010 she may expect to give birth on 24 August 2011 (±14 days). Most doctors do not need to do the calculations, as obstetric calculation discs are readily available.

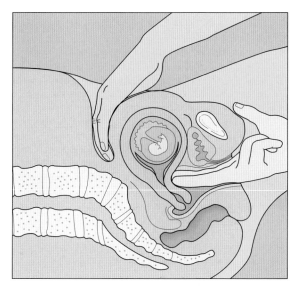

Fig. 1.6 Hegar's sign.

The calculation has to be altered if the woman's menstrual cycle is prolonged, or if she was taking oral contraceptives during the cycle before she became pregnant, as ovulation may have been delayed and conception may have occurred up to 14 days later than expected. In these two circumstances the EDC will be later than calculated, and to obtain greater accuracy of prediction an ultrasound examination at the 18th to 20th week of pregnancy may be needed. Many obstetricians have an ultrasound of the fetus performed routinely at the time of the first visit, to accurately establish the gestation and fetal viability. Women appreciate an early ultrasound of their fetus and hearing its heart beat.

Most women seek to have the pregnancy confirmed during the first 10 weeks, but some delay until later. The uterus becomes palpable early in the second trimester (i.e. from 13 weeks' gestation) on abdominal examination (Fig. 1.7) and fetal heart sounds can be heard using an ultrasonic heart detector at this time. The woman feels her fetus moving from about 18 weeks' gestation.

Once pregnancy has been diagnosed further investigations should be made. These are discussed in Chapter 6.

Evidence of a previous pregnancy

In a few cases the woman may deny that she has been pregnant before, but the doctor is suspicious. This suspicion can grow stronger if:

- The breasts show pigmentation of the areolae.
- The abdominal wall has silver-grey longitudinal lines (striae gravidarum).
- On inspection of the vulva, the perineum shows evidence of damage and repair.

However, a firm diagnosis cannot be given as these signs can be produced by other disorders.

Pseudocyesis

Emotional disturbance, such as an intense desire to have a baby or fear of losing a lover, may lead some women to believe that they are pregnant when they are not. The emotions stop the release of gonadotrophic hormones, with resultant amenorrhoea. The woman's emotions cause her to complain of the symptoms of pregnancy, often in a bizarre order. The breasts become full and may secrete a cloudy fluid; the abdomen becomes enlarged because of fat or flatus. On superficial examination the woman appears to be pregnant; however, vaginal examination shows the uterus to be normal in size. It may be necessary to have an ultrasound examination to convince the woman that she is not pregnant. Once the absence of pregnancy has been confirmed, the woman should be given sympathetic psychiatric attention.

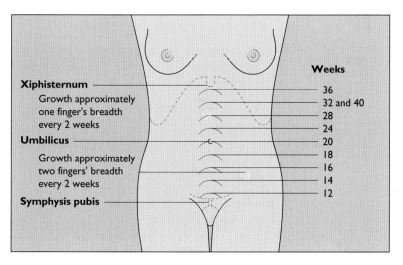

Fig. 1.7 The abdominal markings of uterine growth related to the number of weeks after the last menstrual period.

Xiphisternum
Growth approximately one finger's breadth every 2 weeks
Umbilicus
Growth approximately two fingers' breadth every 2 weeks
Symphysis pubis

Weeks
36
32 and 40
28
24
20
18
16
14
12

Medicolegal aspects and patient–doctor communication

Obstetrics and gynaecology has for some time been perceived as a high-risk speciality for medicolegal claims. The reasons for this appear to be:

1. The pregnant woman's (and her family's) expectation that she will give birth to a perfect baby.
2. The gynaecological patient's expectation that her diagnosis, treatment and operation, if needed, will have a perfect result.
3. The trend of some lawyers using contingency litigation in medicolegal claims.
4. The large amounts of compensation determined by some judges and juries.

What can be done?

The doctor

The doctor should take the following measures to reduce litigation:

First consultation

The doctor should listen carefully to what the patient says and should seek clarification of the issues. The patient (and her partner if she wishes) should be given ample opportunity to ask questions, which the doctor should answer in clear English, if necessary through an appropriate interpreter. They should outline the treatment they intend to follow, stating the benefits and disadvantages (if any) of the proposal. Written information should be made available to the woman and her family whenever possible. Except in emergency situations, treatment or surgery should not be instituted precipitously, giving the patient time to reflect and ask further questions. The conversation should be recorded by the doctor in the notes, dated and signed.

Follow-up visits

At each visit the doctor should follow the procedure outlined above, giving more time for the woman to ask questions to clarify issues she may find obscure. Again the doctor's notes should be completed meticulously, dated and signed, and pathology and ultrasound reports should be seen, evaluated and signed off before they are filed.

Operative procedures in obstetrics and gynaecological surgery

When a consultant or a trainee undertakes an operative procedure, the record of that procedure should be recorded in some detail in the operation notes, preferably by the operating surgeon, signed and dated. When the woman is visited after childbirth or after an operative procedure she should be given time and the opportunity to ask questions, and the answers should be given simply and clearly. All observations should be recorded and signed.

Ultimately, a reduction in litigation will occur if the doctor can communicate well with the patient, being sensitive to her concerns and answering her questions without showing any haste or impatience (Box 1.2).

Box 1.2 Doctor–patient communication

Good communication is essential to patient assessment, treatment, and the avoidance of subsequent medicolegal problems.

To achieve this the doctor should:

- Listen attentively and with empathy to what the patient is saying
- Listen more and talk less, only interrupting the patient to clarify a point
- Avoid being confrontational, condescending, overbearing or judgemental, particularly in sensitive matters such as sexual preferences, practices and abuse
- Avoid using medical jargon, use simple clear and understandable English, and make sure the patient understands the explanation of the obstetric, gynaecological, medical or surgical procedures proposed
- Provide consumer information in a pamphlet or DVD format
- Avoid creating the appearance that he or she wants to conclude the consultation prematurely
- Make a follow-up appointment if there is any doubt that the patient understood clearly, so the issues can be discussed further with the woman and, if she wishes, her partner

Chapter | 2 |

Ovulation and the menstrual cycle

The endocrinological changes that take place to transform a female child into an adolescent who menstruates and ovulates and is capable of conceiving a child, begin several years before puberty, but the most marked changes occur in the 2 years before the girl's first menstrual period (menarche).

Disturbances occurring during the menstrual cycle are discussed in Chapters 28 and 29.

MENARCHE

The underlying major endocrinological change is that the hypothalamus begins to secrete releasing hormones. These lead to the release into the circulation of adrenal androgens and pituitary human growth hormone (hGH). It is hGH that causes the growth spurt which begins 3–4 years before the menarche, and which is maximal in the first 2 years (Fig. 2.1). The physical growth slows down as the first menstruation (menarche) approaches. This is because increasing quantities of oestrogen are secreted by the ovaries and feed back negatively, reducing hGH secretion. Shortly after the secretion of hGH starts, the hypothalamus begins to release gonadotrophin-releasing hormone (GnRH) in an episodic pulsed manner. At first, the pulses are greater in amplitude during sleep, but after 2 years they occur by day and night at about 2-hour intervals. GnRH induces the release of follicle-stimulating hormone (FSH) and luteinizing hormone (LH) from the pituitary gland, which in turn bind to receptors in the ovaries and induce the secretion and release of oestrogen and progesterone into the circulation. The quantity of FSH and LH increases as the girl matures.

Until the age of 8 years, only small quantities of oestrogen are secreted (and less of progesterone). After that age oestrogen secretion begins to rise, slowly at first, but after the age of about 11 years the rise is quite rapid. The FSH levels reach a plateau when the girl is aged about 13. LH levels rise more slowly until 1 year before menarche, at which time a rapid rise occurs (Fig. 2.2). By this time, the GnRH pulses occur every 90 minutes. These hormonal changes persist until after the age of 40, when changes presaging the menopause begin (see Ch. 42).

It is thought that the rapid rise of LH induces the onset of menarche, but other factors are also involved. These include an increase in the fat : lean ratio of body composition, which in turn is related to good nutrition and the absence of debilitating diseases.

Between the early 1800s and the mid 1900s the average age at menarche fell from 15–17 years to 13–13.5 years. There has been little change over the past 30 years the mean age being around 12.5 years with the exception that obese girls tend to enter puberty earlier than those of normal weight. The initial reduction is believed to be due to better childhood nutrition. It is hypothesized that the greater amount of body fat in girls today permits the greater aromatization of androgens to oestrogens.

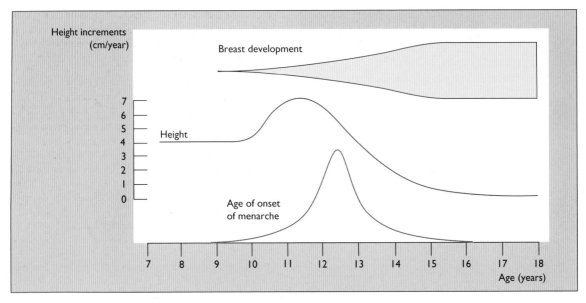

Fig. 2.1 The menarche in relation to growth and breast development in adolescence.

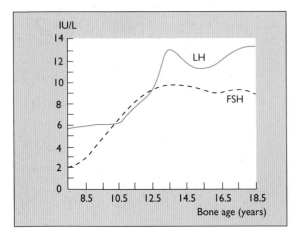

Fig. 2.2 Pubertal changes in levels of FSH and LH in girls.

Rapidly rising levels of oestrogens feed back positively to the hypothalamus and pituitary gland, leading to the LH surge that precedes the menarche.

The menarche may be delayed in women who are of low body weight, such as ballet dancers, women who have anorexia nervosa, or those who are compulsive exercisers.

EFFECTS OF OESTROGEN AND PROGESTERONE ON BODY TISSUES

More than 20 oestrogens have been isolated, the three considered the most important being oestrone, oestradiol and oestriol. Oestrone is a relatively weak oestrogen and interconverts with 17-β oestradiol, which is the most active and the predominant oestrogen in the reproductive years. Oestradiol is rapidly transported in the blood to tissues that have oestrogen-binding receptors. In the blood, 60% is bound to albumin, 37% to sex hormone-binding globulin, and 3% is free. The tissues of the genital tract and the lobular elements of the breasts have the highest concentration of cells containing specific oestrogen-binding receptors, and consequently are most affected by circulating oestradiol.

Once attached to the specific binding sites oestradiol is transferred to the cell's nucleus, where it activates genes, leading to RNA synthesis. This process is regulated to some extent by progesterone, which blocks the formation of new receptors and induces intracellular enzyme production; these enzymes also regulate oestrogen metabolism. Following nuclear gene activation, oestradiol is rapidly converted to the relatively inactive oestriol, which is transported to the liver where it is conjugated with glucuronic acid. The conjugate is then excreted, mostly in the urine. This leaves the cell receptors free to bind more oestradiol.

Oestradiol stimulates the growth of the vulva and the vagina after the menarche, the hormone causing proliferation of both the epithelial and the muscular layers. This oestrogen also stimulates the formation of more blood vessels, which supply the organs. The uterus is particularly stimulated by oestradiol, which increases its vascularity. Oestradiol causes endometrial proliferation, stimulating the growth of the glands and stroma as well as the growth of the muscular layers of the uterus, so that the uterus grows from its prepubertal size to its adult size in the perimenarchal years (Fig. 2.3). The great increase in circulating oestrogen in pregnancy causes the rapid growth of the uterus, and the lack of this hormone after the menopause leads to uterine atrophy.

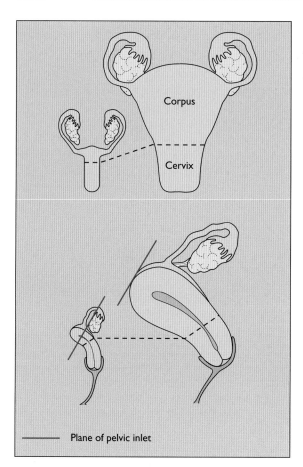

Plane of pelvic inlet

Fig. 2.3 The prepubertal uterus compared with the adult uterus. Note particularly the change in ratio of the corpus and cervix.

Progesterone acts on tissues that have oestrogen receptors, but only if they are first sensitized by oestrogen. Progesterone hinders the maturation of the vaginal epithelial cells and renders the cervical mucus viscous, while also increasing the thickness and succulence of an oestrogen-primed endometrium, preparing it to accept a fertilized egg. Progesterone aids in fat deposition and is thermogenic, raising the body temperature by 0.2–0.5 °C.

MENSTRUATION AND OVULATION

At puberty each ovary contains about 200 000 oogonia surrounded by mantles of theca lutein cells, many of which have developed fluid-filled cavities (antra) to become primary follicles.

From now on until their disappearance at the time of the menopause, and in the absence of pregnancy, severe weight loss or of certain other conditions, between 15 and 20 of these follicles are stimulated to grow each month

by FSH and LH secreted by the anterior pituitary gland. One (occasionally more) of the follicles grows more rapidly than the others and, reaching the ovarian surface, causes the release of an ovum. If an ovum is released and pregnancy does not occur, menstruation follows.

The control of this system is complex and reciprocating. The initial stimulus originates in the hypothalamus with the release of GnRH into the hypophyseal portal vessels. As mentioned, GnRH released in a pulsatile manner reaches the pituitary gland, where it stimulates the growth and maturation of gonadotrophs, which secrete FSH and LH. FSH acts on 10–20 'selected' primary follicles, by binding onto the theca granulosa cells that surround them. The effect of the rising amounts of FSH is to cause fluid to be secreted into the cavity of the follicles, one of which grows more rapidly than the remainder. Simultaneously the theca granulosa cells that surround the selected follicles secrete increasing amounts of oestradiol, which enters the circulation.

The endocrinological effect of the rising levels of oestradiol is that it exerts a negative feedback on the anterior pituitary and the hypothalamus, with the result that the secretion of FSH falls whereas that of oestradiol rises to a peak (Fig. 2.4). Some 24 hours later a sudden large surge of LH and a smaller surge of FSH occur. This positive feedback leads to the release of an ovum from the largest follicle. Ovulation has occurred. (If large amounts of FSH are produced by the anterior pituitary gland, or usually if FSH injections are given, superovulation occurs, seven or more follicles reaching maturity, a technique used in in-vitro fertilization.)

The collapse of the follicle from which the ovum has been released leads to a change in its nature. The theca granulosa cells proliferate, become yellow in colour (luteinized) and are referred to as theca-lutein cells. The collapsed follicle becomes a corpus luteum. The lutein cells of the corpus luteum secrete progesterone as well as oestrogen. Progesterone secretion reaches a plateau about 4 days after ovulation and then rises progressively should the fertilized ovum implant into the endometrium. The trophoblastic cells of the implanted embryo immediately secrete hCG, which maintains the corpus luteum so that the secretion of oestradiol and progesterone continues. On the other hand, if pregnancy fails to occur the theca-lutein cells degenerate and produce less oestradiol and progesterone. This reduces the negative feedback on the gonadotrophs, with a rise in the secretion of FSH. The falling circulating levels of oestradiol (Table 2.1) and progesterone cause changes in the endometrium (see p. 14), which leads to menstruation.

ENDOMETRIAL CYCLE

Menstruation is the periodic discharge from the uterus of blood, tissue fluid and endometrial cellular debris, in varying amounts. The quantity of tissue fluid is the

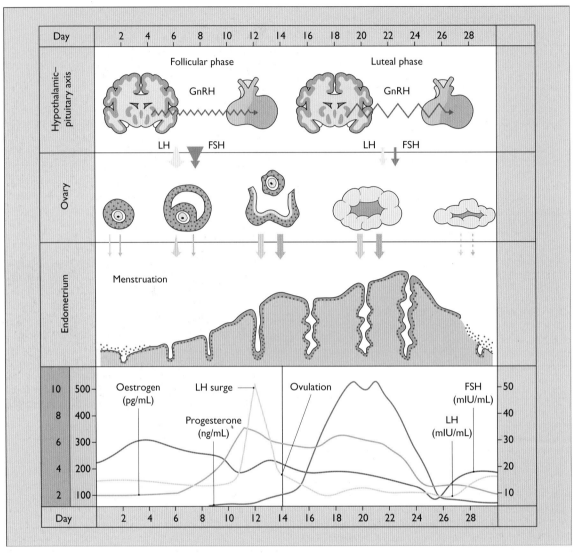

Fig. 2.4 Hormone levels in the normal menstrual cycle – considerable variations are compatible, however, with normal menstrual function. Here, the inter-relationship of ovarian steroids and hypothalamic–pituitary gonadotrophins is shown. After menstruation, rising levels of oestrogen exert a negative feedback, reducing FSH release. Towards midcycle still higher oestrogen levels exert a positive feedback, causing a sudden peak release of LH, which induces ovulation. An increased release in FSH also occurs. Failure of this sequence will lead to anovulation and irregular cycles. In the luteal phase, LH levels must be sufficiently high to maintain the corpus luteum until the conceptus has implanted and commenced hCG secretion, which then maintains corpus luteum function. If conception fails to occur the corpus luteum deteriorates after about 7 days, with the resulting falling levels of progesterone and oestrogen. As a consequence menstruation occurs and FSH levels rise, initiating a new menstrual cycle.

greatest variable. This means that some women who complain of heavy periods do not become anaemic as might be expected (see Ch. 28). The mean blood loss during menstruation is 30 mL (range 10–80 mL). Menstruation normally occurs at intervals of 22–35 days (counted from day 1 of the menstrual flow to day 1 of the next) and the menstrual discharge lasts from 1 to 8 days.

A convenient way to describe the endometrial menstrual cycle is to start just after menstruation ceases and follow the cycle to the next menstruation as it passes through the proliferative and secretory (luteal) phases.

Table 2.1 Plasma oestradiol levels during the menstrual cycle	
	PLASMA OESTRADIOL (pmol/L)
Early follicular phase	75–600
Late follicular phase	110–1500
Periovulatory peak	170–1000
Early and mid-luteal phase	75–1000
Late luteal phase	10–900

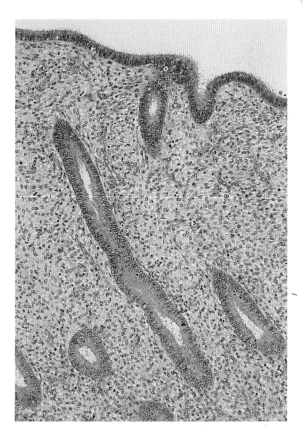

Fig. 2.5 Endometrium – early proliferative phase. Note that the glands are straight, short and narrow. The surface epithelium is thin.

Proliferative phase

As each area of the endometrium is shed during menstruation, regenerative repairs begin, the endometrial surface being reformed by the metaplasia of stromal cells and by an outgrowth of epithelial cells of the endometrial glands. Within 3 days of menstruation ceasing, the repair of the entire endometrium is complete.

In the early proliferative phase the endometrium is thin, the glands few, narrow, straight, and lined with cuboidal cells, and the stroma is compact (Fig. 2.5). The early regenerative phase lasts from day 3 of the menstrual cycle to day 7, when proliferation speeds up. The epithelial glands increase in size and grow down perpendicular to the surface. Their cells become columnar with basal nuclei. The stromal cells proliferate, remaining compact and spindle shaped (Fig. 2.6). Mitoses are common in glands and stroma. The endometrium is supplied by basal arteries in the myometrium which send off branches at right angles to supply the endometrium. At first, as each artery penetrates the basal endometrium it is straight, but in the middle and superficial layers it becomes spiral. This coiling permits the artery to supply the growing endometrium by becoming uncoiled. Each spiral artery supplies a defined area of endometrium.

Luteal phase

If ovulation occurs, as is usual except at the extremes of the reproductive years, the endometrium undergoes marked changes. The changes start in the last 2 days of the proliferative phase, but increase dramatically after ovulation. Secretory vacuoles, rich in glands, appear in the cells lining the endometrial glands. At first the vacuoles are basal and displace the cell's nucleus superficially (Fig. 2.7). They rapidly increase in number and the glands become tortuous. By the sixth day after ovulation the secretory phase is at its peak. The vacuoles have streamed past the nucleus. Some have discharged mucus into the cavity of the gland; others are full of mucus, leading to a saw-toothed appearance (Fig. 2.8). The spiral arteries increase in length by uncoiling (Fig. 2.9).

In the absence of pregnancy, the secretion of oestrogen and progesterone falls as the corpus luteum ages. The fall leads to an increase in endometrial free arachidonic acid and endoperoxidases. These enzymes induce stromal cell lysosomes to synthesize and secrete prostaglandins ($PGF_{2\alpha}$ and PGE_2) and prostacyclin. $PGF_{2\alpha}$ is a powerful vasoconstrictor and causes uterine contractions; PGE_2 causes uterine contractions and some vasodilatation; prostacyclin is a vasodilator, causes muscle relaxation and inhibits platelet aggregation. During menstruation the ratio of $PGF_{2\alpha}$ to the other two prostaglandins increases. This change reduces the blood flow through the endometrial capillaries and leads to a shift of fluid from the endometrial tissues into the capillaries, with a resulting decrease in endometrial thickness. This leads to increased coiling of the spiral arteries and a further decrease in blood flow. The area of endometrium supplied by the spiral artery becomes hypoxic, and ischaemic necrosis occurs. The vasoconstriction occurs in different spiral arteries at different times, alternating

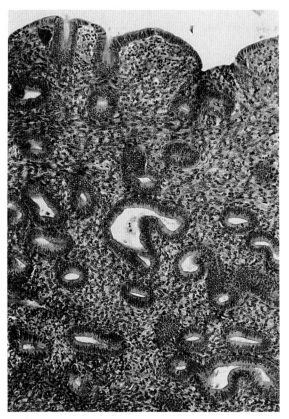

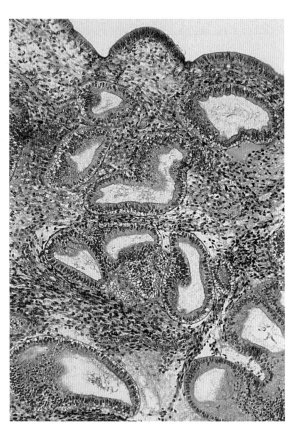

Fig. 2.6 Endometrium – late proliferative phase. The glands have become longer and tortuous and, in a few, early secretory changes may be observed. The stroma remains dense.

Fig. 2.7 Endometrium – early luteal phase. The tortuosity of the glands, and the subnuclear vacuoles, can be seen.

with vasodilatation. The necrotic area of the endometrium is shed into the uterine cavity, accompanied by blood and tissue fluid. Menstruation has begun.

In the past decade molecular biology has identified at least 50 proteins secreted by the endometrium that may be involved in controlling menstruation. For example, endothelin causes marked vasoconstriction of the spiral arteries and consequently reduced blood flow in them. Other proteins promote cell division, which could help in repairing the endometrium.

Menstrual phase

During menstruation the superficial and middle layers of the endometrium are shed, the deep basal layer being spared (Fig. 2.10). The shedding occurs in an irregular, haphazard manner, some areas being unaffected and others undergoing repair, while simultaneously other areas are being shed. The shed endometrium, with tissue fluid and blood, forms a coagulum in the uterine cavity. This is immediately liquefied by fibrinolysins and the liquid,

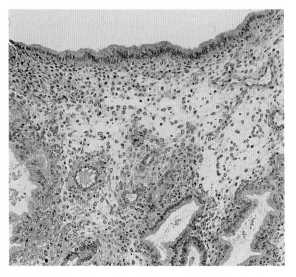

Fig. 2.8 Endometrium – day 6 after ovulation. The glands are now very tortuous, with secretion in the lumen and increasing fluid separating the stromal cells. In a fertile cycle day 6 is when the ovum reaches the uterine cavity.

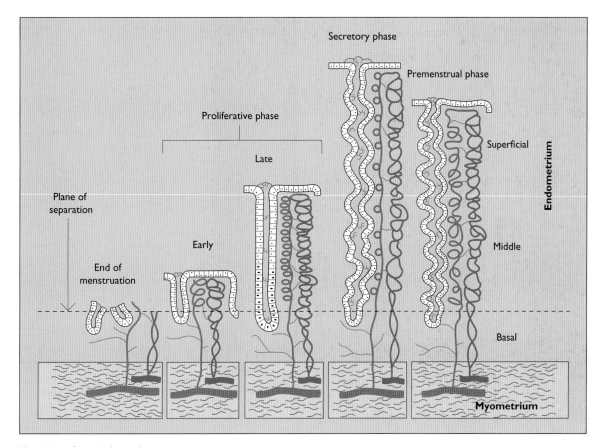

Fig. 2.9 Endometrial vascular patterns.

which does not coagulate, is discharged through the cervix by uterine contractions. If the quantity of blood lost in the process is considerable, there may be insufficient fibrinolysins and clots are expelled through the cervix.

The blood vessels supplying the area beneath the shed endometrium are sealed with a haemostatic plug consisting of aggregated platelets and by fibrin fibres, which infiltrate the platelet aggregations to form a stable occlusive plug. In addition, vasoconstriction occurs. The basal layer of the endometrium regenerates and new epithelium covers the denuded area. When regeneration exceeds necrosis and repair is complete or nearly complete, menstruation ceases and a new menstrual cycle begins.

CERVICAL CYCLE

During the follicular phase the glands lining the clefts of the cervical canal proliferate and secrete a thick mucus, which forms a complex mesh in the cervical canal. Just

before ovulation, the sudden surge of oestrogen changes the character of the cervical mucus, which becomes thin and forms long strands through which helical channels appear. Following ovulation, progesterone alters the nature of the cervical mucus, which again becomes thick and impenetrable.

VAGINAL CYCLE

Cyclic changes occur in the vaginal epithelium which are dependent on the ratio between oestrogen and progesterone. In the follicular phase, superficial and large intermediate cells predominate. As ovulation approaches the proportion of superficial cells increases and few leucocytes can be seen (Fig. 2.11). Following ovulation a marked change occurs as progesterone is secreted. The superficial cells are replaced by intermediate cells and leucocytes increase in number, causing the smear to look dirty (Fig. 2.12).

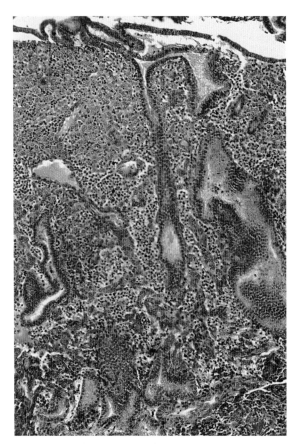

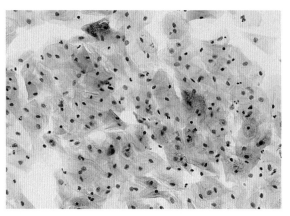

Fig. 2.11 Vaginal exfoliative cytology – late proliferative phase. Note the discrete cells with small nuclei and the clear background.

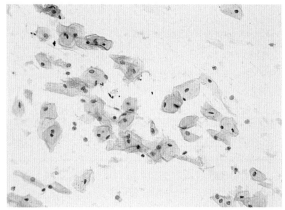

Fig. 2.10 Endometrium – early menstrual phase. The section shows the beginning of focal necrosis in the superficial zone of the endometrium, with small areas of haemorrhage into the stroma and infiltration with neutrophils.

Fig. 2.12 Vaginal exfoliative cytology – luteal phase. The cells have clumped and the background infiltration of leucocytes has begun.

Chapter | 3 |

Conception and placental development

By the time a woman reaches puberty each of her ovaries contains about 200 000 primary oocytes, enclosed in primordial follicles. Each oocyte is separated from the cellular primordial follicle by a clear area, the perivitelline space, and a thickened 'shell', the zona pellucida. Each primordial follicle is capable of growing under the influence of follicle-stimulating hormone (FSH) to form a mature follicle. Each month from about the age of 15 years to the age of 45 years, some 20 of the primordial follicles grow through the stage of vesicular follicles to become mature antral follicles.

In contrast to other body cells, the oocyte has only 23 chromosomes. At some stage of its growth it undergoes a meiotic division of its nucleus and an unequal division of its cytoplasm, to become a secondary oocyte. The smaller cell is expelled into the perivitelline space and is termed a polar body (Fig. 3.1B). The oocyte and its polar body both contain 23 chromosomes.

One of the 20 follicles (occasionally two or more, particularly if the ovaries are hyperstimulated in an in-vitro fertilization programme) outstrips the others, developing a large fluid-filled antrum and migrating to bulge through the thickened surface of the ovary (Fig. 3.2). With the release of the luteinizing hormone (LH) surge by the pituitary at midcycle the follicle bursts, expelling the ovum, which is gathered into the Fallopian tube by the fimbriae that project from its proximal end. The ovum, surrounded by the perivitelline, is contained in a condensed opaque substance 5–10 µm thick called the zona pellucida. Adherent to the zona pellucida are theca granulosa cells derived from the mature follicle.

Once the ovum has been expelled the follicle collapses and turns yellow, forming the corpus luteum (Fig. 3.2). The ovum is now ready to be fertilized should it be reached by a sperm.

Of the 60–100 million sperm ejaculated into the vagina at the time of ovulation, several million will negotiate the helical channels in the cervical mucus to reach the uterine cavity. Several hundred will pass through the narrow entrance to the fallopian tubes, and a few will survive to reach the ovum in the fimbrial end of the Fallopian tube. One sperm may penetrate the zona pellucida of the ovum, its head entering the substance of the ovum. When this occurs a chemical reaction prevents the entry of any other sperm. At the same time the oocyte undergoes another division of its chromosomes and a second polar body is formed (see Fig. 3.1D).

Once inside the cytoplasm of the ovum the sperm's nuclear membrane dissolves, leaving a naked male pronucleus. The ovum, having divided to produce a second polar body, also loses its nuclear membrane. The two naked nuclei approach each other and fuse (see Fig. 3.1E). Fertilization and conception have occurred.

Within a few hours of fertilization, the fused nuclei divide to form two cells (see Fig. 3.2E). Once this has occurred, further cell division proceeds rapidly until, within 3–4 days, a solid mass of cells (the morula) has formed (see Fig. 3.2G, H).

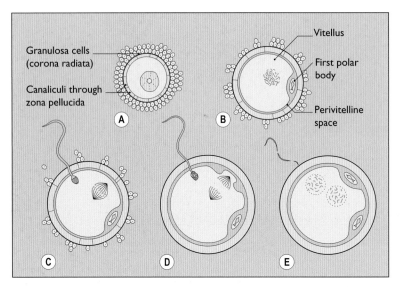

Granulosa cells (corona radiata)

Canaliculi through zona pellucida

Vitellus

First polar body

Perivitelline space

Fig. 3.1 Formation of the ootid and fertilization: (A) primary oocyte; (B) secondary oocyte formed after first maturation division, first polar body pinched off; both oocyte and polar body have undergone reduction division and now each has a haploid number of chromosomes (B, C); (C) second maturation division stimulated by sperm penetrating into vitellus; (D) second polar body forming. The first polar body may also undergo a reduction division; (E) male and female pronuclei formed.

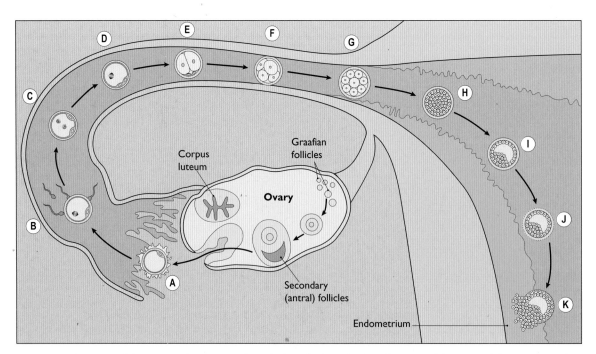

Corpus luteum

Graafian follicles

Ovary

Secondary (antral) follicles

Endometrium

Fig. 3.2 Development of the ovum and its passage through the Fallopian tube into the cavity of the uterus: (A) unsegmented oocyte; (B) fertilization; (C) pronuclei formed; (D) first spindle division; (E) two cell stage; (F) four cell stage; (G) eight cell stage; (H) morula; (I) and (J) blastocyst formation; (K) zona pellucida lost and implantation occurs.

IMPLANTATION

Implantation occurs 8–10 days after ovulation in most healthy pregnancies.

The morula is rapidly propelled along the Fallopian tube to enter the uterine cavity. During its passage, fluid passes through canaliculae in the zona pellucida to create a central fluid-filled cavity in the morula, forming a blastocyst (see Fig. 3.21). On reaching the uterine cavity the zona pellucida becomes distended and thin. It soon disappears, leaving the surface cells of the blastocyst in contact with the endometrial stroma. About 50% of blastocysts adhere to the endometrium. The surface trophoblastic cells of the adhering blastocyst differentiate into an inner cellular layer, the cytotrophoblast, and an outer syncytiotrophoblast.

Knobs of trophoblast rapidly form and invade the endometrial stroma in a controlled manner (Fig. 3.3). By the 10th day after fertilization the knobs of trophoblastic tissue have developed a mesodermal core and have pushed deep into the endometrial stroma (Fig. 3.4). The stromal cells react to the invasion by becoming polyhedral in shape and filled with glycogen and lipid, converting into a decidua, which supplies the energy needed by the invading trophoblast. At the same time a number of deep cells at one pole of the blastocyst differentiate to become an inner cell mass, from which the embryo will develop.

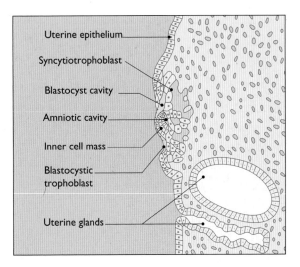

Fig. 3.4 Section of a 8-day human ovum partially implanted in secretory endometrium (× 100). The embryo is represented by the inner cell mass; the blastocyst has collapsed.

By the 9th to 10th day after fertilization the inner cell mass has differentiated into an ectodermal layer, a mesodermal layer and an endodermal layer, in which a small fluid-filled cavity, the amniotic sac, has formed (Fig. 3.5). The further development of the amniotic sac, in which the fetus will float relatively weightless until it is born, is shown in Figure 3.6.

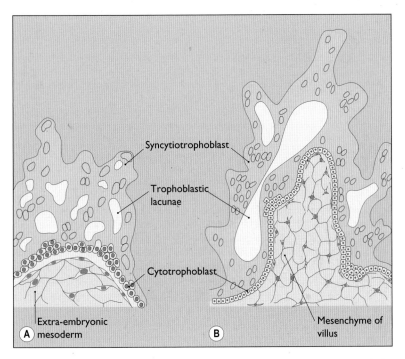

Fig. 3.3 Early stage in development of chorionic villi. (A) Trophoblast projection has occurred, with the development of lacunae and much intermingling with maternal tissue, which for clarity is not shown. No mesoblastic core has yet entered the villus. (B) The mesoblastic core is now developing within the villus.

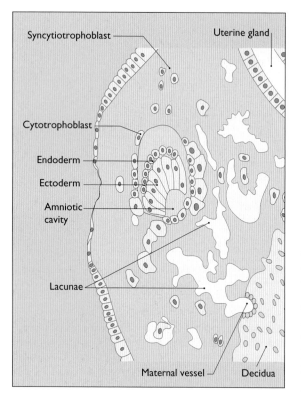

Syncytiotrophoblast

Uterine gland

Cytotrophoblast

Endoderm

Ectoderm

Amniotic cavity

Lacunae

Maternal vessel

Decidua

Fig. 3.5 A section through the middle of the Hertig–Rock 9-day embryo.

The inner cell mass projects into the original blastocystic cavity, the walls of which are formed from cytotrophoblast, and the cavity is filled with mesoderm (Fig. 3.7). Quickly, the surface layer of ectoderm divides to surround a fluid-filled cavity in the mesoderm – the yolk sac (see Fig. 3.6A–C).

With further development the yolk sac shrinks in size and a second fluid-filled cavity, the amniotic sac, surrounds the growing embryo (see Fig. 3.6D, E).

FORMATION OF THE PLACENTA

Meanwhile, the trophoblastic syncytium has penetrated more deeply into the decidua. As well as invading the endometrial stroma the syncytium secretes human chorionic gonadotrophin (hCG), which aids in maintaining the function of the corpus luteum to secrete oestrogen and progesterone. In some areas of the decidua the syncytium has surrounded and invaded the walls of the interdecidual portions of the uterine spiral arteries to convert them from being relatively thick-walled to thin-walled vessels, permitting a greater flow of blood. These vessels are fragile and break to form small blood lakes, or lacunae. In normal pregnancies the process is complete by 20–22 weeks'

gestation. Failure of the process to occur normally may be a factor in the development of pre-eclampsia.

With further proliferation the knobs of trophoblast become finger-like and blood vessels appear in their mesodermal core. These vessels will soon link up with blood vessels forming in the embryonic mesoderm. The finger-like projections are termed chorionic villi. The chorionic villi proliferate and erode more vessels, so that the lacunae increase in size. Blood flows into them under pressure, to create large blood-filled spaces in which the proliferating chorionic villi float.

By the 19th day after fertilization the entire conceptus is covered by growing chorionic villi, some attached to the decidua (anchoring villi) but most floating freely in the blood lakes. At this stage further penetration of the decidua ceases, by immunological or chemical mechanisms, and a collagen layer appears through which the spiral arteries and veins pass. As the blood supply to the chorionic villi is greatest on the deep surface of the conceptus the villi grow profusely here, resembling leafy trees (chorion frondosum). The chorionic villi covering the remainder of the conceptus degenerate, forming the chorion laeve. The chorion frondosum forms the placenta, which is the functional union between the conceptus and the maternal tissues. Connection between the fetal and placental circulation is established by day 35, and by the 70th day the placental development is complete (Fig. 3.8).

The placenta is composed of about 200 trunks, some large, some of medium size, but most small, which divide into limbs, branches and twigs, covered with chorionic villi. Each of the main trunks forms a cotyledon, 10 being large, 40 medium, and the rest small and of little functional significance.

As the blood lakes coalesce, a large blood-filled space is created in which the villi covering each fetal cotyledon float, moved by the motion of the blood. The roof of the space is formed by chorion (the chorionic plate) and its base by trophoblast and decidua (the decidual plate). Septa of varying heights and sizes grow from the decidual plate to separate each fetal cotyledon, each forming an intervillous space. Each intervillous space is supplied by a number of separate arteries, which enter the space at the base of the septa. During maternal systole arterial blood spurts into the space, like a fountain, at a pressure of 80 mmHg. The pressure of the blood pushes the villi aside and the blood hits the chorionic plate and then flows laterally and downwards, bathing the villi, to escape slowly through the veins in the decidual plate (Figs 3.9 and 3.10).

It has been estimated that the maternal blood flow through the placenta increases from 300 mL/min at 20 weeks' gestation to 600 mL/min at 40 weeks. The total surface area of the villi has been estimated to be 11 m², and the placenta at 40 weeks weighs one-sixth of the weight of the baby.

Each villus has a complex anastomosis of capillaries (Fig. 3.10), so there is ample opportunity for the exchange of gases and nutrients. The exchange is enhanced by the vascular resistance in the vessels of the chorionic villi (Fig. 3.11).

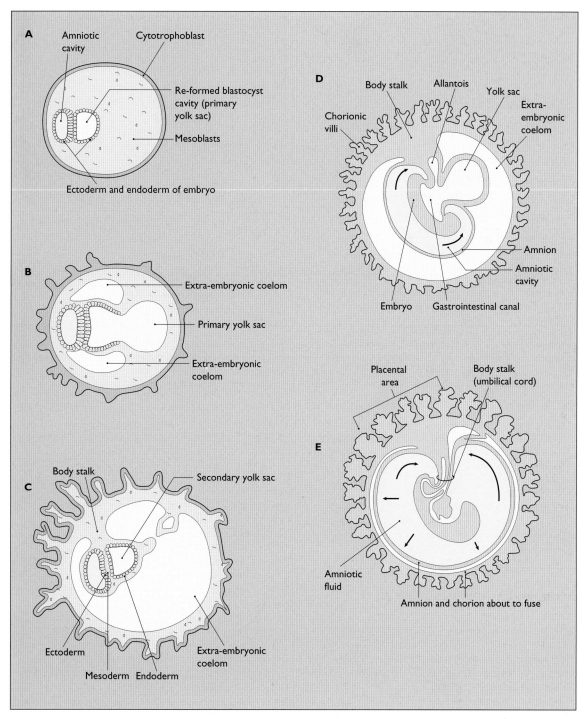

Fig. 3.6 Formation of the amniotic cavity. (A) Formation of the inner cell mass, and the development of the amniotic cavity and the primary yolk sac. (B) Spaces appear in the mesoblast to form the extra-embryonic coelom. (C) The primary yolk sac diminishes in size as the extra-embryonic coelom enlarges. (D) The amniotic sac develops and begins to occupy the extra-embryonic coelom. (E) By the 45th day the amniotic sac has surrounded the embryo, which is suspended in the protective liquor amnii.

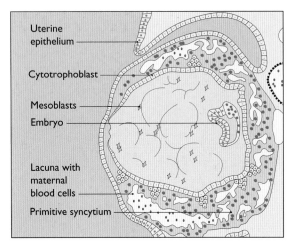

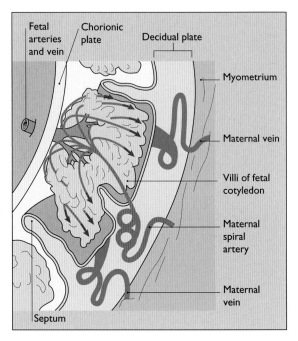

Fig. 3.7 Section of an 11½-day human embryo (Barnes embryo). The blastocystic trophoblast has differentiated into primitive syncytium and cytotrophoblast. Mesoblast has differentiated from the inner surface of the latter and almost fills the original blastocyst cavity. Lacunae have appeared in the actively growing syncytium, and maternal blood cells have seeped into several of them. Buds appear at intervals on the syncytium; these are the forerunners of chorionic villi.

Fig. 3.9 An intervillous space. A fetal cotyledon can be seen, in which the fountain effect of the maternal arterial blood is demonstrated. The blood cascades over the tree-like villi to escape through the maternal veins.

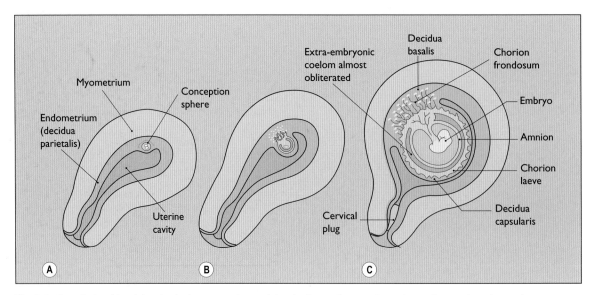

Fig. 3.8 The relationship of the chorionic sac, amnion and developing embryo to the endometrium and uterine cavity at successive stages in early pregnancy. (A) 3 weeks, (B) 5 weeks and (C) 10 weeks after the last menstrual period.

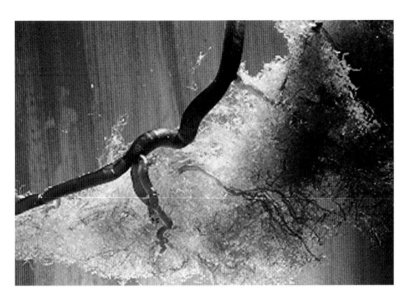

Fig. 3.10 Cast of placental vasculature showing the branching of the vessels.

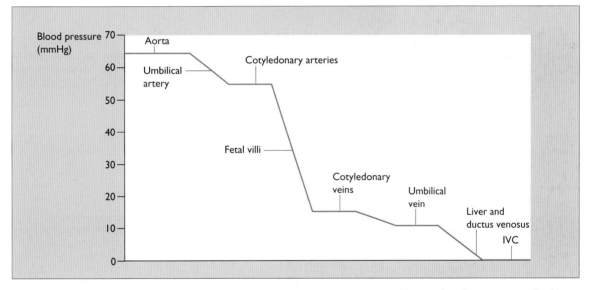

Fig. 3.11 The fall in blood pressure from the aorta through the umbilical circulation and liver to the inferior vena cava (IVC) in the mature fetal lamb.

The increasing blood flow as pregnancy advances compensates for ageing changes that occur in the placenta, and for the development of placental infarcts.

FUNCTION OF THE PLACENTA

The placenta acts for the fetus as:

- An organ of respiration
- An organ of nutrient transfer and excretion
- An organ of hormone synthesis.

It also acts as an immunological barrier protecting the fetus (formed from paternal as well as maternal genes) from rejection by the mother's immune system.

Transport mechanisms through the placenta

Transport of substances through the placenta takes place by:

- Passive transport
  - simple diffusion
  - facilitated diffusion

- Active transport
  - enzymatic reaction
  - pinocytosis.

These mechanisms require the expenditure of energy, and the rate of placental metabolism has been calculated as comparable to that of the liver or kidney. The transfer of substances is shown in Table 3.1.

Respiratory function

The extensive vasculature in the villi and the relatively slow passage of maternal blood through the intervillous space permits a good exchange of oxygen and carbon dioxide between the fetal and the maternal blood by passive diffusion. The exchange is further enhanced by the maternal blood entering the intervillous space having a 90–100% saturation and a Po_2 of 90–100 mmHg. After the metabolic needs of the placenta have been met the fetal erythrocytes take up the oxygen, which is 70% saturated and has a Po_2 of 30–40 mmHg, sufficient to meet all fetal needs. Carbon dioxide, like oxygen, diffuses passively across the placenta (Fig. 3.12).

Hydrogen ions, bicarbonate and lactic acid diffuse across the placenta, the acid–base status of mother and fetus thus being closely related. As the transfer takes place slowly, the fetus is able to buffer any additional acidity from its reserves, unless maternal acidosis is aggravated by dehydration or ketoacidosis, as may occur in late labour, when fetal acidosis may result.

The efficiency of these exchanges depends on a good maternal blood supply to the spiral arteries and a well-functioning placenta. Should the maternal blood supply to the arteries be reduced, as may occur in severe hypertensive states (see Ch. 14), placental ageing (see Ch. 19), uterine hyperactivity or cord compression (see Ch. 20), fetal keto-acidosis may occur independently of maternal acidosis.

Nutrient transfer

Most nutrients are transferred from mother to fetus by active transfer methods, involving enzyme processes. Complex nutrients are broken down into simple components before transfer and are reconstituted in the fetal chorionic villi. Glucose is particularly important as it is the major source of energy for the growing fetus, supplying over 90% of its requirements (10% deriving from amino acids). The quantity of glucose transferred increases after the 30th gestational week. Towards the end of pregnancy about 10 g of glucose per kilogram weight is retained daily, and the excess over metabolic requirements is converted into glycogen and fat. The glycogen is stored in the liver and the fat is deposited around the heart and behind the scapula. In the last quarter of pregnancy 2 g of fat are synthesized daily, and thus by 40 weeks' gestation 15% of the fetal body weight is fat. This provides an energy store of 21 000 kJ and provides for the metabolic functions and the regulation of body temperature in the days after birth. In preterm and dysmature babies the energy stores are lower, which may cause problems (see Ch. 19).

Table 3.1 Transfer of substances through the placenta

MATERNAL BLOOD	INTERVILLOUS SPACE	PLACENTAL TRANSFER METHODS		
		Passive	Active	Pinocytosis
H$_2$O, O$_2$, CO$_2$, urea, Na, K	⟶	+		
Glucose	Facilitated by carrier molecule		+	
Polysaccharides	Mono- and disaccharides		+	
Protein ⟶	Amino acids		+	
Fat	Free fatty acids		+	
Vitamin A ⟶	Carotene	+		
Vitamin B complex, vitamin C	⟶		+	
Iron, phosphorus ⟶	⟶		+	
Antibodies	Only IgG	+		+
Erythrocytes	⟶	±		+

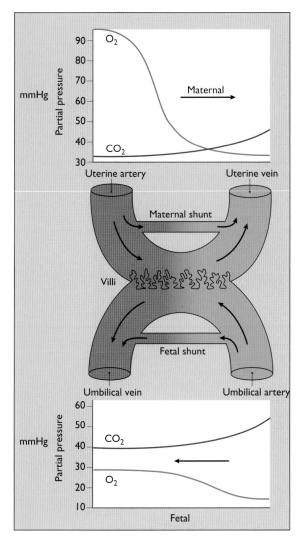

Fig. 3.12 Schematic representation of placental gas exchange. It can be seen that fetal blood has a much lower partial pressure of oxygen than adult blood; the fetus in utero has been described as living in conditions of oxygenation resembling those at the top of Mount Everest.

Oddly, lipids, as free fatty acids, are poorly transferred. Those transferred are resynthesized into phospho- and other lipids and are stored in fetal adipose stores until the 30th gestational week. After this time the fetal liver becomes capable of synthesizing lipids and now takes over.

Drug transfer

The transfer of drugs through the placenta is no different from that of nutrients, and all pass through to some extent. The rate is governed by the solubility of the ionized molecules in fat and the thickness of the trophoblast.

In the second half of pregnancy the trophoblast becomes thinner, whereas the placental area increases in size; drugs therefore pass through more rapidly.

The greatest risk to the developing fetus of the teratogenic effect of a drug is during organogenesis, that is, from 17 to 70 days postconception (31–84 days postmenstrual age). After this time the risk of major birth defects is almost negligible.

Illegal drugs (narcotics, cocaine and amphetamines) taken by the mother pass through the placenta and may affect fetal development. The extent of their effect is difficult to determine, as most drug abusers also smoke and drink alcohol. The fetus tends to be growth restricted, may have congenital abnormalities and is likely to be born preterm, and if the mother takes narcotics the infant may have withdrawal symptoms (see pp. 51–52).

Hormone synthesis

The placenta synthesizes a number of hormones, the function of which, in many cases, is not understood. The main hormones produced are human chorionic gonadotrophin, human placental lactogen, oestrogen and progesterone.

Human chorionic gonadotrophin

Human chorionic gonadotrophin (hCG) is synthesized from the early days of placentation. Its blood level reaches a peak between the 60th and 80th days of pregnancy, when 500 000–1 000 000 IU are secreted each day. The amount secreted then falls to between 80 000 and 120 000 IU/day, a level which is maintained until term (Fig. 3.13). The peak is higher and lasts longer in multiple pregnancy and in gestational trophoblastic disease. After childbirth the level falls rapidly. Initially the function of hCG is to maintain the corpus luteum's secretion of progesterone and

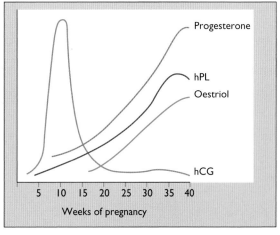

Fig. 3.13 Oestriol, progesterone, hCG and hPL (human placental lactogen) plasma levels in pregnancy.

oestrogen. Once the placenta takes over this function, the level of hCG declines. Human chorionic gonadotrophin may also regulate oestrogen production by the placenta and suppress maternal immunological reactions directed against the fetus.

Oestrogen

In pregnancy the main source of oestrogen is the placenta. The synthesis of oestrogen requires the intervention of the fetus, as the placenta lacks specific enzymes (C17, 20-desmolase and 16-hydroxylase), which are required in the synthesis of oestrogen from acetate and cholesterol. Of the three classic oestrogens, oestriol (E_3), oestradiol (E_2) and oestrone (E_1), the placenta produces more oestriol and retains it selectively. The result is that compared to a non-pregnant circulating $E_3 : E_2 : E_1$ ratio of $3 : 2 : 1$, in pregnancy the ratio is $30 : 2 : 1$. This means that over 90% of the oestrogen secreted in pregnancy is oestriol, and the level rises progressively throughout pregnancy (Fig. 3.13).

Actions of oestrogen

At the cellular level oestrogen, mainly in the form of oestradiol, enhances RNA and protein synthesis. Oestrogen alters the polymerization of acid mucopolysaccharides, which has the effect of increasing the hygroscopic properties and reducing the adherence of collagen fibres in connective tissue. This effect is most marked in the cervix, which becomes swollen and soft in pregnancy. Oestrogen also aids the growth of uterine muscle, both by its enzymatic action on the muscle fibres and by increasing the blood flow.

In the breast, oestrogen increases the size and mobility of the nipple and causes duct and alveolar development. It may also play a part in causing water retention in pregnancy.

Progesterone

In pregnancy, progesterone is secreted initially by the corpus luteum but, by the 35th gestational day, the placental cytotrophoblast takes over all significant production from maternally supplied precursors, mainly cholesterol. At this stage of pregnancy the plasma progesterone level is 50 ng/mL. From now on the level rises in a linear manner to reach 150 ng/mL by term (see Fig. 3.13).

Actions of progesterone

In pregnancy the main action of progesterone is to cause muscle relaxation, and because the uterus has a large number of progesterone receptors its effect is most marked on the myometrium. Progesterone also relaxes the lower oesophageal sphincter, the gastric muscles, the intestines and the ureters. These effects account for some minor disturbances of pregnancy, for example heartburn, delay in stomach emptying, ureteric dilatation and reduced peristaltic activity leading to constipation.

Progesterone regulates the storage of body fat to some extent and is hyperthermic, leading to a rise in body temperature of 0.5–1.0°C. It may have a hypnotic effect on brain cells and may be responsible for the placidity experienced by many pregnant women. Progesterone is also implicated in the hyperventilation some women experience.

Protein hormones

The placenta secretes a number of pregnancy-specific hormones, of which human placental lactogen (hPL), or human chorionic somatomammotropin, is the best understood. Its secretion is the reverse of that of hCG: when hCG falls from its peak, hPL continues to rise (see Fig. 3.13). The most important pregnancy-preserving function of hPL is to mobilize free fatty acids from maternal body stores. This lipolytic effect reduces utilization of maternal glucose, which is then diverted for fetal energy needs. Human placental lactogen also stimulates insulin secretion, but inhibits its effects at peripheral sites, and aids in the transfer of amino acids to the fetus.

IMMUNOLOGY OF THE TROPHOBLAST

The fetus is an allograft, but paradoxically is not rejected by the maternal immune system. The explanation for this is unclear. One hypothesis is that the trophoblast secretes antigen that bind to sites on the trophoblast. Bound to these sites, it induces the production of fetal immunosuppressor cells. A further mechanism may be that hCG partially blocks maternal immunological responses. These mechanisms prevent the 'foreign' cells of the conceptus from being recognized and rejected.

Chapter | 4 |

Embryo and fetus

Once implantation has occurred the embryo develops rapidly. A neural primitive streak develops in the second week after fertilization; during the third week the fetal heart develops and links up with the primitive vascular system; during the fourth week the gut has formed; and by the sixth week the urogenital sinus has formed.

By the seventh week after fertilization most of the organs have formed and the embryo becomes a fetus. The early growth of the fetus is shown in Table 4.1.

NUTRITION

Fetal growth is determined by many factors, both genetic and environmental. Of the latter, adequate placental perfusion and placental function are crucial. Maternal nutrition is not a limiting factor except in cases of extreme starvation, although chronic undernutrition may be associated with anaemia and may lead to a low-birthweight baby.

The fetus, insulated in its protective amniotic sac and relatively weightless, directs most of the energy supplied to it to growth. The energy is derived mainly from glucose. Only small amounts of lipids, as free fatty acids, cross the placenta until the fourth quarter of pregnancy. Any excess carbohydrate, after the growth and metabolic energy needs of the fetus have been met, is converted into lipids, and this conversion increases as term approaches.

From the 30th gestational week the fetal liver becomes increasingly efficient and converts glucose into glycogen, which is stored in the fetal heart muscle, the skeletal muscle and the placenta. Should fetal hypoxia occur the fetus is able to obtain energy from the heart muscle and placenta for anaerobic glycolysis (see Ch. 20).

Free fatty acids are formed and stored in brown and white adipose tissue. Brown fat is deposited around the fetal neck and behind the scapulae and the sternum and around the kidneys. It is metabolized to provide energy to maintain the infant's body temperature after birth. White adipose tissue forms the subcutaneous cover of the body of a term fetus, but in preterm babies the layer may be thin. It acts as an insulator and as a lipid store.

The fat stores of an 800 g fetus (24–26 weeks' gestation) constitute 1% of its body weight; by the 35th week fat constitutes 15% of fetal body weight.

As the placenta clears the blood of bilirubin and other metabolic products that require a transferase activity, the fetal (and neonatal) liver is deficient in certain transferases. The result is that unless the deficiencies are corrected in the early neonatal period, bilirubin may accumulate in the neonate's blood, which is of some consequence in haemolytic disease of the newborn (see p. 129–130).

Amino acids cross the placenta by active transfer and are converted into protein. Protein synthesis exceeds protein breakdown, and the fetus uses some of the breakdown amino acids for resynthesis.

Table 4.1 Characteristics indicating maturity of the fetus

PERIOD OF GESTATION (WEEKS FROM THE 1ST DAY OF THE LAST PERIOD)	PERIOD OF GESTATION (WEEKS FROM FERTILIZATION)	LENGTH OF FETUS (CROWN TO RUMP (cm))	CHARACTERISTICS
8	6	2.3	Nose, external ears, fingers and toes are identifiable but featureless, head is flexed on the thorax
12	10	6.0	External ears show main features, eyelids fused, neck has formed, external genitals formed but undifferentiated
16	14	12.0	External genitals can be differentiated, skin transparent red
20	18	15.0	Skin becoming opaque, fine hair (lanugo) covers body
24	22	21.0	Eyelids separated, eyebrows, eyelashes and fingernails present, skin wrinkled due to lack of subcutaneous fat
28	26	25.0	Eyes open, scalp hair growing

The fetus also synthesizes a specific protein, α-fetoprotein (AFP) in its liver. The peak of AFP is reached between the 12th and 16th gestational weeks, after which a decline occurs until term. The protein is secreted in the fetal urine and swallowed by the fetus, to be degraded in its gut. If the fetus is unable to swallow, as in cases of anencephaly, the level of AFP in the amniotic fluid rises.

CARDIOVASCULAR SYSTEM

The circulatory pattern of the fetus is shown in Figure 4.1. It should be noted that over 50% of the cardiac output passes through the umbilical arteries to perfuse the placenta. The cardiac output increases to term, at which time about 200 mL/kg per minute is usual. The heart rate lies between 110 and 150 bpm to maintain this output. The fetal blood pressure also increases through the pregnancy and, after the 36th week, has a mean of 75 mmHg systolic, 55 mmHg diastolic.

Haemopoiesis commences in the villous capillaries, but from the second trimester liver production becomes dominant. The red cell count, the haemoglobin level and the packed cell volume increase as pregnancy advances. Most of the erythrocytes contain fetal haemoglobin (HbF). At 15 weeks' gestation all the cells contain HbF; by the 36th week 70% of the erythrocytes contain HbF, and 30% adult haemoglobin, but there are wide variations. Cells containing HbF are able to absorb more oxygen at a given P_{O_2}. They are more resistant to haemolysis but less resistant to trauma than cells containing adult haemoglobin.

LUNGS

In the early embryo the lungs are made up of epithelial tubes surrounded by mesoderm. With further development the epithelium becomes folded and glandular to form primitive alveoli. By the 22nd gestational week a capillary system has developed and the lungs are capable of gas exchange.

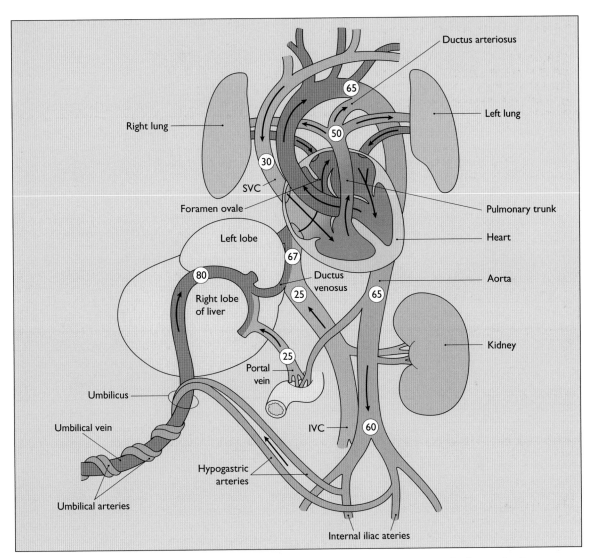

Fig. 4.1 Normal circulation in the fetus in utero. IVC, inferior vena cava; SVC, superior vena cava. The figures give the approximate oxygen saturation of the blood at given points in the circulatory system.

By term, three or four generations of alveoli have developed and been replaced. Their epithelium, which has a cuboidal appearance, becomes flattened with the first breath. By the 24th week, fluid fills the alveoli and the passages. There are two principal alveolar cell types, the flatter type I pneumocytes, which facilitate gas exchange, and the cuboidal type II pneumocytes that by the 24th week begin to secrete a surface-active lipoprotein surfactant. Surfactant facilitates lung expansion at birth and helps the air-containing lung to maintain its normal volume. However, until the 35th week the amount of surfactant may be insufficient for

some babies to expand their lungs after birth, and hyaline membrane disease may develop.

The fetus makes respiratory movements (breathing) from early in pregnancy. At first they are sporadic, but by mid-pregnancy the movements become regular and increase in frequency as the pregnancy advances. Respiratory activity results in the inspiration of amniotic fluid into the bronchioles but no further, as the fluid secreted into the alveoli is under higher pressure. The reduction in fetal breathing movements when the fetus is subjected to chronic hypoxia can be observed during ultrasound examination. Acute episodes of hypoxia in late pregnancy or during the birth may stimulate gasping. This fetal gasping draws the amniotic fluid, which often contains meconium, deeper into the lungs.

GASTROINTESTINAL TRACT

In the uterus the fetal intestinal tract is relatively quiet. Some of the swallowed amniotic fluid, and the cellular material it contains, enters the gut, where it is acted upon by the enzymes and bacteria to produce meconium. The meconium remains in the gut unless an episode of severe hypoxia leads to contractions of the gut, at which time the meconium is expelled to mix with the amniotic fluid.

RENAL SYSTEM

The fetal kidney develops from the metanephros, and new glomeruli continue to be formed until the 36th gestational week. Urine is secreted and expelled into the amniotic fluid from the 16th week and probably earlier. Its rate of flow increases as term approaches.

IMMUNE SYSTEM

In early pregnancy the fetus has a poor capacity to produce antibodies in response to invasion by maternal antigens or by bacteria. From the 20th week (perhaps earlier) it becomes able to mount an immune response to a challenge. The fetal response is supplemented by the transfer of maternal antibody molecules (provided that they are not too large in size) to the fetus, which provide it with passive protection that may persist for some weeks after birth.

MUSCULAR SYSTEM

Almost weightless in its amniotic capsule, the fetus makes movements from an early age. As the pregnancy advances the fetal movements become stronger, and occur more often. Bouts of activity are followed by periods when the fetus seems to be sleeping. These movements strengthen the fetal muscles and a count of them gives an indication of fetal wellbeing (see p. 153).

ENDOCRINE ACTIVITY

The fetal hypothalamus secretes corticotrophin-releasing hormone (CRH) by the 13th week, thyrotrophin-releasing hormone (TRH), gonadotrophin-releasing hormone (GnRH) and somatostatin by the 15th week, and growth hormone-releasing hormone (GhRH) by the 18th week after fertilization.

Growth hormone (GH) can be released by the fetal pituitary by the 7th week and luteinizing hormone (LH) and follicle-stimulating hormone (FSH) by 9 weeks. Although adrenocorticotrophic hormone (ACTH) is detectable by the 10th week the pituitary–adrenal axis remains immature and the adrenal gland only becomes sensitive to ACTH late in pregnancy. This is possibly because the main source of ACTH is the placenta.

Thyroid-stimulating hormone (TSH) is released from the 14th week, but T_3 and T_4 levels remain low throughout pregnancy. Immediately after birth there is a surge of TSH, which leads to a rapid transient rise in T_3 and T_4 and a fall in reverse T_3.

The posterior lobe of the fetal pituitary gland secretes oxytocin from the second trimester and levels rise during labour. Arginine vasotocin is detectable from the 9th week but its function is not understood. Arginine vasopressin is secreted from the 12th week and plays a key role in cardiovascular function under stress conditions.

Antinatriuretic factor (ANF) is released from the atria (predominantly from the right) in response to pressure changes; this helps regulate blood volume by increasing glomerular filtration. Another key component for fetal cardiovascular homeostasis is the renin–angiotensin–aldosterone system. Fetal renin levels are 20 times greater than adult levels, and renin is released in response to a fall in blood volume. Aldosterone is detectable from the second trimester. Aldosterone increases renal sodium reabsorption and has a negative feedback effect on renin release.

Insulin is present in the fetal pancreas by the 10th week, but pancreatic release of insulin is relatively insensitive until 28 weeks. The two growth factors IGF-1 and IGF-2 increase with gestation, especially from 33 weeks, and are related to fetal placental lactogen levels.

Chapter | 5 |

Physiological and anatomical changes in pregnancy

HORMONAL CHANGES

Most of the anatomical changes that occur in pregnancy are due to the hormones secreted by the placenta. These hormones and their effects on the woman's body are described in Chapter 3. In addition, other endocrine glands synthesize hormones, in different quantities during pregnancy compared with the non-pregnant state. These changes are briefly described below.

Pituitary gland

In pregnancy the pituitary gland increases in size by 50%. The secretion of follicle-stimulating hormone (FSH) and luteinizing hormone (LH) falls to very low levels, whereas that of adrenocorticotrophic hormone (ACTH), melanocyte hormone and prolactin increases. Prolactin levels, for example, increase until the 30th gestational week and then more slowly to term. Prolactin may be a factor in the fall of FSH and LH to very low levels by the eighth week of pregnancy.

Adrenal gland

Total corticosteroids increase progressively to term. This could, to some extent, account for a pregnant woman's tendency to develop abdominal striae, glycosuria and hypertension.

Thyroid gland

The thyroid gland enlarges during pregnancy, occasionally to twice its normal size. This is due mainly to colloid deposition caused by a lower plasma level of iodine, consequent on the increased ability of the kidneys to excrete during pregnancy. Oestrogen stimulates an increased secretion of thyroxine-binding globulin. In consequence both T_3 and T_4 levels rise. These raised levels do not indicate hyperthyroidism, as both the thyroid-stimulating hormone (TSH) and the free thyroxine levels are in the normal range. When tests are made to determine thyroid function these changes must be taken into account.

GENITAL TRACT CHANGES

Uterus

The effect of the hormonal stimulation is most marked upon the tissues of the genital tract, and the uterine muscle fibres grow to 15 times their prepregnancy length during pregnancy, whereas uterine weight increases from 50 g before pregnancy to 950 g at term (Fig. 5.1). In the early weeks of pregnancy the growth is by hyperplasia, and more particularly by hypertrophy of the muscle fibres, with the result that the uterus becomes a thick-walled spherical organ. From the 20th week growth almost ceases and the uterus expands by distension, the stretching of the muscle fibres being due to the mechanical effect of the growing fetus. With distension the wall of the uterus becomes thinner and the shape cylindrical (Fig. 5.2). The uterine blood vessels also undergo hypertrophy and become increasingly coiled in the first half of pregnancy, but no further growth occurs after this, and the additional length required to match the continuing uterine distension is obtained by uncoiling the vessels.

The uterus is derived from the two Müllerian ducts and the myometrium is made up of a thin external, largely longitudinal, layer; a thin inner, largely circular layer; and a thick, intricately interlaced middle layer, which comprises two spiral systems of interdigitating muscles derived from the two Müllerian ducts. The proportion of muscle to connective tissue is greatest in the fundal area and diminishes as the lower segment of the uterus and cervix is approached, the lower half of the cervix having no more than 10% of muscle tissue.

The effect of the uterine distension is to stretch both interdigitating spiral systems and to increase the angle of crossing of the fibres, in the thinner lower segment area

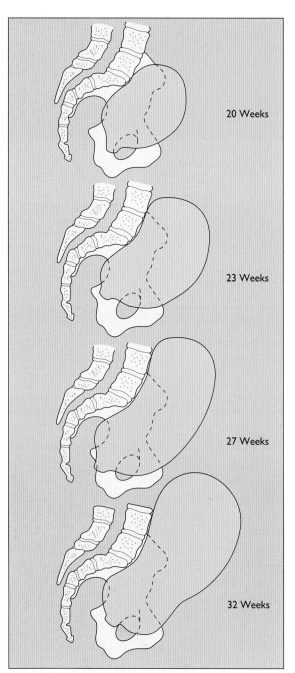

Fig. 5.2 Enlargement of the uterus in normal pregnancy.

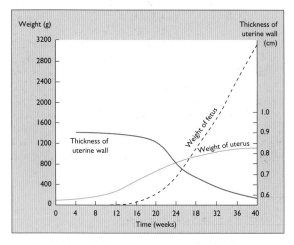

Fig. 5.1 Relation of the weight of the uterus and the thickness of the uterine wall to the weight of the fetus at varying times in normal pregnancy.

where the fibres cross at an angle of about 160° and are less stretched. Incision of the myometrium in this zone is anatomically more suitable, and experience of lower segment caesarean section confirms that healing is better (Fig. 5.3).

The lower uterine segment is that part of the lower uterus and upper cervix lying between the line of attachment of

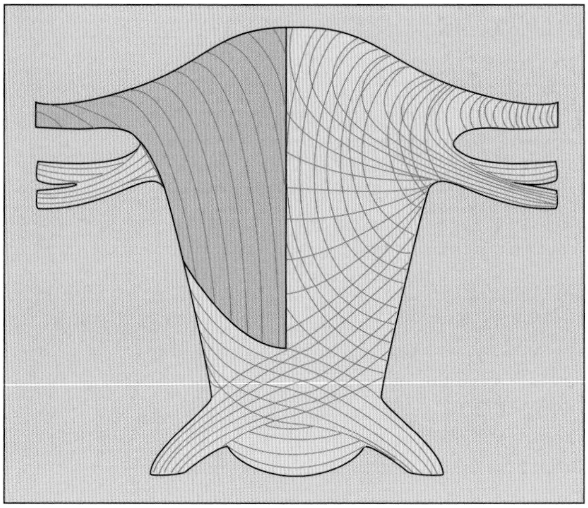

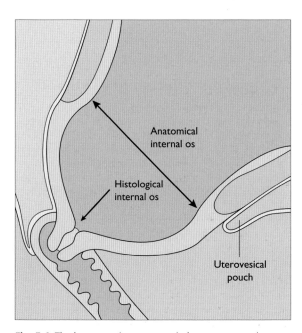

Fig. 5.3 Representation of the obliquity of decussation and interweaving of myometrial fibres. The obtuse angle of decussation in the lower segment can be seen.

the peritoneum of the uterovesical pouch superiorly and the histological internal os inferiorly. It is that part of the uterus where the proportion of muscle diminishes, this muscle being replaced increasingly by connective tissue (mainly collagen fibres), which forms 90% of the cervical tissues (Fig. 5.4). Because of this the lower uterine segment becomes stretched in late pregnancy as the thickly muscled fundus draws it up from the relatively fixed cervix.

Anatomical internal os

Histological internal os

Uterovesical pouch

Fig. 5.4 The lower uterine segment in late pregnancy (see also Fig. 7.8).

Cervix

The cervix becomes softer and swollen in pregnancy, with the result that the columnar epithelium lining the cervical canal becomes exposed to the vaginal secretions. This change in the cervix is due to oestradiol, which increases the hygroscopic properties of the cervical connective tissue and loosens the acid mucopolysaccharides (glycosaminoglycans) of the collagen-binding ground substance.

Prostaglandins act on the collagen fibres, especially in the last weeks of pregnancy. At the same time, collagenase is released from leucocytes, which also helps in breaking down collagen. The cervix becomes softer and more easily dilatable – the so-called ripening of the cervix. In this way the cervix is more easily able to dilate in labour.

Vagina

The vaginal mucosa becomes thicker, the vaginal muscle hypertrophies, and there is an alteration in the composition of the surrounding connective tissue, with the result that the vagina dilates more easily to accommodate the fetus during parturition. The changes, initiated by oestrogen, occur early in pregnancy and there is increased desquamation of the superficial vaginal mucosal cells with increased vaginal discharge in pregnancy. Should pathogens, whether bacterial, fungal (such as candida) or parasitic (such as trichomonads), enter the vagina they can more easily establish themselves and, consequently, vaginitis is more frequently found in pregnancy.

CARDIOVASCULAR SYSTEM

The changes that occur during pregnancy to the blood volume, the plasma volume and the red cell mass are shown in Figure 5.5 and Table 5.1. The plasma volume increases to fill the additional intravascular space created by the placenta and the blood vessels. The red cell mass increases to meet the increased demand for oxygen. Because the increase in the red cell mass is proportionately less than the increase in the plasma volume, the concentration of the erythrocytes in the blood falls, with a reduction in the haemoglobin concentration. Although the haemoglobin concentration falls to about 120 g/L at the 32nd week, a larger total haemoglobin is present than when not pregnant. Concurrently the number of white blood cells increases (to about 10 500/mL), as does the blood platelet count.

Cardiovascular dynamics

To deal with the increased blood volume and the additional demand for oxygen in pregnancy the cardiac output increases by 30–50% (Fig. 5.6). Most of the increased output is due

Table 5.1 Plasma volume, red cell volume, total blood volume and haematocrit in pregnancy

	NON-PREGNANT	WEEKS OF PREGNANCY		
		20	30	40
Plasma volume (mL)	2600	3150	3750	3850
Red cell mass (mL)	1400	1450	1550	1650
Total blood volume (mL)	4000	4600	5300	5500
Body haematocrit (%)	35.0	32.0	29.0	30.0
Venous haematocrit (%)	39.8	36.4	33.0	34.1

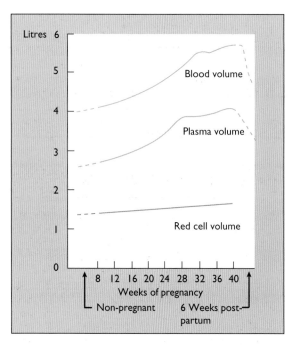

Fig. 5.5 Blood changes in pregnancy.

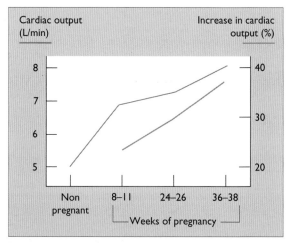

Fig. 5.6 Cardiac output in pregnancy.

Regional distribution of the blood

The uterus receives the greatest proportion of the blood flow, which is vital to perfuse the placenta properly, reaching 500 mL/min by late pregnancy. Renal blood and plasma flow increase to 400 mL/min above non-pregnant levels by the 16th week of pregnancy, and remain at this high level to term. Blood flow through the capillaries of the skin and mucous membranes increases, reaching a maximum of 300–400 mL/min by the 36th week. The increased skin blood flow is associated with peripheral vasodilatation. This is the reason why pregnant women 'feel the heat', sweat easily and often profusely, and may complain of nasal congestion.

RESPIRATORY SYSTEM CHANGES

Breathing remains diaphragmatic during pregnancy, but because of the restricted movement of the diaphragm after the 30th week, pregnant women breathe more deeply,

to an increased stroke volume, but the heart rate increases by about 15%. The increased cardiac output is balanced by a decrease in the peripheral resistance (Fig. 5.7). For these reasons, blood pressure falls in early pregnancy rising back to prepregnancy levels by the third trimester.

In common with other blood vessels, the veins of the legs become distended. The leg veins are affected particularly in late pregnancy because of the obstruction to venous return caused by the higher pressure of the venous blood returning from the uterus and the mechanical pressure of the uterus on the vena cava. This may lead to varicosities in the leg veins (and occasionally the vulval veins) of susceptible women.

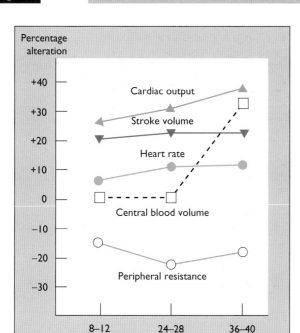

Fig. 5.7 Cardiovascular dynamics: percentage alterations over non-pregnant levels occurring in pregnancy.

increasing tidal volume and ventilation rate, thus permitting an increased mixing of gases and an increased oxygen consumption of 20%. It is thought that this effect is due to the increased secretion of progesterone. It may lead to overbreathing and a lower arterial P_{O_2}. In late pregnancy the lower rib cage flares out to some extent and may not return to its prepregnancy state, causing some concern to figure-conscious women.

ALIMENTARY SYSTEM CHANGES

In the mouth the gums may become 'spongy', probably because of intracellular fluid retention, a possible progesterone effect. The lower oesophageal sphincter is relaxed, which may permit regurgitation of gastric contents and cause heartburn. Gastric secretion is reduced and food remains longer in the stomach. The intestinal musculature is relaxed, with lower motility, which permits a greater absorption of nutrients but may lead to constipation.

RENAL SYSTEM CHANGES

The smooth muscle of the renal pelvis and ureters relaxes, causing their dilatation. This increases the capacity of the renal pelvis and ureters from 12 mL to 75 mL and increases the chance of urinary stasis. The bladder musculature relaxes, which also encourages urinary stasis. In consequence, urinary tract infection is more common in pregnancy. The muscles of the internal urethral sphincter relax and this, together with the pressure of the uterus on the bladder, may cause some degree of incontinence.

The renal blood flow increases to the 16th week of pregnancy and then levels off. The glomerular filtration rate increases by 60% in early pregnancy and remains at the new level until the last 4 weeks of pregnancy, when it falls. As tubular reabsorption is unaltered, the clearance of many solutes is increased. Up to 300 mg of protein per 24 hours may be excreted, which is normal. The increased glomerular filtration rate, together with the natriuretic effect of progesterone, would cause an increased loss of sodium were it not for increased production of renal renin and, in consequence, angiotensin.

IMMUNE SYSTEM CHANGES

Human chorionic gonadotrophin can reduce the immune response of pregnant women. In addition, serum levels of IgG, IgA and IgM decrease from the 10th week of pregnancy, reaching their lowest level at the 30th week and remaining at this level to term. These changes may account for the anecdotal increase in the risk of infection among pregnant women.

WEIGHT GAIN IN PREGNANCY

The better absorption of nutrients from the gut, the reduction of muscle tone and a reduction in thyroid activity produce a quiescence in the maternal metabolism. The body adapts to preserve and nourish the growing fetus.

During pregnancy a woman inevitably gains weight. A healthy person may expect to gain 12.5 kg (range 9–15 kg) in pregnancy, of which 9 kg is gained in the last 20 weeks. The 'ideal' weight gain is only a guide, and an allowance should be made for individual variations. However, a woman whose prepregnancy weight is in the normal range (body mass index (BMI) 19–24.9) or who is overweight (BMI 25–29.9) should avoid excessive weight gain (more than 15 kg), as she may find it difficult to regain her prepregnancy weight after the birth. This is of concern to many women, who want to be reassured that they will regain their body shape and prepregnancy weight as soon as possible after the baby has been born.

After the birth there is a great variability in weight loss. Six weeks after the birth an average woman weighs 3 kg more than her prepregnancy weight. Six months after the birth she will weigh about 1kg more than she weighed before she became pregnant.

The situation is different for obese and underweight women, both during pregnancy and after birth. An obese woman (BMI >30) should be encouraged to limit her weight gain during pregnancy, as she has an increased risk that pre-eclampsia may occur and that she will have a large baby. She should have a glucose tolerance test performed to exclude gestational diabetes mellitus, and she should be advised to eat a sensible but not a very low-energy diet. An underweight woman (BMI <18) should avoid becoming pregnant until she has gained weight, as she has a 20% chance of giving birth to a low-birthweight baby.

Elements of weight gain in pregnancy

Weight gain in pregnancy is caused by several factors:

- The products of conception – the fetus, placenta and amniotic fluid
- The maternal factors – the uterus and breasts, the increased blood volume, the increased stores of fat, water retention.

Fetus, placenta and amniotic fluid

In the first 20 weeks of pregnancy fetal weight gain is slow; in the second 20 weeks it increases more rapidly. The weight gain of the placenta shows the reverse of that of the fetus (Fig. 5.8). The amniotic fluid increases rapidly from the 10th week, being 300 mL at 20 weeks, 600 mL at 30 weeks, and peaking at 1000 mL at 35 weeks. After this a small decline in the total quantity of amniotic fluid occurs.

Maternal factors

The weight of the uterus increases throughout pregnancy. It is more rapid in the first 20 weeks, when myohyperplasia is occurring, than in the second 20 weeks when most of

Table 5.2 The elements of weight gain (g) in pregnancy at 40 weeks	
INCREASING ELEMENT	**WEIGHT GAIN (g)**
Fetus	3300
Placenta	600
Uterus	900
Breasts (glandular tissue)	400
Blood	1200
Fat deposited	2500
Fluid (extracellular)	2600
Total	11000

the enlargement is due to stretching of the muscle fibres. The breasts increase in weight throughout pregnancy owing to deposition of fat, increased retention of fluid, and growth of the glandular elements. The blood volume also increases throughout the pregnancy (see Fig. 5.5). The amount of fat deposited in adipose tissues depends on the amount of fat and carbohydrate in the diet. A gain of 2.5–3.0 kg of fat is usual, of which 90% is deposited in the first 30 weeks. The fat contains 90–105 MJ of energy, which can be released after birth for various activities, including breastfeeding. In a normal pregnancy the total body fluid increases by 6–8 L, of which 2–4 L is extracellular. Most of the fluid is retained before the 30th week, but a pregnant woman who has no clinical oedema retains 2–3 L of extracellular fluid in the last 10 weeks of pregnancy.

The elements of weight gain in pregnancy and their weight at 40 weeks are shown in Table 5.2.

Energy

The resting metabolic rate (RMR) in pregnancy is 10–15% higher than in non-pregnant women. The extra energy required in the 40 weeks of pregnancy for the increased RMR, the growth of the fetus and placenta, the increase in size of the uterus and breasts, and the extra fat is about 250 MJ. This works out at about 0.9 MJ a day – an amount provided by two slices of bread and 100 mL of milk. A pregnant woman does not need to eat for two!

There are, however, exceptions to this statement. Poor women in developing countries, particularly where starvation is not uncommon, benefit by having food supplements during pregnancy. These supplements aid modestly in increasing the birthweight of the baby and giving her or him a greater chance of survival.

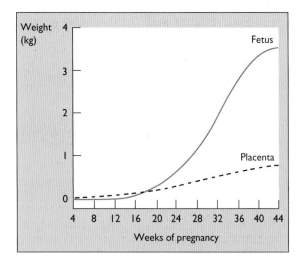

Fig. 5.8 Fetal and placental weight curves compared at various gestational periods.

Chapter | 6 |

Antenatal care

AIMS OF ANTENATAL CARE

The aims of antenatal care are to ensure that:

- The mother reaches the end of the pregnancy as healthy as, or even healthier than, she was before she became pregnant.
- Any physical or psychological problems arising during the pregnancy are detected and treated.
- Any complication of pregnancy is either prevented or detected early and managed adequately.
- The mother gives birth to a healthy baby.
- The mother has the opportunity to discuss her anxieties and fears about the pregnancy.
- The mother is informed about any proposed procedures, the reason for the procedure and the probable outcome.
- The couple are prepared for the birth and for child rearing, including receiving information about diet, childcare and family planning.

PRECONCEPTION ADVICE

Ideally all women planning to become pregnant should be seen before conception. This visit gives the opportunity to review her personal and family history and to optimize control of conditions, such as hypertension or diabetes, before pregnancy.

It is also an opportunity to outline her antenatal care options and to discuss the tests she will be offered during the pregnancy, for example, screening for chromosome anomalies. If there is a history of congenital or genetic abnormalities referral to a genetics clinic can be arranged. If the woman is overweight or underweight she can be given appropriate dietary and exercise advice and be offered referral to a dietitian. The immune status of the woman can also be explored, particularly relating to her ABO group and Rhesus factor, and immunity to rubella, hepatitis B and C and varicella.

All women should be advised to take 0.4 mg of folate in the weeks before becoming pregnant and for the first 3 months of pregnancy to reduce the risk of a neural tube defect. Women with a past history of spina bifida or anencephaly should increase their daily intake of folate to 4 mg/day. Women who smoke should be strongly encouraged and supported to quit, for the reasons detailed later. If her partner also smokes he should also be encouraged to access a QUIT programme.

ANTENATAL CARE PROVIDERS

The providers of antenatal care may be a general practitioner, an obstetrician or a midwife. In many centres antenatal care is now provided by a team comprising midwives, hospital-based obstetricians and community general practitioners, each member of the team contributing their particular skills and expertise. The antenatal care may take place in a doctor's rooms, in a hospital clinic, or in a clinic conducted by a midwife. The opportunity should be available for an expectant mother to choose which facility she would prefer, but she should know that, if a complication should arise, she would be transferred, if necessary, quickly and efficiently, to a facility staffed by experienced obstetricians.

Whichever facility a pregnant woman has chosen she should have the opportunity to talk to a health professional about matters that concern her during the pregnancy in an unhurried way and have her questions answered by an informed, communicative doctor and midwife.

PSYCHOLOGICAL PREPARATION FOR MOTHERHOOD

Some women appear confident that their pregnancy will proceed normally and that the birth of the baby will be easy. Most women, however, have concerns about the pregnancy and the process of childbirth. In the early weeks many women fear that the pregnancy may terminate as

a miscarriage. Later in pregnancy many women fear that the baby will be malformed or retarded, or that childbirth will be dangerous and painful. A few women are concerned that after the birth they will not be able to regain their prepregnancy body shape. These fears may not be expressed unless the woman feels confident that she is able to ask her doctor about them and expect to receive a reasoned answer. Fears about the difficulty and pain of childbirth can be reduced by simple explanations of the nature and course of labour.

Women who obtain social and psychological support during pregnancy are less likely than those who do not, to have negative feelings about their pregnancy and the forthcoming birth. They are more likely to feel that they are 'in control' during the pregnancy, to have a worry-free childbirth, to communicate more effectively with their doctor or nursing staff, and to be more satisfied with the care they receive.

Many women are helped by antenatal classes, run either in conjunction with antenatal clinics or privately. The importance of providing written information in the woman's primary language cannot be overstated.

DIET IN PREGNANCY

Many pregnant women are confused about what they should eat during pregnancy to make sure that they and their baby are properly nourished. What should a pregnant woman eat? To a large extent this will depend on her cultural background, her usual eating behaviour and her income level. As a general principle, women should be advised to eat a well-balanced diet that includes a sufficient amount of each of the five core food groups. It should be low in fat and high in fibre, with sufficient fresh fruit and vegetables, as is suitable for the general population and for her family. Although many women will eat slightly more during pregnancy there is no good evidence that they should drastically alter or increase their food intake. Table 6.1 shows the mean daily intake or RDI (recommended daily intake) that women should try to achieve. Table 6.2 shows what a pregnant woman should try to eat each day, translated into the foods a household buys.

Most pregnant women who eat a sensible diet do not need vitamin supplements, with the exception of folate. It is now recommended that a woman who intends to become pregnant should take folate 0.5 mg a day for 3 months prior to conception and during the first trimester. Generally high-folate foods should be encouraged, such as plenty of fresh fruit and vegetables, and fortified breakfast cereals, as well as a folic acid supplement, as it is generally difficult to obtain this extra folate without a supplement. Women carrying a multiple pregnancy should continue taking folate throughout.

Healthy women living in the industrialized countries whose haemoglobin is within the normal range and

Table 6.1 Recommended daily intakes		
	RDA	**SEE NOTE**
Protein	51 g	*
Thiamin	1.0 mg	*
Riboflavin	1.5 mg	*
Niacin	14–16 mg niacin equivalents	*
Vitamin B_6	1.0–1.5 mg	*
Total folate	400 µg	†
Vitamin B_{12}	3.0 µg	*
Vitamin C	60 mg	*
Zinc	16 mg	*
Iron	32–36 mg	‡
Iodine	150 µg	*
Magnesium	300 µg	*
Calcium	1100 µg	*
Phosphorus	1200 µg	*
Selenium	80 µg	*
Vitamin A	750 µg retinal equivalents	
Vitamin E	7.0 mg α-tocopheral equivalents	
Sodium	920–2300 mg	
Potassium	1950–5460 mg	

*Indicates an increased requirement compared to non-pregnant female 19–54 years

†Daily requirement is doubled to 400 µg daily. RDI = 200 µg in a non-pregnant female 19–54 years

‡RDI is expressed as a range to account for differences in bioavailability in foods. RDI is for second and third trimesters

Table 6.2 A healthy diet		
Carbohydrate foods	=	4–6 servings
1 serving	=	2 slices bread
	=	1 cup cooked rice, pasta, noodles
	=	1 cup porridge or $1\frac{1}{3}$ cup cereal flakes
Protein foods	=	$1\frac{1}{2}$ servings
1 serving	=	100 g cooked meat or chicken
	=	$\frac{1}{2}$ cup cooked dried beans or peas
	=	2 small eggs
	=	120 g fish fillet or $\frac{1}{2}$ cup tinned fish
	=	$\frac{1}{3}$ cup nuts
Milk and dairy foods	=	3 servings
1 serving	=	250 mL or 1 cup of milk
	=	40 g or 2 slices cheese
	=	1 carton/200 g yoghurt
Fruit	=	4 servings
1 serving	=	1 piece of fruit
	=	$\frac{1}{2}$ cup juice
	=	1 cup canned fruit
Vegetables	=	5–6 servings
1 serving	=	$\frac{1}{2}$ cup cooked vegetables
	=	1 cup salad vegetables
	=	1 potato
	=	$\frac{1}{2}$ cup cooked dried beans/lentils
Extras	=	$0–2\frac{1}{2}$ servings
1 serving	=	$\frac{1}{2}$ chocolate bar
	=	1 slice cake
	=	1 packet chips (crisps)

who eat a sensible diet usually do not require iron supplements. However, many women routinely supplement their diet with iron, as they may find it difficult to eat enough iron-rich foods and are at risk of iron deficiency. A protective factor in pregnancy is that dietary iron absorption is also increased. Iron-rich foods, such as red meat, legumes/pulses, wholegrain breads and cereals and fortified breakfast cereals, should be encouraged as well as including vitamin C-rich foods with those foods containing iron to aid in the absorption of iron. High-risk women in developed countries, such as: women on a limited budget; women with fad food behaviours or eating disorders; vegan/vegetarian women; and most women living in the developing countries require iron supplementation. This is discussed in Chapter 15.

Excess vitamin A during pregnancy may also be harmful to the fetus, so care must be taken not to exceed the recommended daily intake of vitamin A. The best advice is for women to avoid vitamin supplements that contain vitamin A and other rich sources of vitamin A, such as liver. If they want to take a supplement they should be advised to choose a specific pregnancy multi-vitamin that does not contain vitamin A.

Calcium requirements are increased from 800 to 1100 mg calcium per day. This is usually met quite easily by an intake of three servings of calcium-rich foods daily. As with iron, the absorption of calcium from the diet is increased during pregnancy. Occasionally a woman may choose or be prescribed additional calcium.

Vitamin D stores may be inadequate in women who have restricted exposure to sunlight, who have a diet low in oily fish, eggs and meat or who are obese. These women should be advised to take 10 µg of vitamin D daily.

Another important food issue in pregnancy is for women to practise good food hygiene and food safety. This includes basic advice such as storing, preparing and cooking foods at the appropriate temperatures, and avoiding foods that may not be cooked thoroughly, i.e. foods from takeaway shops, meat pies and salads. The avoidance of uncooked foods such as soft cheese and raw fish is also prudent. The rationale for this is to ensure that all food is uncontaminated by food-borne bacteria, particularly *Listeria*, which may be harmful for the fetus.

ANTENATAL SCREENING

A great deal of prenatal care is spent in detecting potentially dangerous conditions early; screening is one strategy used. In its simplest form blood pressure measurement is a screening strategy, and is discussed later. Currently, much interest is being shown in screening for congenital defects, such as Down syndrome, neural tube defects and single gene defects, using DNA probes (Box 6.1).

Screening for genetic defects

Screening for Down syndrome and certain other genetic defects (for example cystic fibrosis, thalassaemia, haemophilia, Huntington's disease, some muscular dystrophies)

> **Box 6.1 Possible indications for genetic diagnostic tests in first half of pregnancy**
>
> - Pregnancies in women over 35 years of age
> - Pregnancies at increased risk for fetal neural tube defects (i.e. previously affected child)
> - Previous pregnancy resulting in the birth of a chromosomally abnormal child, or one with multiple malformations
> - Known chromosomal abnormality in either parent
> - History of sex-linked disease (e.g. thalassaemia, haemophilia, Duchenne muscular dystrophy)
> - Couples at risk for detectable inborn errors of metabolism

can be carried out by chorionic villus sampling or amniocentesis. Before using these methods, an ultrasound examination of the fetus is made to exclude gross abnormalities (Figs 6.1–6.3).

Chorionic villus sampling

A sample of chorionic tissue is removed from the placental edge between the 9th and 11th weeks of pregnancy by introducing a needle transabdominally and advancing it to the edge of the placenta under ultrasound guidance. About 20 mg of chorionic tissue is sucked into a syringe. The karyotype of the sample is determined within 48 hours.

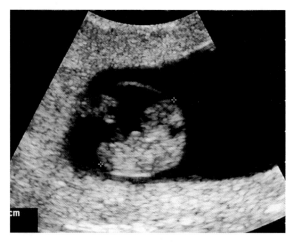

Fig. 6.1 Ultrasound scan showing a normal fetus at 8 weeks' gestation.

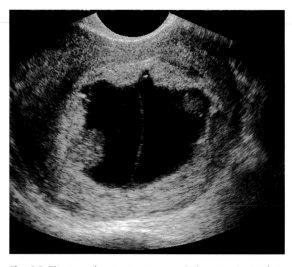

Fig. 6.2 The scan shows an empty amniotic sac at 11 weeks' gestation. The patient aborted 1 week later.

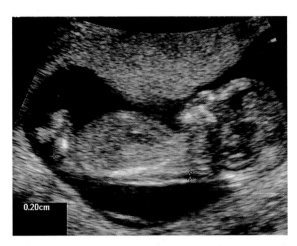

Fig. 6.3 Scan of a normally developing fetus at 12 weeks' gestation. The measurement of nuchal thickness is within the normal range, indicating a very low risk of Down syndrome.

Amniocentesis

The procedure is carried out at about the 15th week of pregnancy. A needle is thrust through the abdominal wall and into the amniotic sac, guided by ultrasound to avoid the placenta and fetus, and a sample of amniotic fluid is removed. This is centrifuged and the fetal cells obtained are cultured for 3 weeks. They are then harvested and a karyotype is made.

Chorionic villus sampling or amniocentesis?

The choice between chorionic villus sampling (CVS) and amniocentesis is controversial. CVS is performed in the first quarter of pregnancy and a preliminary karyotype result using FISH is obtained within 24–48 hours, so that parental anxiety about the result is reduced. However, the karyotyping is slightly less accurate than with amniocentesis because of potential contamination with cells of maternal origin, and the risk of abortion following CVS is slightly higher (1–3% above the background rate compared with 0.5–1% following amniocentesis). Concern has been expressed that CVS may be followed in late pregnancy by oligohydramnios and limb defects. A multicentre study of over 140 000 patients has shown no increase in these defects when CVS is compared to amniocentesis. On the other hand, the karyotype is only obtained 2 weeks after amniocentesis, which increases the psychological stress on the parents, and if the fetus is abnormal and termination of pregnancy is suggested, the process is more painful and psychologically disturbing.

Down syndrome and trisomy 18

Although the risk of Down syndrome and other trisomies, such as trisomy 18, is age related (Table 6.3), because the majority of babies are born to mothers under 35 most centres now offer screening to all women. Three screening regimens are commonly employed. The first calculates the risk using pregnancy-associated plasma protein A and free β-hCG levels at 9–13 weeks' gestation, with the aim to take the serum sample at 10 weeks'. The second measures the nuchal thickness of the fetus between 11 weeks 0 days and 13 weeks 6 days: in about 80% of fetuses with Down syndrome there is increased fluid accumulation behind the neck (see Figs 6.4 and 6.5). The risk is then calculated using the nuchal thickness measurement combined with maternal age. The third method combines the levels of β-hCG, α-fetoprotein (AFP) and free unconjugated oestriol measured between 15 and 20 weeks. Oestriol and AFP levels are lower in fetuses with Down syndrome and β-hCG levels are raised. In some centres inhibin A levels are also used, as this increases the detection rate from 65% to 75–80%.

The combination of first trimester and nuchal translucency screening raises the detection rate from 70 to 90% without affecting the false positive rate of 5%.

If the risk of Down syndrome is calculated to be more than 1/200–250 the woman is then offered CVS if the gestation is between 11 and 14 weeks, or an amniocentesis if the gestation is more advanced.

Screening for open neural tube defects

Open neural tube defects (NTD) occur in two to five pregnancies per 1000. Because of the screening programme for Down syndrome and the use of second-trimester ultrasound scans, additional screening is not necessary

Counselling the patient

It is most important that the implications and details of these screening programmes are carefully explained to the couple, including the false positive and false negative rates. The counsellor must ensure that they clearly understand the difference between screening and diagnostic tests.

If an abnormal result is obtained they must then explain the possible consequences and the choices open to the parents. To reduce the couple's anxiety they must be given sufficient time to absorb the information and have their questions clearly answered, avoiding medical jargon. The counsellor must inform, but not influence, the woman or her partner, who alone are responsible for making the decision whether to terminate or to continue the pregnancy.

Medical imaging in pregnancy

The development of ultrasound imaging, particularly using newer technologies, for example real-time ultrasound and colour Doppler imaging, has made a considerable impact on the care of the pregnant woman.

The role of ultrasound examination in obstetrics is shown in Box 6.2. Examples of ultrasound imaging are shown in Figures 6.4–6.11.

Table 6.3 The incidence of Down syndrome (T21) and trisomy 18 (T18) according to maternal age and gestational age. Note the fall between early pregnancy and birth, which is due to spontaneous pregnancy loss and to selective termination of pregnancy.

MATERNAL AGE (YEARS)	10 WEEKS		12 WEEKS		16 WEEKS		20 WEEKS		40 WEEKS	
	T 21	T18	T21	T18	T21	T18	T21	T18	T21	T18
20	1/983	1/1993	1/1068	1/2484	1/1200	1/3590	1/1295	1/4897	1/1527	1/18013
25	1/870	1/1765	1/966	1/2200	1/1062	1/3179	1/1147	1/4336	1/1350	1/15951
30	1/576	1/1168	1/626	1/1456	1/703	1/2103	1/759	1/2869	1/895	1/10554
33	1/352	1/715	1/383	1/891	1/430	1/1287	1/464	1/1755	1/547	1/6458
35	1/229	1/465	1/249	1/580	1/280	1/837	1/302	1/1142	1/356	1/4202
37	1/140	1/284	1/152	1/354	1/171	1/512	1/185	1/698	1/218	1/2569
39	1/82	1/167	1/89	1/208	1/100	1/300	1/108	1/409	1/128	1/1505
40	1/62	1/126	1/68	1/157	1/76	1/227	1/082	1/310	1/97	1/1139
42	1/35	1/71	1/38	1/89	1/43	1/128	1/46	1/175	1/55	1/644
44	1/20	1/40	1/21	1/50	1/24	1/72	1/26	1/98	1/30	1/359

From Snijders et al. Fetal Diagn Ther 1995;10:356–7 and Snijders et al. Ultrasound Obstet Gynecol 1999;13:167–70 © John Wiley and Sons Limited. Reproduced with permission

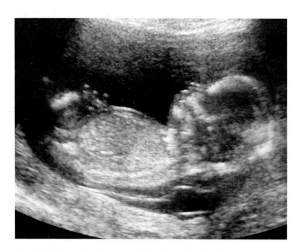

Fig. 6.4 Scan showing an enlarged nuchal thickness. CVS was then performed and established the diagnosis of Down syndrome.

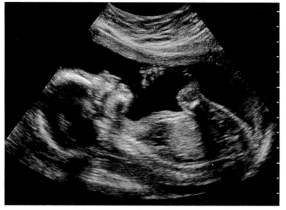

Fig. 6.5 The profile of a normal 18-week fetus.

ANTENATAL DEPRESSION

Between 5 and 10% of women develop depression at some time during their pregnancy, as judged by psychometric scales such as the Edinburgh Postnatal Depression Scale (EPDS). The vulnerable women tend to be primigravid, to have poor social support, to have either a partner who is unemployed or none at all, to be ambivalent about being pregnant or to be anxious about the health of their fetus. Vulnerable women require empathetic support from their attending health professionals and time to talk about their feelings when they are seen at an antenatal clinic or in a doctor's rooms. These women are also likely to develop postnatal depression (see pp. 187–188).

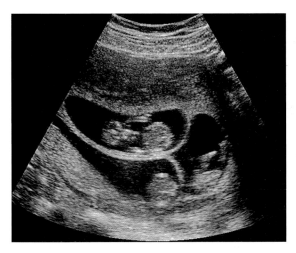

Fig. 6.6 Triplets in three separate amniotic sacs at 12 weeks' gestation.

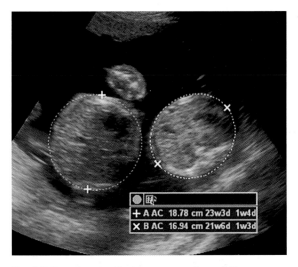

Fig. 6.7 Scan showing the transverse sections of the abdomens of twins at 23 weeks' gestation.

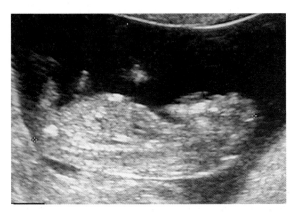

Fig. 6.8 Scan showing a fetus at 12 weeks with anencephaly.

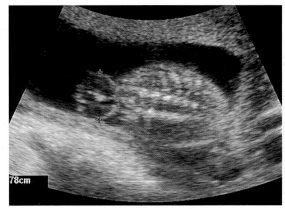

Fig. 6.9 Scan at 18 weeks' gestation showing the failure of fusion of the spine in a fetus with spina bifida.

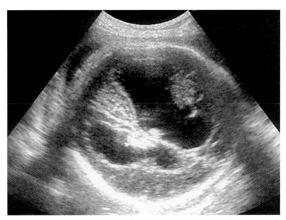

Fig. 6.10 Scan of the head of a fetus at 34 weeks who had developed hydrocephalus and ventriculitis following acute cytomegalovirus infection.

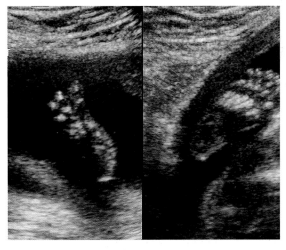

Fig. 6.11 Scan showing a fetus with three toes on the left foot; the right foot is developing normally.

Two examinations require further discussion: blood pressure and weight, and whether the patient should be weighed at each antenatal visit.

Blood pressure

A significant rise in blood pressure from the baseline in early pregnancy provides an early warning that the patient may develop gestational hypertension or the more severe pre-eclampsia (see Ch. 14). For this reason the woman's blood pressure should be measured at each antenatal visit.

In a normal pregnancy the blood pressure tends to remain at a constant level until the last quarter, when a rise of less than 10 mmHg may occur. By convention a systolic pressure of more than 140 mmHg and a diastolic pressure of more than 90 mmHg are considered to indicate hypertension. However, a rise from the baseline measurement of >30 mmHg systolic pressure and more than 15 mmHg diastolic should be noted and a further reading made a few days later.

Problems in recording blood pressure, which may make the readings erroneous, occur in pregnant as well as in non-pregnant patients. These are associated with, for example, the posture of the woman, the size of the cuff, the accuracy of the sphygmomanometer, the time of day and the emotional state of the patient ('white coat hypertension').

To reduce these variables, blood pressure recording equipment should be calibrated regularly, cuffs checked and the blood pressure taken with the patient seated or reclining with her arm at heart level. The brachial artery should be palpated and an appropriately sized cuff inflated until the pulsation disappears. Elevations of 2 mmHg should be recorded, and if the rise is significantly above the baseline a further reading should be taken after an interval.

The systolic pressure is easy to record. The disappearance of sounds Korotkoff (K) 5 is the most accurate marker of intra-arterial diastolic blood pressure. There is a greater concordance between observers when K5 is used to identify the diastolic pressure in pregnant women. If the sounds can be heard down to zero then the muffling or K4 should be recorded.

Weighing the pregnant patient

It has been customary to weigh a pregnant patient at each antenatal visit as it was believed that a small weight gain (or no gain) between visits is associated with restricted fetal growth, and that a weight gain of more than 1 kg a week in the second half of pregnancy is an early marker for the possible development of pre-eclampsia. Careful studies show that the measurement of weight gain is a poor predictor that these problems will develop, and that therefore regular weighing to detect these problems is of limited benefit in low-risk women. However, with the epidemic of obesity in many societies, regular weighing can be used to help women minimize abnormal weight gain.

CARE OF THE PREGNANT WOMAN

With this background information it is now possible to discuss the care of a pregnant woman. As mentioned in Chapter 1, most women have a good idea that they are pregnant when they visit a medical practitioner to confirm the diagnosis. At this visit the doctor will inquire about the present pregnancy, the history of previous pregnancies, family history, previous illnesses or infections (including genital herpes, varicella and HIV/AIDS) and other matters and will examine the woman as already described.

A weight gain of less than 4 kg may be expected before the 20th week of pregnancy; after that a gain of not more than 0.5 kg a week should occur.

Women who are obese (body mass index >30) at the onset of pregnancy require additional prenatal care, as they are more likely to develop gestational diabetes, pre-eclampsia, may have a difficult labour and are at increased risk of thromboembolism and late fetal death. Women who are at low weights before pregnancy (body mass index <19) are more likely to miscarry and have growth-restricted babies.

Routine testing of the urine for protein and glucose

Again it has been the routine to test the pregnant woman's urine at each visit for protein and glucose, but there is debate about its value in the *uncomplicated low-risk pregnancy*. It is important that at the first antenatal visit the urine is careful examined for markers of infection, renal disease and heavy glycosuria in **all** women. Women at risk of developing pre-eclampsia, e.g. women with diabetes or strong family history of hypertensive disorders, should have regular urine testing for protein.

Laboratory tests

Several laboratory tests are made at the first antenatal visit, either by the health professional consulted or, if the woman is referred to a hospital antenatal clinic or to an obstetrician as a private patient, at the referral visit (Box 6.3).

FREQUENCY OF ANTENATAL VISITS

In 1929 there was, in Britain, increasing concern that the maternal mortality rate had not fallen since 1880 (when it was 5 per 1000 live births). This led to the formation of a committee which recommended that a pregnant woman should visit an antenatal clinic every 4 weeks to the 28th week of pregnancy, then every 2 weeks to the 36th week, and thereafter weekly until delivered. Much discussion has arisen recently regarding whether this 80-year-old recommendation is still appropriate. The number of visits can be safely reduced from the traditional 14 to 7–10 without increasing the risk of adverse perinatal outcomes. Using such a schedule the woman is first seen between weeks 7 and 10, and then between 12 and 15, 18 and 20, 26 and 28, and at 32, 34–36, 38, 40 and 41 weeks. If at any time abnormalities are detected the frequency of visits is adjusted accordingly.

Whatever schedule is adopted, a pregnant woman should be asked at each antenatal visit if she has any problems she wishes to discuss and if she is feeling fetal movements. She should have her blood pressure measured, her urine tested for protein where indicated, and

---

Box 6.3 Routine laboratory tests at the first or early antenatal consultation

At first antenatal visit

Blood:	Haemoglobin concentration (normal range 10.5–15.0 g/L)
	Haematocrit (PCV) (normal > 35)
	MCV* and MCH† (especially if patient Southern European, Asian or African because of possible thalassaemia)
	Iron store status
	ABO and Rhesus group. Rhesus antibodies
	All patients, irregular antibodies
	VDRL or similar test (to exclude syphilis)
	Hepatitis B surface antigen (HBsAG)
	Antirubella antibodies
	HIV antibodies
Vaginal smear:	If symptomatic
Urine:	Urinalysis
	Midstream sample for bacteriuria culture

At subsequent antenatal visits

All women repeat the irregular antibody test at 28 weeks' gestation.
Haemoglobin: check between 32 and 36 weeks and/or measure serum ferritin.

*MCV = mean cell volume;
†MCH = mean cell haemoglobin

---

the height of her fundus estimated (see Fig. 1.7, p. 7) or measured with a tape measure (Fig. 6.12) to evaluate the growth of the fetus. Once the fundus of the uterus can be palpated abdominally the fetal heart can be detected with a hand-held Doppler and women find it reassuring to hear the fetal heart at each visit. If an abnormal heart rhythm or rate is heard a formal ultrasound assessment of the fetal heart should be performed.

In addition, after the 28th week the health professional customarily palpates the woman's abdomen to determine the growth, presentation and position of the fetus. The technique used is discussed later in this chapter.

PREPARATION FOR BREASTFEEDING

During pregnancy the health professional should encourage the woman to breastfeed her infant. The benefits of breastfeeding should be discussed:
- Breast milk provides the ideal nutrition for infants and contributes to their healthy growth and development.

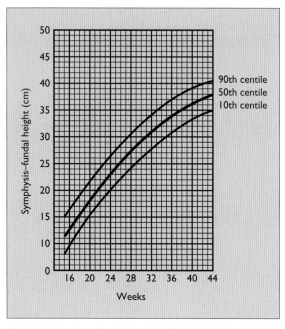

Fig. 6.12 Gestational age estimated from symphysis–fundal height.

- For most women breastfeeding provides a sense of satisfaction and pleasure.
- Exclusive breastfeeding contributes to a woman's health by increasing the space between pregnancies.
- Breastfeeding reduces the chance that the baby will develop infections, particularly gastrointestinal infections, thereby lowering infant mortality.

The health professional may provide the woman with a pamphlet about the breastfeeding support groups in her area.

Should the woman choose not to breastfeed, for whatever reason, the health professional should avoid making her feel guilty and should discuss the importance of preparing the breast-milk substitute according to the manufacturer's directions.

GROWTH OF THE FETUS DURING PREGNANCY

As mentioned above, fetal growth can be determined roughly by the height of the fundus or the distance between the symphysis pubis to the top of the uterus. A more accurate assessment of the fetal growth and weight can be obtained by ultrasound imaging (Fig. 6.13), but this is only required in some pregnancies, for example if the doctor suspects that the fetus is either growth restricted or macrosomic or when medical complications associated with abnormal growth are present. Until about the 28th week of pregnancy the position of the fetal head (or buttocks) relative to the mother's pelvis is of little clinical importance. After that time it becomes increasingly important, and should be monitored by the doctor or midwife. For the purposes of communication descriptive terms are used:

- The **lie** of the fetus refers to the relationship of its long axis to the mother. By the 38th week the fetus may have a longitudinal lie or an oblique or a transverse lie (Fig. 6.14).
- The **presentation** of the fetus relates to the fetal part that occupies the lower part of the uterus over the

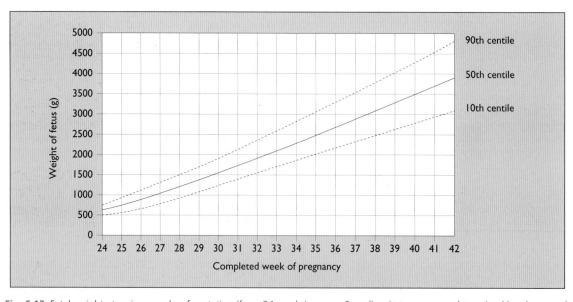

Fig. 6.13 Fetal weight at various weeks of gestation (from 24 weeks) among Scandinavian women as determined by ultrasound.

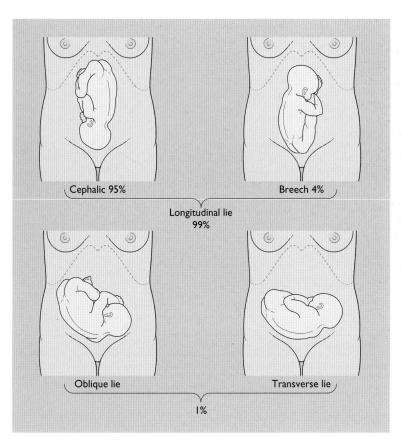

Fig. 6.14 The lie and presentation of the fetus.

pelvic brim. If the fetal head presents it is termed a cephalic presentation; if the buttocks present it is a breech presentation; if a shoulder presents it is termed a shoulder presentation.

- The **presenting part** of the fetus is that portion of the fetus which is presenting against the cervix in the first stage of labour, or against the vagina in the second stage. If the presentation is cephalic, the presenting part is usually the posterior part of the fetal head, the vertex or occiput, but it may be the face or the brow.
- The **attitude** of the fetus is defined as the relation of various fetal parts to other parts. Normally the fetus lies with all its joints flexed, but in some breech presentations the legs are extended along its body.
- The **position** of the presenting part of the fetus is of little clinical significance until labour is established. It refers to the relationship of the presenting part to the bony pelvic walls, and will be discussed in Chapter 8.

Technique of abdominal examination

The patient assumes a reclining position, having emptied her bladder. The abdominal examination to the fetus is made by four 'manoeuvres', which are shown in Figures 6.15–6.18. The information is recorded in the patient's antenatal records.

Assessment of the shape and size of the maternal pelvis

There is little practical benefit in clinically assessing the shape and size of the pelvis before labour. Unless there is a history of a fractured pelvis involving its lateral wall, radiological assessment (X-ray pelvimetry) is rarely used in current practice, as it has not been shown to be a clinically useful predictor of successful vaginal birth.

AGE AND REPRODUCTIVE PERFORMANCE

Teenage pregnancy

More teenagers are becoming sexually active at an earlier age than in previous decades. Studies in northern Europe and North America have shown that by the age of 17 years 50% of teenaged women have had sexual intercourse, and

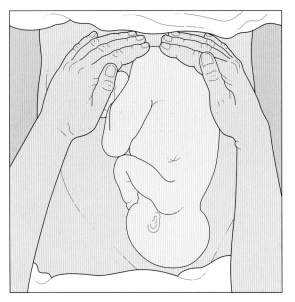

Fig. 6.15 First manoeuvre – fundal palpation. The height of the fundus is estimated and the fundal area gently palpated in an attempt to identify which pole of the fetus (breech or head) is occupying the fundus.

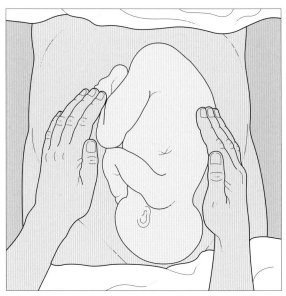

Fig. 6.16 Second manoeuvre – lateral palpation. The examiner's hands slip gently down the sides of the uterus with quick palpation to try to identify on which side the firm back of the fetus or the soft belly and knobbly limbs can be detected.

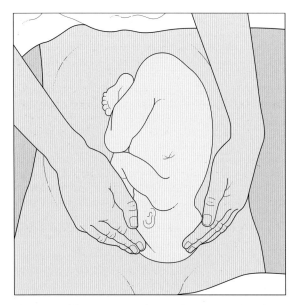

Fig. 6.17 Pelvic manoeuvre. The examiner turns to face the patient's feet and slides his hands gently on the lower part of the uterus, pressing down on each side to determine the presenting part. If it is the fetal head it can be ballotted between the fingers.

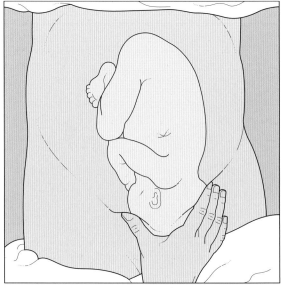

Fig. 6.18 Pawlik's manoeuvre. This is not always necessary and must be performed gently. The presenting part is moved between the fingers and thumb of the examiner's hand, to determine whether it is the fetal head or breech and the degree of descent into the maternal pelvis.

that by the age of 20 years the proportion has risen to 70%. Only one woman in four uses contraceptives in the first 4–6 months of starting sexual intercourse. Improved education associated with the increased use of contraception has resulted in a decline and now a stabilization in the number of young women who become pregnant. In Australia and the UK, 5% of teenaged women, and in the USA 9% of teenaged women, become pregnant each year. Of these, 45–50% obtain an induced abortion, 5% miscarry, and the remainder continue the pregnancy and give birth.

Women under the age of 18 have an increased risk of developing complications of pregnancy and childbirth, being more likely to develop pre-eclampsia or anaemia, and to give birth to a low-birthweight baby. The reasons appear to be:

- Low socioeconomic status
- A nutritionally poor diet
- Alcohol and drug abuse
- A lack of antenatal care.

The problems can be avoided if the adolescent accepts the need for and receives antenatal care from helpful health professionals and social workers. If this occurs the proportion of adolescent pregnant women developing complications in pregnancy is no greater than among women aged 20–35.

Pregnancy in older women

In the past two decades the proportion of women choosing to delay their first pregnancy until they are in their 30s has doubled in most developed countries. Such women tend to belong to the upper socioeconomic groups, to be well educated and to have a career. In Australia births to women aged 30 years in 2006 accounted for 55% of all births compared with 42% in 1994. For women aged 35 years or more this rose to 21.5% from 12.7% over the same time interval. The median age at first birth similarly rose from 25 to 30 years of age. These 'older primigravidae' have an increased risk of having essential hypertension and of developing pre-eclampsia, gestational diabetes and antepartum haemorrhage. They are also more likely to have a baby with Down syndrome, but they have no increased risk of a preterm birth or of fetal growth restriction.

The duration of the first stage of labour in women aged over 34 years is 60 minutes longer than women aged 20–24 years and the second stage 35 minutes longer. Overall they have an increased chance of giving birth by caesarean section or by forceps or ventouse. In Australia, women aged 35 or more are almost three times more likely to be delivered by caesarean section than are women under 20. This may be because the joints are less flexible and myometrial contractions less efficient. Coupled with this is the increased incidence of associated medical complications. In part this may be due to the obstetrician's concern that the woman's fecundity is reduced, and to the desire to obtain a 'perfect' baby.

Provided pregnant women over the age of 35 receive antenatal care, a sound genetic diagnosis and counselling early in pregnancy, the outcome in terms of a live healthy mother and a live healthy child is excellent.

PREPARING FOR CHILDBIRTH

A woman who knows what to expect in childbirth is better able to cooperate and to find the experience less painful. Antenatal classes are available in many hospitals, and are provided by private obstetric physiotherapists for childbirth training. Childbirth training has broadened in recent years, along with the expansion of the original technique of psychoprophylaxis first developed in Russia. Psychoprophylaxis is based on the belief that fear and anxiety about pain and danger in childbirth, learned before the woman becomes pregnant and during pregnancy, sink deeply into her memory and produce a 'conditioned reflex'. Because of this, every time a woman thinks of childbirth a mental image of pain and danger is conjured up, with the result that she enters labour anxious and tense. The tension and fear may increase the pain and delay the birth of the baby. Psychoprophylaxis seeks to eliminate the 'conditioned reflex' and to replace the negative image of childbirth with a more positive one. This is achieved by education during pregnancy in the hope that knowledge and insight will change the woman's perceptions of labour. Psychoprophylaxis also seeks to alter the brain's perception of pain and to convert it into a sensation of discomfort, which can be relieved by muscular activity. This is based on the concept of 'pain dissociation': pain becomes less intense if the woman keeps her mind busy by concentrating on something else. The suggested mental activity usually involves concentrating on a learned pattern of breathing, counting breaths, focusing on a particular point in the room, or consciously commanding the body to release its tension. However, it is very difficult for most women to maintain control and remain calm during the particularly painful stages of labour. The distraction techniques of psychoprophylaxis alone are therefore unrealistic and unsatisfactory for many women during childbirth.

As anthropologists, psychologists, physiotherapists and midwives have become increasingly active in the development of prepared childbirth, new strategies for pain management have been developed which offer more than the original psychoprophylaxis concept.

The social environment in which the baby will be born, and its effect on the woman, is now becoming an important consideration. Many women want their partner or some other 'support person' to be with them during childbirth. The presence of an informed loved one during labour gives the woman familiar and personal support to reduce the clinical environment of a delivery ward.

The discomfort and pain of childbirth are reduced if the attending nursing and medical staff treat the woman as an intelligent individual, who has needs and who can make choices, and who is perceived as a woman having a baby rather than as a patient requiring medical attention. Some hospitals are trying to make the place of birth as non-clinical as possible by providing a supportive environment with floor mattresses, functional beds, soft fabrics and colours, and a shower. These can reduce a woman's anxiety and enable her to cope more efficiently with the process of childbirth.

Techniques of auditory and visual imagery or 'mindfulness' provide an additional means of managing pain in labour. Instead of dissociating from her pain (as in psychoprophylaxis) the woman uses the sensations of labour to assist her in creating an image of what is happening inside her body, allowing herself to feel the pain and let it go. For example, she may visualize her cervix opening each time she has a contraction; the baby's head moving deeper into her pelvis; or the baby opening her vagina in the second stage of labour.

Another development has been the use of relaxation techniques. In psychoprophylaxis, relaxation is taught as a method of control. The woman uses quiet, controlled breathing to convince herself that she is not experiencing pain. More recently, relaxation has been used by the woman as a method of 'letting go' and so reducing the pain. She may move and rock to achieve relaxation; she may stamp her feet, or bang her fists to release stress and diffuse the pain. She may discover that for her, the most effective form of pain control is a combination of floor positions, rhythmic groaning and belly rocking.

The proponents of active involvement in childbirth believe that, if possible, the woman should be given a free choice in the position she wishes to adopt and the movements she wishes to make during labour and the birth of the baby. The woman may choose to lie on her side, to squat, or to position herself on her hands and knees. She may prefer to be supported in a nearly upright position, with her partner in front of or behind her. In this technique there is much less focus on breathing as an exercise or pattern, and more on breathing as a method that helps the woman 'go with the flow'.

It is important to find out the woman's preferred mode of behaviour, and to encourage her to use it in childbirth. A woman who is 'tactile', for example, will probably respond well to massage, hot packs applied to her back, and showers, and will tend to move about a good deal during labour. Other women prefer 'visualization', or eye-to-eye focusing, or will respond to key words such as 'relax', 'go soft', 'let go'. A third group of women are able to relieve the pain of labour more effectively by using auditory strategies. They respond to their support person 'pacing' them during a contraction, and to giving themselves positive messages.

When a woman responds to the pain in a way she naturally prefers, her behaviour ceases to be due to a technique or a method. This reduces the anxiety that comes from having to perform a technique with which she is not comfortable, and which she fears she may not perform well.

The philosophy adopted by numbers of childbirth educators is to provide information and to give the woman permission to be herself. Some women prefer neither to attend classes nor to employ a private childbirth educator. For them, training videotapes are available which enable the woman and her partner to learn at home.

SIGNS THAT LABOUR IS ABOUT TO START

The signs that indicate that labour is soon to start or has started are described on page 68. An expectant mother should have these signs described to her or have access to a book that describes them, so that she can be comfortable knowing when she is probably in labour. A question asked by many women during an antenatal visit concerns whether they will be given drugs to relieve the pain of labour. They should be reassured that analgesics are readily available should they be requested. This matter is discussed on pages 82–84.

Many women are fearful that they will be left alone during the course of childbirth. Today, many women want their husband or partner or a 'significant other person' to be with them through the childbirth process, and most hospitals agree to this.

ANTENATAL INFORMATION

Certain matters affecting the mother during pregnancy should be discussed at the early visits.

Dental care

An early visit to the dentist is advised so that any dental care required can be carried out in the first half of pregnancy.

Employment

In the current economic conditions many pregnant women choose to or have to work. Provided she does not become too tired, that her enlarging abdomen does not interfere with the job and that industrial conditions in the office, factory or store are appropriate, work during pregnancy will harm neither the mother nor the fetus.

Exercise

Exercise is to be encouraged if this is the usual habit of the mother, but need not be insisted upon if she is usually sedentary. She should take walks and other light exercise if she wishes. The woman should neither become a fanatic for exercise nor refrain from all physical activity. If she enjoys swimming, she may continue to swim. Contact and high-impact sports do pose potential risks for the pregnant woman as they may lead to abdominal trauma, falls or excessive stress on joints. Scuba diving should be avoided because of reported fetal birth defects and fetal decompression disease. In general, she should not alter her regimen of exercise just because she is pregnant, unless the exercise is very strenuous and may raise her body temperature significantly.

Immunization

Pregnant women are particularly susceptible to influenza, vaccination should be encouraged. If the woman is about to travel overseas, antityphoid or cholera inoculations may be given. All pregnant women who have not been immunized against poliomyelitis, or whose immunity has lapsed, should be immunized in early pregnancy.

Sex during pregnancy

Many doctors fail to discuss sex during pregnancy, and many women feel inhibited about asking. Because of this many couples are inadequately informed, and have considerable misconceptions.

Studies have shown that many pregnant women have reduced sexual desire and activity, especially in the early weeks and after the 30th week. The reason for this decline in libido is unclear. Some women find sexual intercourse uncomfortable; others fear that coitus and orgasm may damage the fetus or bring on premature labour. Others see themselves as unattractive, or find the physical awkwardness of coitus in late pregnancy inhibiting.

It is appropriate to talk with the couple. There is no evidence that coitus, cunnilingus or masturbation, whether leading to orgasm or not, have any damaging effect on the fetus, or induce labour prematurely. All forms of sexual enjoyment are permissible in pregnancy, with the proviso that, during cunnilingus, the man should be warned not to blow, forcing air into the woman's vagina, as this has led to air embolism in pregnancy.

Many pregnant women want additional closeness from their partner, and he should be supportive and gentle at all times. In late pregnancy coitus with the man on top may be uncomfortable, but other positions are not, and non-coital sexual satisfaction may be preferred. Coitus can continue, if the couple wish, up to term without any damage to mother or baby. The principal medical contraindications to coitus are ruptured membranes and known placenta praevia.

Smoking

The deleterious effects of smoking on reproductive health are well established and women who smoke should be given every encouragement and support to quit. Currently 30% of women in their early 20s in Australia are regular smokers, and pregnancy provides a strong motivation for many to stop or at least to substantially reduce their consumption. Compared with non-smokers, women who smoke have a between 10 and 40% lower probability of conception per cycle and an increased risk of both primary and secondary infertility. It is also important to advise the woman and her family of the risks to the fetus and baby of passive smoking.

Following conception smokers have twice the risk of miscarriage, and a small increased risk of an ectopic pregnancy.

Smoking is a major contributor to perinatal morbidity and mortality (see Table 6.4). One-third of sudden infant deaths (SID) are attributable to cigarette smoking.

One reason for the damaging effect of smoking in pregnancy is that smokers have a reduced intervillous blood flow and higher blood levels of carbon monoxide.

Nicotine replacement therapies, such as gum and patches, have had limited trials in pregnancy, but because of nicotine's effect on placental and fetal blood flow, including cerebral blood flow, their use is still controversial. If she does opt to use nicotine patches then she should be advised to remove them at night

Encouraging and supporting smokers to quit smoking is the single most effective way to reduce premature birth. The '5 As' approach is recommended as the minimum approach to aid the woman to quit and stay quit – see Box 6.4.

Table 6.4 Increased risks associated with cigarette smoking	
	RELATIVE RISK (RR)
Preterm premature rupture of membranes (PPROM)	2.0–5.0
Premature delivery	1.2–2.0
Placental abruption	1.4–2.4
Placenta praevia	1.5–3.0
Intrauterine growth restriction	1.5–10.0
Perinatal mortality	1.3

Recreational drugs

Alcohol

Heavy alcohol consumption in pregnancy (more than 120 g, or 12 standard drinks a day) is associated with:

- Fetal growth restriction
- Developmental delay and neurological complications in the baby
- Fetal alcohol syndrome (facial characteristics: low-set ears, elongated midface, small head and upturned nose, skeletal and cardiac malformations). The incidence of FAS is multifactorial and compounded by smoking and other drug abuse, poor diet and social deprivation.

A consumption of seven standard drinks in a week and no more than two in any one day spread over at least 2 hours does not appear to have any damaging effects on the fetus or mother. Nevertheless, a pregnant woman should be advised to limit her consumption of alcohol especially during the first trimester, as there is concern about the long-term effects on the neurodevelopment of the child, particularly with numerical problem-solving and reading proficiency, which is dose dependent.

Heroin and other opiates

The major risks are:

- Intrauterine growth restriction (IUGR)
- Premature labour
- Drug withdrawal for the neonate
- Other social deprivation issues
- Medical diseases, e.g. hepatitis B and C and HIV.

Most specialist drug clinics prefer to convert the addict to methadone or to continue buprenorphine if she is already stabilized on it, using the lowest dose that prevents craving.

During labour the fetus should be monitored, especially if there is IUGR. Following delivery the neonate should be carefully monitored for signs of drug withdrawal (restlessness, tremors, high-pitched screaming, yawning and sweating).

Cocaine

Heavy use of cocaine (coke, crack) is associated with:

- IUGR
- Placental abruption
- Stillbirth
- Premature rupture of the membranes and delivery
- Need for neonatal resuscitation
- Intraventricular haemorrhage
- Developmental delays.

As with alcohol these complications are compounded by the abuse of other drugs and poor lifestyle.

Amphetamines

Heavy use of amphetamines (speed, crystal, uppers, meth) is associated with:

- Cleft palate
- Hypertension and pre-eclampsia
- IUGR
- Premature delivery.

Cannabis

Heavy cannabis consumption has been linked to subtle differences in cognitive processes, reduced memory and verbal scale performance and sleep disturbance in 3-year-olds, reduced height at 6 years of age and increased hyperactivity at age 10. The woman should be encouraged to stop using it before conception and during pregnancy.

Chapter | 7 |

Physiological and anatomical changes in childbirth

Labour and childbirth is the process whereby the fetus and placenta are expelled from the uterus by coordinated myometrial contractions. The reason why labour starts remains obscure in spite of much research and many theories. When this is elucidated it should be possible to prevent premature labour, with its increased perinatal mortality and morbidity.

For labour to commence two things have to occur: the onset of coordinated uterine contractions and the softening of the uterine cervix. The critical factor for the increase in uterine activity is the rise in intracellular calcium, which activates phosphorylation of myosin and the creation of cross-bridges with actin, which results in the contraction of the myometrial cell. The cervical changes are due to a breakdown in collagen owing to the release of metalloproteinases and an increase in the water content. Prostaglandins and leukotrienes are involved in these physiological changes.

The fetus then has to negotiate the birth canal, propelled by contractions of the uterus. Factors that can delay or prevent this are:

- The shape and size of the bony and soft tissues of the woman's pelvis (the passages)
- The size of the fetus (the passenger)
- The quality and frequency of the uterine contractions (the powers).

THE PASSAGES

Bony pelvis

The bony pelvis is made up of four bones, the two innominate bones, the sacrum and the coccyx, united at three joints. When a woman stands erect, the pelvis is tilted forward. The pelvic inlet makes an angle of about 55° with the horizontal. The angle varies between individuals and between races; for example, black Africans have a lesser angle. An angle of more than 55° may make the descent of the fetal head into the pelvis difficult (Fig. 7.1).

The 'true' pelvis is bounded by the pubic crest, the iliopectineal line and the sacral promontory. An 'ideal obstetric' pelvis is described in Box 7.1 and the brim is shown in Figure 7.2. The true pelvis is cylindrical in shape, with a bluntly curved lower end, and is slightly curved anteriorly. Anteriorly the pubic bones form its boundary, measuring 4.5 cm. Posteriorly, the curve of the sacrum forms its

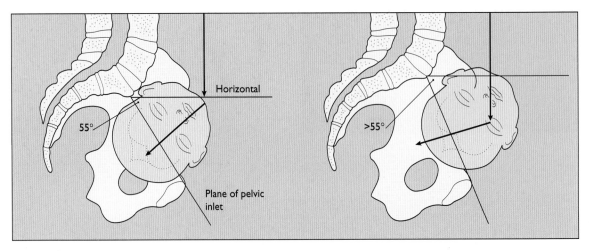

Fig. 7.1 Effect of the inclination of the pelvic brim on the engagement of the fetal head.

Box 7.1	**The ideal obstetric pelvis**
Brim	Round or oval transversely
	No undue projection of the sacral promontory
	Anterior–posterior diameter 12 cm
	Transverse diameter 13 cm
	The plane of the pelvic inlet not less than 55°
Cavity	Shallow with straight side-walls
	No great projection of the ischial spines
	Smooth sacral curve
	Sacrospinous ligament at least 3.5 cm
Outlet	Pubic arch rounded
	Subpubic angle > 80°
	Intertuberous diameter at least 10 cm

boundary, measuring 12 cm. Laterally its walls narrow slightly distally (Fig. 7.3). The walls are penetrated by the obturator foramen anteriorly and the sciatic foramen laterally, which is divided into two parts by the sacrospinous and sacrotuberous ligaments.

For descriptive purposes the true pelvis can be divided into four zones. These are shown in Figure 7.4. The measurements of the zone of the inlet are shown in Figure 7.2. The zone of the cavity is wedge-shaped in profile and almost round in section. It is the most roomy part of the true pelvis, the anterior–posterior diameter measuring 13.5 cm and the transverse diameter 12.5 cm.

The zone of the midpelvis passes through the apex of the pubic arch, the spines of the ischia, the sacrospinous ligament and the tip of the sacrum. It is the smallest zone and its most important diameter is the ischial–bispinous diameter, which measures 10.5 cm. If this zone is contracted the fetal presenting part may not be able to rotate and may become arrested.

The zone of the outlet (Fig. 7.5) does not usually interfere with the birth unless the pubic rami are narrow, which reduces the intertuberous diameter. In these cases delay may occur and the soft tissues of the perineum may be torn and damaged.

The axis of the birth canal corresponds to the direction the fetal presenting part – usually the head – takes during its passage through the birth canal (Fig. 7.6).

Factors influencing pelvic shape and size

Minor alterations in pelvic shape have been found in many women receiving routine radiological pelvimetry, but only in a few instances has the abnormality been found to delay the birth. Smaller women tend to have a smaller bony pelvis, but also tend to have smaller babies. More severe alterations occur in populations where rickets or osteomalacia are found, but are uncommon in the developed countries today.

Soft tissues of the female pelvis

These include the uterus, the muscular pelvic floor and the perineum. The anatomical details are described in Chapter 43.

Uterus

The uterus in pregnancy can be divided into three parts:

- The upper uterine segment
- The lower uterine segment
- The uterine cervix.

Upper uterine segment

This portion of the uterus consists of the fundus and that part of the uterus lying above the reflection of the vesico-uterine fold of peritoneum. During pregnancy it undergoes the greatest degree of myometrial hyperplasia and hypertrophy. In labour it provides the strong contractions that push the fetus along the birth canal.

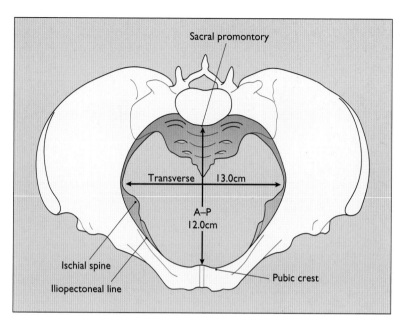

Fig. 7.2 The 'ideal obstetric' pelvis: pelvic inlet. A–P = anterior–posterior.

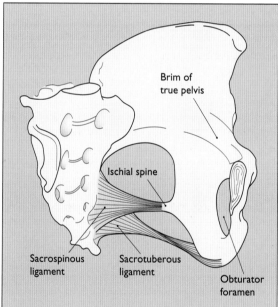

Fig. 7.3 The pelvic cavity. The right innominate bone has been removed in order to show the extent of the cavity.

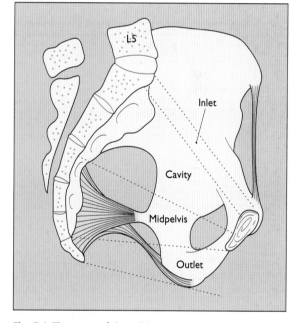

Fig. 7.4 The zones of the pelvis.

Lower uterine segment

This portion of the uterus lies between the vesico-uterine fold of the peritoneum superiorly and the cervix inferiorly. During pregnancy the upper part of the cervix is incorporated into the lower uterine segment, which stretches to accommodate the fetal presenting part (Fig. 7.7). In late pregnancy, as the upper segment muscle contractions increase in frequency and strength, the lower uterine segment develops more rapidly and is stretched radially to permit the fetal presenting part to descend (Fig. 7.8). In labour the entire cervix becomes incorporated into the stretched lower uterine segment.

Cervix uteri

In late pregnancy the cervix becomes softer because of chemical changes in the collagen fibres, and shorter as it is incorporated into the lower uterine segment. It also

55

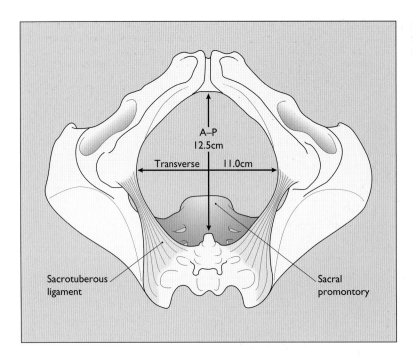

Fig. 7.5 The female pelvic outlet viewed from below. A–P = anterior–posterior.

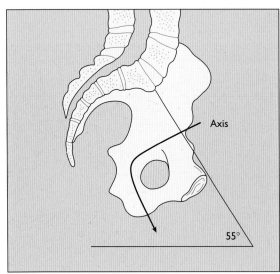

Fig. 7.6 Inclination of the pelvic brim and the axis of the birth canal. The plane of the pelvic brim makes an angle of about 55° with the horizontal in the erect patient, and the plane of the outlet about 10° with the horizontal. The axis of the birth canal is angled, the alteration in direction occurring at the pelvic floor.

undergoes a variable degree of dilatation. Collectively, these changes are termed cervical 'ripening'. The changes may occur abruptly or gradually at any time after the 34th week of pregnancy, but usually occur nearer term, especially in primigravidae. At the 34th gestational week the cervix is 2 cm or more dilated in 20% of primigravidae and in 40% of multigravidae, and the proportion increases towards term (Fig. 7.9).

At the onset of labour the cervix of a primigravida is ripe, and is either partly, or not, effaced (i.e. incorporated into the lower uterine segment).

Formation of the birth canal during labour

When myometrial contraction and retraction have led to full dilatation of the cervix the fetal head descends into the vagina, which expands to encompass it (Fig. 7.10). Normally an apparent space, the vaginal muscle has hypertrophied and the epithelium become folded during pregnancy so that it can accommodate the fetus without damage. As the fetal head descends it encounters the pelvic floor and the leading point is directed forwards by the gutter formed by the levatores ani. The fetus must now pass through the urogenital diaphragm. The levator muscles stretch and are displaced downwards and backwards, so that the anus receives the full force of the descending head and, dilating, gapes widely to expose the anterior rectal wall. Pressure is also exerted on the lower part of the vagina and the central portion of the perineum, and as the head is born the tissues may tear.

The descent of the fetus from the uterus and out into the world is straight to the level of the ischial spines; it then moves in an anterior curve around the lower border of the symphysis pubis. If the pubic arch is wide, the head will stem close behind the symphysis and the perineum will not be so stretched. If the angle is narrow the head is forced back, the direction of the curve is more obtuse and perineal damage is likely.

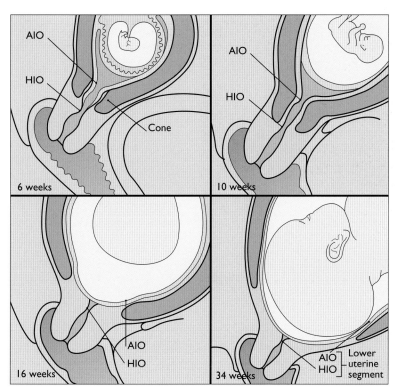

Fig. 7.7 Formation of the lower uterine segment based on the observations of CP Wendell-Smith. Cone, the condensation of muscle at the junction of the body of the uterus and the cervix; AIO, anatomical internal os; HIO, histological internal os.

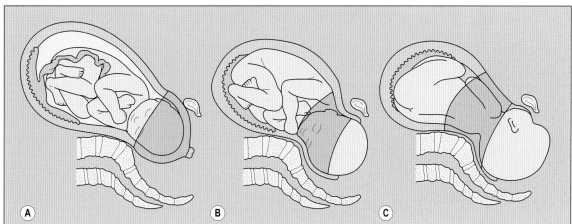

Fig. 7.8 (A) The lower uterine segment in late pregnancy. (B) The lower uterine segment in late labour. It is dilated circumferentially and has thinned but is shorter. (C) In obstructed labour the dilated and thinned lower uterine segment stretches and is in danger of rupture.

THE PASSENGER

The fetus may influence the progress of childbirth by its size and its presentation. Of all the fetal parts, the head is the least compressible and pliant. However, because of the ability of the skull bones to override each other the fetus is able to negotiate the birth canal provided

that the fetus is not too big and the uterine contractions are sufficiently strong.

Anatomy of the fetal skull

The face of the term fetus is relatively small in relation to the cranium, which makes up most of the head. The cranium is made up of five bones held together by a membrane,

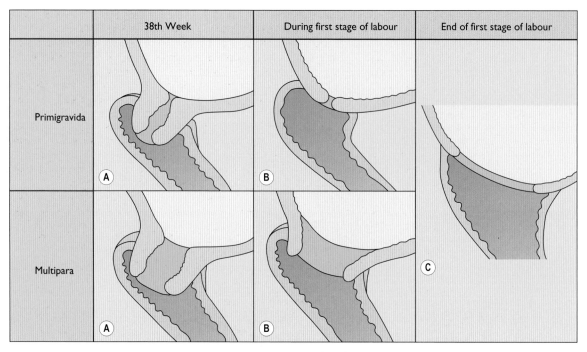

	38th Week	During first stage of labour	End of first stage of labour
Primigravida	A	B	
Multipara	A	B	C

Fig. 7.9 Progressive effacement and dilatation of the cervix in late pregnancy and labour. **Primigravida.** (A) Little or no effacement or dilatation has occurred. (B) Effacement has occurred but dilatation is not yet marked. (C) The cervix is fully effaced and dilated. **Multipara.** (A) Dilatation has begun but no effacement has yet occurred. (B) Effacement and dilatation are occurring simultaneously. (C) The cervix is fully effaced and dilated.

Fig. 7.10 Birth canal of a patient in the second stage of labour.

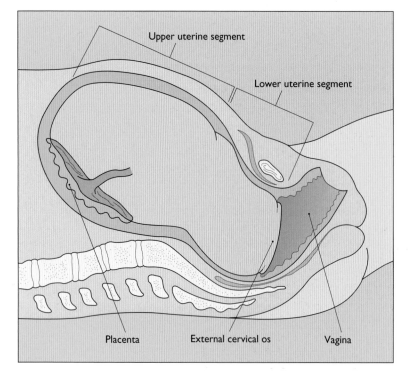

Upper uterine segment

Lower uterine segment

Placenta   External cervical os   Vagina

which permits their movement during birth and in early childhood. The bones are the two parietal bones, the two frontal bones and the occipital bone (Fig. 7.11). The membranous areas between the bones are called sutures. The coronal suture separates the frontal bones from the parietal bones. The sagittal suture separates the two parietal bones, and the lambdoid suture separates the occipital bone from the parietal bones (Fig. 7.12). The anterior fontanelle is the diamond-shaped area of the junction of the sagittal and the two coronal sutures. The posterior fontanelle is the smaller Y-shaped area at the junction between the sagittal suture and the two lambdoid sutures. The configuration of the posterior fontanelle permits the occipital bone to be displaced under the two parietal bones during childbirth, thus reducing the volume of the fetal skull. This is called moulding. During moulding, the parietal bones may also slip under each other (Fig. 7.13).

Regions of the fetal skull have been designated to aid in the description of the presenting part felt at vaginal examination during labour. The occiput is the area lying behind the posterior fontanelle. The vertex is the area of the skull lying between the anterior and posterior fontanelle and between the parietal eminences. The bregma is the area around the anterior fontanelle. The sinciput is the area lying in front of the anterior fontanelle: this can be divided into two parts, the brow, which is the area between the anterior fontanelle and the root of the nose, and the face, which is the area below the root of the nose.

The region of the skull that presents in labour depends on the degree of flexion of the head. The diameters are shown

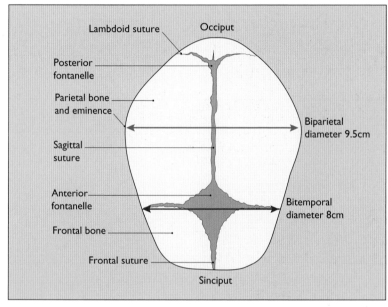

Fig. 7.11 Fetal skull from above, showing important obstetrical diameters.

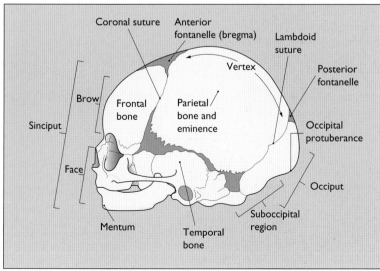

Fig. 7.12 Fetal skull from the side, showing landmarks.

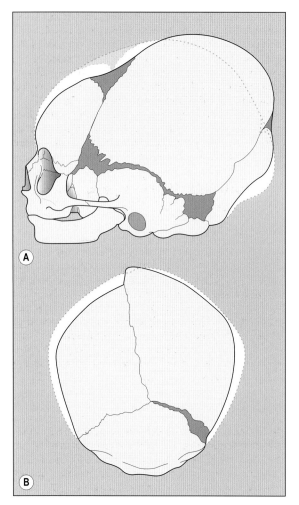

(A)

(B)

Fig. 7.13 Moulding of the fetal skull. (A) Lateral view. (B) Posterior view. The dotted line shows the shape before moulding.

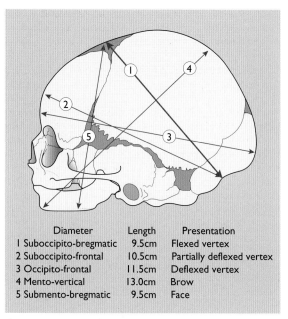

	Diameter	Length	Presentation
1	Suboccipito-bregmatic	9.5cm	Flexed vertex
2	Suboccipito-frontal	10.5cm	Partially deflexed vertex
3	Occipito-frontal	11.5cm	Deflexed vertex
4	Mento-vertical	13.0cm	Brow
5	Submento-bregmatic	9.5cm	Face

Fig. 7.14 Diameters of the fetal skull.

in Figure 7.14, along with degrees of flexion or deflexion of the head on presentation to the maternal pelvis.

In labour, after the amniotic sac has ruptured, releasing amniotic fluid, the dilating cervix may press firmly on the fetal scalp, reducing both lymphatic and venous return from it. This may cause a tissue swelling beneath the skin called a caput succedaneum (Fig. 7.15). It is soft and boggy to the touch and disappears within a few days of birth.

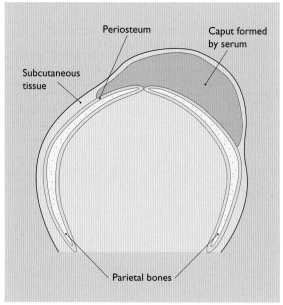

Fig. 7.15 Caput succedaneum.

THE POWERS

The myometrium is formed from interdigitating muscle fibres of the two Müllerian ducts. The middle parts of the ducts adhere and the central septum is lost to form a single hollow organ – the uterus. The myometrium has three layers:

- An outer longitudinal thin layer
- A thick middle spiral layer, the size of which diminishes towards the cervix and occupies only 10% of the cervical tissue
- A thin circular inner layer. Each muscle fibre is made up of bunches of fibrils, which in turn are made up of spindle-shaped cells averaging 200 mm in length and 7 mm in diameter. These cells are composed

of smaller contractile fibres comprising interdigitating chains of actin and myosin, surrounded by a permeable membrane.

Characteristics of myometrial contractions

The uterus, although composed of many individual muscle fibres, functions as a single hollow muscular organ. The myometrium is never completely relaxed. It has a resting tone of between 6 and 12 mmHg. From early until late pregnancy the uterus contracts at intervals; the contractions (Braxton Hicks contractions) are painless. Each contraction causes a rise in intrauterine pressure of varying amplitude or intensity. This has two elements: a rapid rise to a peak and a slower return to the resting tone. For descriptive purposes the intensity of the contraction multiplied by the frequency of the contractions (per 10 minutes) provides a measure of uterine activity, which is expressed in Montevideo units (Fig. 7.16). With the development of tocography, a different measure of uterine activity can be obtained. With a cardiotocograph linked to a computer, the area under the contraction can be measured and expressed in kilopascals per 15 minutes. These two methods of measuring uterine activity relate fairly closely to each other.

Spread of uterine contractions

A uterine contraction starts from a pacemaker located at the junction of the Fallopian tube and the uterus on one side. The contractile wave passes inwards and downwards from the pacemaker at a rate of 2 cm per second to involve the entire uterus in the contraction. In a normal labour the intensity and incremental phase of the contraction is greater in the upper uterine segment, as the muscle is thicker and there is a greater amount of actinomyosin to contract. This permits the contraction to be coordinated, the maximal intensity occurring in the upper part of the uterus, with a reducing intensity as the wave passes down towards the cervix; the peak of the contraction occurs simultaneously in all parts of the uterus. The phenomenon is known as the triple descending gradient (Fig. 7.17).

The intensity and frequency of the uterine contractions varies during labour, increasing as labour progresses. It has been found that uterine activity is greater if the woman walks about during early labour.

Myometrial activity in pregnancy and labour

Pregnancy

Up to the 30th week of pregnancy uterine activity is slight, small localized contractions of no more than 5 mmHg occurring at intervals of 1 minute. Every 30–60 minutes a contraction of higher amplitude (10–15 mmHg) arises which spreads to a wider area of the uterus and may be palpated (Fig. 7.18A). These palpable contractions occur with increasing frequency and intensity after the 30th week and are referred to as Braxton Hicks contractions (Fig. 7.18B). After the 36th week uterine activity increases progressively until labour starts (Fig. 7.18C).

Onset of labour

This is difficult to determine with accuracy, and consequently difficult to define. At best it can be said to be the time after which uterine contractions cause the progressive dilatation of the cervix beyond 2 cm, and painful contractions usually occur at least every 10 minutes (Fig. 7.18D).

Labour

In true normal labour the intensity and frequency of the contractions increase, but there is no rise in the resting tone. The intensity increases in late labour to 60 mmHg and the frequency to two to four contractions every 10 minutes, or 150–200 Montevideo units. The duration of the contraction also increases from about 20 seconds in early labour to 40–90 seconds at the end of the first stage, and in the second stage (see Fig. 7.18E). Contractions are most effective when they are coordinated, with fundal dominance, have a maximum intensity of 40–60 mmHg, last 60–90 seconds, recur with a 2–4-minute interval between the peaks of consecutive contractions, and the uterus has a resting tone of less than 12 mmHg. More frequent contractions of higher intensity diminish the oxygen exchange in the placental bed and may lead to fetal hypoxia and clinical signs of fetal distress. The efficiency of contractions is greater when the mother walks about or lies on her side during the first stage of labour, and this position also improves the placental blood supply.

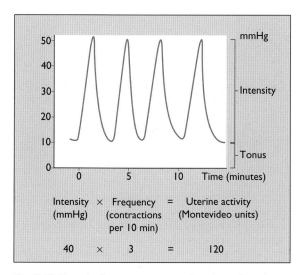

Fig. 7.16 Quantitative measurements of tracings of uterine contractions.

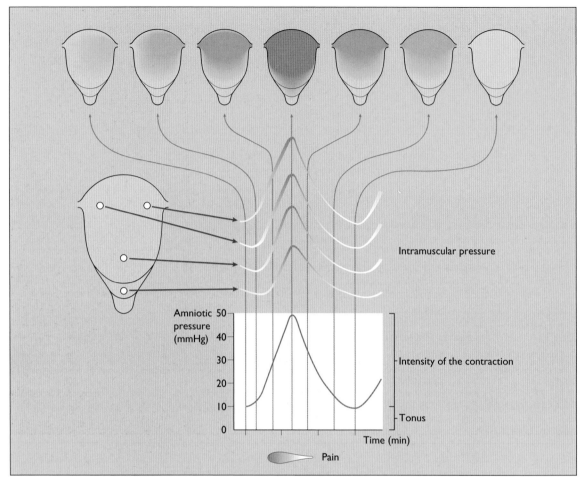

Fig. 7.17 Normal wave of contraction passing over the uterus shown diagrammatically. The small uteri show how the wave starts and spreads, finally fading. The large uterus shows the four points at which the intramyometrial pressure was recorded with microballoons. The contraction phase is shown by the thick ascending line. Note how the peak of contraction occurs in all parts of the uterus simultaneously.

The coordinated contractions of labour cause a permanent shortening of the muscle fibres, and as this is maximal in the upper part of the uterus a distending tension is placed upon the less muscular lower part, and more particularly upon the scantily muscled cervix. The cervix therefore dilates circumferentially with each contraction, closing in at the end of the contraction; however, because of the retraction of the muscle in the upper uterus, a permanent but slight dilatation occurs with each contraction.

In the second stage of labour, voluntary contraction of the diaphragm and abdominal muscles, added to the uterine contraction, propels the baby downwards through the dilated vagina and overcomes the resistance of perineal muscles to its advance (see Fig. 7.18F). At the height of each bearing-down effort the total force exerted on the fetus is approximately 2 kg/cm² and this is resolved into two components: one, a force propelling the head downwards, and the other, a dilating force,

which stretches the birth canal against the resistance of the pelvic and perineal muscles. (If the membranes are intact the resultant propelling force is less, as the amniotic fluid balances it in part.) Because the pelvic floor muscles form an inclined groove, and as the head is ovoid, the additional pressure leads to the rotation of the occiput through 90° to lie anteriorly.

Uterine activity continues unaltered after expulsion of the fetus and leads to the expulsion of the placenta from the upper uterine segment, between 2 and 6 minutes after the birth of the baby. Once the placenta has left the upper segment uterine activity diminishes, but contractions of an intensity of about 60–80 mmHg still occur regularly for 48 hours after delivery, the frequency decreasing as time passes (see Fig. 7.18G–J). These contractions, and those of the third stage, are usually painless, but painful contractions disturb some patients. Further painful contractions may occur with suckling, owing to a reflex release of oxytocin.

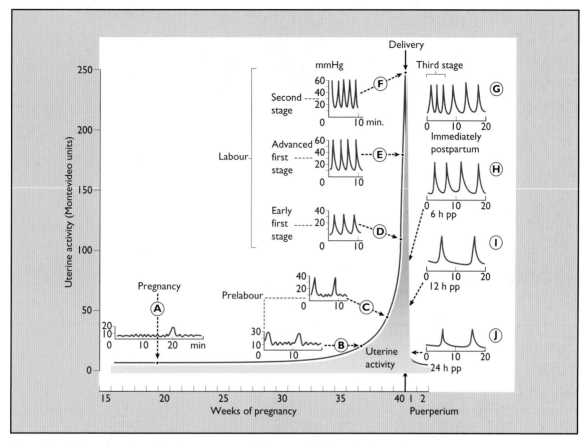

Fig. 7.18 Evolution of uterine activity in pregnancy and labour. For further explanation of A–J see text.

Pain of uterine contractions

The pain of uterine contractions is, in part, due to ischaemia developing in a myometrial fibre. Because there are more fibres and the contractions are stronger in the upper uterine segment, pain is felt more strongly in the cutaneous distribution of cutaneous nerves T12 and L1. At the beginning of the contraction only slight pain is felt; it increases as the contraction grows stronger (Fig. 7.19).

Many women in labour complain of backache, which may be severe. It occurs during cervical dilatation when the lower uterine segment contracts more strongly than usual, or when the triple descending gradient fails to arise. In the second stage of labour the pain is due to uterine contractions and to the stretching of the vaginal, pelvic and perineal tissues. This pain is felt in the back, in the pelvis and down the thighs.

The perception of pain during labour is increased if the woman is apprehensive and has little knowledge of the process of childbirth. One of the reasons for childbirth training (see p. 49) is to reduce fear and improve the mother's understanding of childbirth.

EFFECT OF CHILDBIRTH ON THE MOTHER

Energy expenditure

Labour is appropriately named for it is a period of considerable expenditure of energy, mainly on the contractions of the uterus, but to some extent on increased cardiac activity. The energy is provided initially from metabolism of glycogen from the glycogen–water pool in muscles. In current obstetric practice women in labour are denied food, and thus the pool is rapidly depleted and energy is obtained by the oxidation of stored body fat. This may lead to the accumulation of ketones in the blood, predominantly D-3-hydroxybutyric acid and to a lesser extent lactic and pyruvic acids. In consequence, a mild metabolic acidosis develops. This is most marked in the expulsive stage of labour, when a fall in the blood pH is usual, although it remains in the normal range of 7.3–7.4. This is compensated for by a mild respiratory alkalosis, resulting from hyperventilation, which is common during this time.

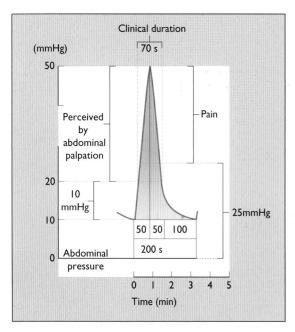

Fig. 7.19 Pain in labour. The initial part of the contraction is painless and not perceived by abdominal palpation. The duration of the contraction observed clinically (70 seconds) is shorter than the duration of myometrial activity (200 seconds).

The mild ketoacidosis is of little practical importance, provided that the woman enters labour in a good nutritional condition and the birth occurs in less than 12 hours.

This extra expenditure of energy leads to increased heat production, and sweating occurs with a loss of body fluid.

Body temperature

The body temperature rises slightly during childbirth, but remains lower than 37.8 °C, unless the woman becomes ketoacidotic, at which point it may rise above this level.

Cardiovascular changes

The cardiac output increases by 12% over the prelabour readings between contractions and by 30% during contractions. The increased cardiac output is effected by an increase in stroke volume and heart rate. The mean arterial pressure rises by about 10%, and in the expulsive stage of labour the rise may be greater. These changes further increase cardiac work in response to a uterine contraction. The right atrial pressure rises and may reach 40–50 mmHg in late labour, and the cardiopulmonary blood volume increases at the same time. Following the birth a further rise in cardiac output occurs. Because bradycardia is usual at this time, the rise is due to an increase in stroke volume. The effect lasts for 3–4 days.

For these reasons childbirth may pose a hazard to a woman who has uncompensated heart disease or who is severely anaemic.

Blood loss during childbirth

Clinical estimates of blood loss during childbirth show that a mean of 400 mL is lost. This may be an underestimate. In a healthy woman this loss is of no clinical significance, as it is less than the increase in blood volume that occurs in pregnancy.

Gastrointestinal tract

In labour gastric emptying is delayed and partly digested food may remain in the stomach for more than 12 hours. Intestinal motility is also delayed.

EFFECT OF CHILDBIRTH ON THE FETUS

The entry of a child into the world is not gentle. Unlike other mammals, humans have developed a large head which has to traverse a relatively small bony birth canal, propelled by uterine contractions. During a contraction the uterus exerts a force on the fetus of $1 \, kg/cm^2$, and during the expulsive stage the force doubles when voluntary expulsive efforts are added to the uterine contractions.

The effect of this force is mainly on the fetal head, and so moulding of the fetal skull may occur. Normally the baby is unharmed, but if moulding is great because of cephalopelvic disproportion, an inexpert delivery of the baby by forceps or vacuum extraction may lead to intracranial oedema or damage.

During childbirth the fetus suffers some degree of hypoxia. If the fetus has obtained a good supply of glucose during pregnancy this causes few problems, but if the fetus is growth restricted because of insufficient supplies of nutrients from the mother it may enter labour with diminished glycogen reserves and may be unable to compensate for the reduction of glucose and oxygen during an abnormal or prolonged labour. This means that it may have to use anaerobic methods of obtaining energy, with resulting acidaemia, which may affect the fetal heart rate as it attempts to compensate for the relative hypoxia. The fetal heart rate is the result of a balance between the tachycardia produced by sympathetic nerve stimulation and the bradycardia produced by vagal nerve stimulation. Normally, the vagus is dominant and exerts a slowing effect on the fetal heart, which beats at a rate of 140 ± 20 times per minute. If fetal hypoxia occurs, the altered composition of the blood leads to a rise in sympathetic and vagal tones, which differ in effect. The sympathetic effect becomes dominant in mild hypoxia. Its onset is delayed, but if the hypoxia persists it leads to fetal tachycardia. This persists for 10–30 minutes after the cause of the hypoxia has ceased. Vagal stimulation occurs if hypoxia is moderate or severe in degree. Bradycardia occurs rapidly, lasts as long as the hypoxia, and then resolves rapidly.

Course and management of childbirth

CHOICES IN CHILDBIRTH

In most developed countries nearly all women give birth in hospital. In contrast, in the developing countries, particularly in the rural areas where 75% of the population live, most women have their babies at home. Health authorities attempt to select those who would be more safely delivered in hospital and arrange for the transfer of other women to hospital should problems arise.

With the trend towards hospital birth in the developed countries, some groups of women question whether this is always appropriate, claiming that on admission to hospital a pregnant woman loses her autonomy, may not be told about proposed procedures, and can be treated impersonally by busy attending staff. In other words, a normal event is medicalized. Several international organizations have addressed the issues raised by women and made recommendations, which are summarized in Box 8.1.

The criticisms advanced by women's groups have had an effect on obstetric practice and the childbirth choices now provided in many places (Box 8.2).

Prepared participatory childbirth

In this approach the parents undertake childbirth training, learning about the processes of childbirth and how to accept the pains of uterine contractions (see pp. 49–50). Labour is managed by trained staff, and the principles mentioned earlier are observed by both staff and patients. The birth takes place in a quiet environment and the baby is given to the mother at once so that she may offer suckling and celebrate the birth.

Women can have a prepared participatory childbirth in a normal hospital delivery room, but for some it is more satisfactory if there is a birthing centre.

Birthing centre

A birthing centre is usually attached to a hospital so that the patient can be treated by an experienced obstetrician should complications arise. An individual suite in a birthing centre is furnished like a bedroom, containing a firm double bed, chairs and furnishings, with the necessary equipment for medical care and infant resuscitation discreetly hidden. The father of the child or a significant other person remains with the woman in labour, providing support. The woman may have hired her own nurse–midwife (accredited by the hospital) or is looked after by a hospital nurse–midwife or a doctor. After the birth the baby remains with its parents so that bonding and celebration may take place. Early discharge is usual, and the mother is followed up at home by district nurse–midwives. Experience with established birthing centres shows that women choosing this form of childbirth require fewer inductions of labour and less analgesia, have a greater number of spontaneous deliveries, fewer episiotomies and fewer hypoxic babies than do women delivering in conventional delivery units.

They are carefully selected, of course. About 5% of women choosing a birthing centre will require medical intervention, and most of these are then transferred to the delivery floor.

Actively managed childbirth

The development of the partogram and the appreciation that most women have delivered within 12 hours of admission to hospital has led to another approach: actively managed labour.

On admission to the delivery unit, the diagnosis of labour is either confirmed or rejected. If the woman is in labour, the time of admission is designated as the start of labour. A partogram is started and the progress of labour is marked on it (Fig. 8.1). Vaginal examinations are made every 2–4 hours and the cervical dilatation is recorded on the partogram. Action lines, printed on transparent plastic, are superimposed on the partogram (Fig. 8.2). In the active stage of labour the slowest acceptable rate of cervical dilatation is 1 cm/h. If the cervical dilatation lies to the right of the appropriate action line the membranes are ruptured and an incremental dilute oxytocin infusion is established in nulliparous women (and some multiparous women), provided that a single fetus presents as a vertex and there are no signs of fetal distress.

Progress in the second stage of labour is judged by the descent of the fetal head and its rotation. One hour is allowed for the fetal head to reach the pelvic floor (the first or passive phase) and a further hour for the birth to be completed (the second or active phase). If there is delay in the passive phase then oxytocic augmentation is instituted. Delay in the active phase dictates close fetal monitoring and, where indicated, an operative vaginal delivery. Proponents of actively managed labour claim that the incidence of a labour lasting

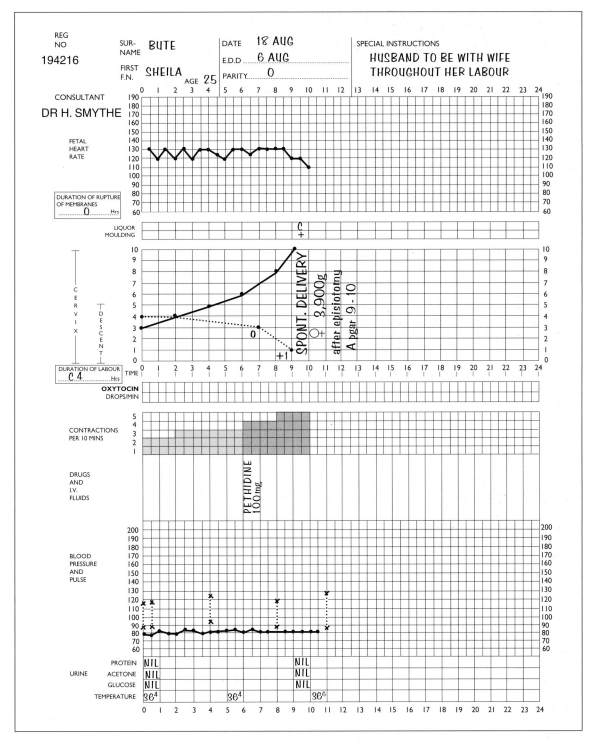

Fig. 8.1 A partogram.

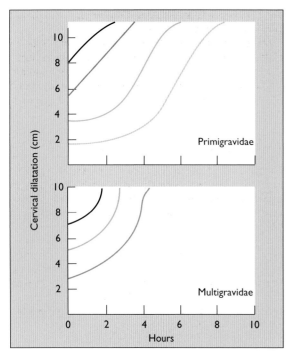

Fig. 8.2 Action lines for the partogram (Studd stencil). The lines show the slowest acceptable rate of cervical dilatation, commencing with the degree of dilatation on admission to the delivery unit.

more than 12 hours is less than 3%; the caesarean section rate is 7–12% and the forceps rate is 8%. Opponents point out that only three randomized studies have been carried out, and that in these studies there was no reduction in the caesarean section or forceps rate.

Elective caesarean section

A small but increasing number of women, particularly those over the age of 35, inform their obstetrician during pregnancy that they wish to be delivered by caesarean section. The obstetrician should listen to the woman and discern the underlying reasons for her request. For some it may be a fear of the pain of labour, for others to avoid any risk of pelvic floor damage during delivery, or a perception that abdominal delivery removes all risks for the baby. It is particularly important that the risks of caesarean versus vaginal delivery are carefully explained (Box 8.3). If the woman confirms that she wishes to be delivered by caesarean section, the obstetrician should either agree to her wish or arrange for a consultation with another colleague.

Home birth

Women choosing this type of delivery must receive good prenatal care; must be screened for any medical or obstetric abnormality; must accept transferral to a hospital if an abnormality arises during pregnancy or childbirth; and must have an experienced midwife. Even then home birth is less safe than giving birth in a midwife-controlled birthing centre.

ONSET OF LABOUR

In the weeks before labour starts the painless uterine contractions, which have been becoming increasingly frequent, merge into a prodromal stage of labour which may last up to 4 weeks. During this time the lower uterine segment expands to take the fetal head, which enters the upper pelvis. This relieves the pressure on the upper part

---

Box 8.3 Effects of caesarean section compared with vaginal birth

Increased	No difference	Decreased
Abdominal pain	Blood loss >1000 ml	Perineal pain
Bladder and ureteric injury	Infection-wound or endometritis	Urinary incontinence
Need for laparotomy or D&C	Genital tract injury	Uterovaginal prolapse
Hysterectomy	Back pain	
ICU admission	Dyspareunia	
Thromboembolism	Postnatal depression	
Length of hospital stay	Neonatal morbidity (excluding breech)	
Readmission	Neonatal intracranial haemorrhage	
Placenta praevia	Brachial plexus palsy	
Uterine rupture	Cerebral palsy	
Maternal death		
Stillbirth in future pregnancies		
Secondary infertility		
Neonatal respiratory morbidity		

Adapted from Caesarean Section, National Collaborating Centre for Women's and Children's Health. 2004. RCOG Press www.rcog.org.uk. Full details of absolute and relative risks can be obtained from full guideline.

of the abdomen ('lightening') but increases the pressure in the pelvis. Consequently, constipation and urinary frequency become apparent, and some patients complain of increased pressure in the pelvis and an increased mucoid vaginal discharge.

False labour

As term approaches many women complain of painful uterine contractions, which may seem to indicate the onset of labour. However, despite the contractions, progressive dilatation of the cervix fails to occur – this condition is termed false labour.

In it, the triple descending gradient of uterine activity fails to become established. A reverse gradient of uterine activity is present, the lower part of the uterus contracting nearly as strongly as the upper part. Because of this, cervical dilatation fails to occur and the pain of the uterine contractions is often felt as low backache.

Clinically, the painful contractions occur more often at night, but their frequency and intensity do not increase as time passes. A woman who complains of this pattern of uterine activity needs an explanation and, if the pains are distressing, requires treatment with analgesics, and perhaps a hypnotic so that she can enjoy a good night's sleep.

Often the pains of false labour recur on a number of days and, in some cases, the reverse gradient of activity changes and true labour starts.

Onset of true labour

True labour may start and progress rapidly, or the start may be slow, with contractions only occurring at long intervals – the so-called sluggish uterus, or, in a more modern idiom, prolongation of the quiet (latent) phase of labour.

If the woman is becoming distressed that labour is not progressing, a more effective pattern of uterine activity can be obtained by performing an amniotomy and by starting an intravenous infusion of oxytocin. This regimen should only be instituted if there is no cephalopelvic disproportion and if the cervix is partly or wholly effaced, 2 cm dilated and soft.

The onset of labour is difficult to time with any degree of accuracy, and may be heralded by the following signs:

1. The false labour pains may become coordinated and regular, or painful contractions may alert the patient that labour has started.
2. A discharge of mucus mixed with some blood may occur. This is due to the effacement and dilatation of the cervix, allowing the 'plug' that previously filled it to be released. The blood comes from minute lacerations in the cervical mucosa. The passage of the mucus and blood is known as the 'show'.

The transition into labour is gradual, but labour may be said to have begun when the cervix is at least 2 cm dilated and contractions become painful and regular, with diminishing intervals between each one.

Because of the difficulty in establishing the time of onset of labour with any degree of accuracy, many obstetricians mark its onset from the time the woman is admitted to hospital. This has advantages if the graphic method of recording the progress of labour (the partogram) is adopted.

Duration of labour

The duration of labour is not easy to determine precisely as its onset is often indefinite and subjective (Box 8.4). In studies of informed women whose labour started spontaneously there was a wide variation in the duration of labour, as can be seen in Table 8.1.

Labour is usually shorter when the patient knows something of the physiology of normal labour, is in good physical and mental health at the onset of labour, and has confidence in her attendants. Delivery within 16 hours may be expected in 90% of nulliparous women (para 0), and the same proportion of multiparous women (para 1+) will deliver within 12 hours.

PROGRESS AND MANAGEMENT OF LABOUR AND BIRTH

The management of labour begins when the woman seeks admission to hospital, which she does when she believes or knows that she is in labour. As labour is a time of anxiety and stress, the attitude of the member of staff who

---

Box 8.4 Duration of labour

Several factors influence the duration of labour. These include the age of the woman, her parity, her knowledge of the process of childbirth, and the size of the fetus and its position in the uterus. Labour seems to last longer in nulliparous women, particularly older primigravidae, and if the baby presents in the occipitoposterior position.

Table 8.1 Duration (and range) of labour (in hours)

	NULLIPARAE	MULTIPARAE
1st stage	8.25 (2–12)	5.5 (1–9)
2nd stage	1 (0.25–1.5)	0.25 (0–0.75)
3rd stage	0.25 (0–1)	0.25 (0–0.5)
	9.5 (2.25–14)	6 (1–10.25)

admits her is most important. The care of the woman during her labour and childbirth may be conducted by a midwife (see also p. 66), or by midwives in partnership with an obstetrician or a general practitioner.

Admission

On admission the woman's antenatal records are obtained and scrutinized for any past medical or obstetric problems, to check the history of the current pregnancy, and to make sure that the appropriate laboratory tests have been made. A history of the present labour is obtained, the frequency and strength of the uterine contractions are noted, and information is obtained about a 'show' of blood or mucus and whether or not the membranes have broken.

A general examination is made by a midwife or a doctor, the blood pressure, pulse and temperature being recorded. The abdomen is palpated to determine the presentation of the fetus and the position of the presenting part in relation to the pelvic brim (see Fig. 6.17). A vaginal examination may be carried out, with aseptic precautions, to determine the effacement and dilatation of the cervix and the position and station of the presenting part. The station of the presenting part is the level of the lowest fetal bony part (head or breech) in relation to an imaginary line joining the mother's ischial spines. It is measured in centimetres above or below the ischial spines (Fig. 8.3). If the amniotic sac (the membranes) has ruptured this is noted. Evidence does not support the common practice of performing a routine 20-minute cardiotocogram (CTG) on admission in low-risk women. The 'admission CTG' is associated with higher intervention rates, i.e. augmentation of labour, epidural analgesia and operative delivery, without a clear improvement in neonatal outcome. The woman is transferred from the admission room to a bed in a delivery room (if she has not already been admitted to it) and a partogram is started which shows the progress of labour at a glance.

First stage of labour

The first stage of labour begins, as mentioned earlier, at an imprecise time. For convenience, labour is estimated to start when the patient says that the pains are becoming regular, or on her admission to hospital when the signs of labour are evident. It ends with the full dilatation of the cervix.

At the beginning of the first stage of labour the fetal presenting part (usually it is the head, so this term will be used in the rest of this chapter instead of the presenting part) has descended into the true pelvis to some extent. In a normally shaped pelvis the position of the occiput is in the transverse diameter of the pelvis in 75% of cases, in the oblique in 14% of cases, in the direct anterior position in 3% of cases, and in a posterior diameter in 8% of cases (Fig. 8.4).

The first stage of labour can be divided into a latent (quiet) phase and an active phase. In the early part of the latent phase the uterine contractions are relatively painless, occur at intervals of 5–10 minutes, and do not usually distress the patient. As the latent phase progresses the contractions become stronger and more frequent, but dilatation of the cervix is relatively slow. Towards the end of the phase the membranes may rupture spontaneously.

The active phase starts when the cervix is 3–4 cm dilated. The cervix dilates more rapidly in the active phase and the process is considered to be normal if it dilates at a rate of 0.5–1.0 cm/h. Towards the end of the active phase, when the cervix is 9 cm dilated, many women complain of very painful contractions and may have a desire to push.

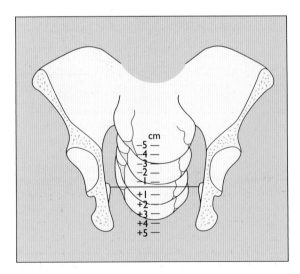

Fig. 8.3 Station of the head.

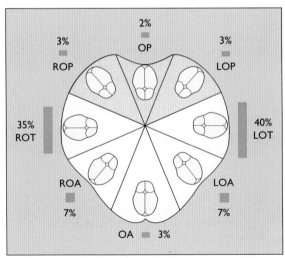

Fig. 8.4 The positions of the vertex at the onset of labour and their relative frequency; the shaded positions are associated with a more difficult labour and delivery. OP, occipitoposterior; OT, occipitotransverse; OA, occipitoanterior.

As it is unwise to push at this stage, a vaginal examination should be carried out to establish whether the cervix is fully dilated.

The duration of the latent and active phases is shown in Figure 8.5. If they last for more than 12 hours in a nulliparous woman, or more than 9 hours in a multiparous woman, the cause should be investigated (see Ch. 21).

During the active part of the first stage of labour, the fetal head descends more deeply into the maternal pelvis and flexes (Figs 8.6–8.8).

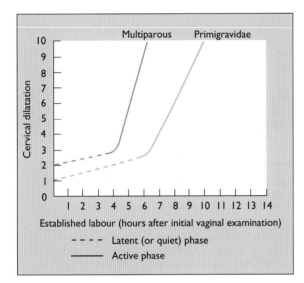

Fig. 8.5 The phases of labour.

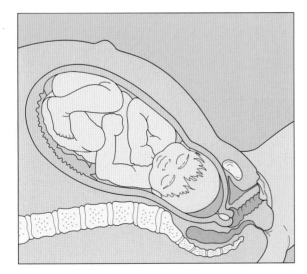

Fig. 8.6 Late pregnancy. The fetal head has engaged in the transverse diameter of the pelvic brim and some flexion of the head on the chest has occurred. The cervix is soft but is not yet effaced, and the amniotic membranes are intact.

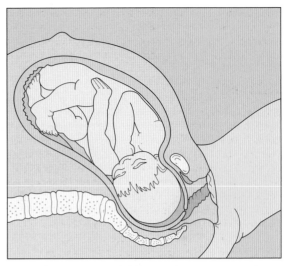

Fig. 8.7 Early labour. There has been further flexion of the fetal head and it has moved more deeply into the true pelvis, causing pressure on the bladder and rectum. The cervix has become effaced but has not yet begun to dilate, and the membranes are intact.

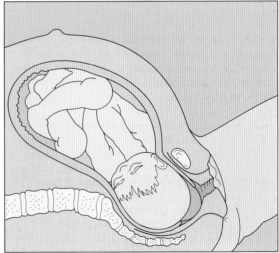

Fig. 8.8 Late first stage of labour. The cervix is now 7 cm dilated and further flexion of the fetal head has occurred. The membranes are still intact.

Management of the first stage of labour

The patient should be made as comfortable as possible and should choose whether she prefers to remain in bed, walk about, sit on a chair and so on. If there is a common room on the delivery floor she may prefer to go there to be with other women. If the head has not descended into the pelvis she should remain in bed, but should be propped up on pillows with a back rest so that the full weight of her uterus does not press on the descending aorta and inferior vena cava, impeding the flow of blood to the uterus and its return to the heart.

It is customary to withhold solid food during labour as the contents of the stomach remain there, and if a general anaesthetic is required for a forceps or a caesarean delivery the acid stomach contents may be regurgitated and inhaled, causing Mendelson's syndrome. Today, few inhalational anaesthetics are given during childbirth, and it is known that fasting does not reduce the acidity of the stomach contents. There seems no good reason why a woman at low risk of an operative procedure requiring general anaesthesia should not be permitted, if she wishes, to eat a low-residue, low-fat diet (such as tea, fruit juice, toast, lightly cooked eggs or biscuits). Food eaten during labour may reduce the chance of maternal ketoacidosis.

Intravenous infusions are not usually required in the first 12 hours of labour, regardless of the presence of ketosis. The patient's lips can be kept moist and she may suck ice. If intravenous fluids are deemed necessary the infusion rate should be 250 mL/h. Glucose infusions providing more than 25 g of glucose during labour should be avoided as they may cause fetal hyperinsulinaemia and neonatal hypoglycaemia.

Specific care in the first stage

The following steps should be followed:

- Support and comfort the patient and inform her about the progress of labour.
- Complete the partogram:
  1. Check pulse, temperature and blood pressure every 2 hours.
  2. Monitor the frequency, strength and intensity of the uterine contractions.
  3. Monitor the fetal heart rate once active labour has started, every 15 minutes in the first stage and every 5 minutes in the second stage of labour. The normal variation is 120–160 bpm. If the rate remains below 100 bpm between contractions, and particularly if meconium is passed, 'fetal distress' may be imminent and the situation should be assessed (see Ch. 20). Although the fetal heart is usually monitored between contractions, a more informative way is to auscultate the heart immediately after a contraction. In some hospitals continuous fetal heart monitoring is practised using a Doppler transabdominal transducer.
  4. When labour has been established, perform a vaginal examination every 4 hours to determine the dilatation of the cervix and the descent of the fetal head (or breech).
  5. Discuss with the patient her need for analgesics or epidural anaesthesia (see p. 83).
- Determine the position of the head in relation to the maternal pelvis, dividing the pelvis into 45° segments.

Right refers to the right side of the woman, left to her left side. If the vertex presents, the occiput is the point of reference; if the breech presents, the sacrum is the point of reference; if the face presents, the chin is the point of reference. In Figure 8.4 the positions and frequency of vertex presentations are shown.

Second stage of labour

The second stage of labour begins when the cervix is fully dilated, to complete the formation of the curved birth canal, and ends with the birth of the baby. The second stage of labour is the expulsive stage, during which the fetus is forced through the birth canal. The uterine contractions become more frequent, recurring at 2–5-minute intervals, and are stronger, lasting 60–90 seconds. The fetal head descends deeply into the pelvis and, on reaching the gutter-shaped pelvic floor, rotates anteriorly (internal rotation) so that the occiput lies behind the symphysis pubis (Fig. 8.9). Anterior rotation occurs in 98% of cases, although in 2% of cases the head rotates posteriorly, with the result that the occiput lies in front of the sacrum.

The uterine contractions are now supplemented by voluntary muscle contractions. Simultaneously with the uterine contraction the patient holds her breath, closes her glottis, braces her feet and, taking a breath, holds it, grunts and contracts her diaphragm and her abdominal muscles to force the fetus lower in her pelvis. The energy expended causes her pulse to rise, and she sweats. As the uterine contraction diminishes and ceases, she relaxes and often dozes.

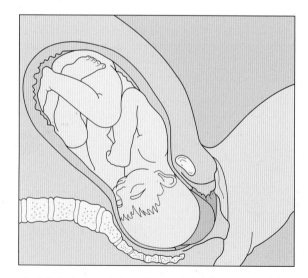

Fig. 8.9 Early second stage. The cervix is fully dilated and the head is beginning to rotate at the level of the ischial spines. Rotation is through 90°, so that the occiput of the fetal head lies in the anterior segment of the pelvis and the sagittal suture in the anterior–posterior diameter of the pelvis. The membranes are intact and bulge in front of the head.

As the fetal head is pushed deeper into the pelvis the patient may complain of intense pressure on her rectum or pains radiating down her legs, caused by pressure on the sacral nerve plexus or obturator nerve. Some 15 minutes later the anus begins to open, exposing its anterior wall, and the head can be seen inside the vagina. With each contraction the fetal head becomes a little more visible, retreating a little between contractions but advancing slightly all the time (Fig. 8.10).

The head now presses on the posterior wall of the lower vagina and the perineum becomes thinner and stretched, its skin tense and shining. The woman complains of a 'bursting' feeling and a desire to push even without a uterine contraction. Soon a large part of the head can be seen between the stretched labia, and the parietal bosses become visible. The further sequence of the birth is shown in Figures 8.11 and 8.12, and is now described. With an extra effort the baby's head is born, extending at the neck so that the forehead, the nose, the mouth and the chin appear in sequence. Mucus streams from the baby's mouth and nose. After a short pause, the head rotates into a transverse diameter (external rotation). This brings the shoulders into the anterior–posterior diameter of the lower pelvis. The shoulders are born next, the anterior shoulder stemming from behind the symphysis and the posterior shoulder rolling over the perineum, followed by the baby's trunk and legs. The baby gasps once or twice and cries vigorously. The uterus contracts to a size found at 20 weeks' gestation.

Management of the second stage of labour

In the second stage of labour the active cooperation of the expectant mother is needed, to add the voluntary muscle contractions of her diaphragm and abdominal muscles to the involuntary uterine contractions, which together increase the downward pressure on the fetus. As the contractions are more painful the woman may need more analgesics, or if she has had an epidural anaesthetic it may need 'topping up'. Some women find relief by back massage or by moving into another position, including sitting up.

Throughout the second stage of labour a medical attendant should be present, helping and encouraging the woman to bear down with each uterine contraction and to relax in between. The woman may choose to push with either an open or closed glottis as there is no significant difference in duration of the second stage, neonatal outcome or damage to the birth canal. As there is much energy expenditure the patient usually sweats and will feel more comfortable if she can have cool face cloths to wipe away the sweat.

During the second stage of labour most women prefer to recline on a bed at 45° to the horizontal, supported, if she wishes, by their partner. Some women choose to sit up, squat or kneel until the baby's head is visible at the vulva.

The woman's contractions are recorded and the fetal heart is auscultated every 5 minutes or after every contraction during the active phase of pushing. If the fetal heart rate falls below 100 bpm and the bradycardia persists for more than 2 minutes, action should be taken to determine the cause. This will include a vaginal examination to make sure that the umbilical cord has not prolapsed. The position of the patient should be changed, as this may affect the fetal heart rate.

Traditionally, the second stage of labour is terminated by vacuum extraction or forceps if it has lasted 2 or more hours, as the likelihood of spontaneous delivery after this is very small. If the woman has an epidural analgesic the second stage may be prolonged to 3 hours without any increased risk to the fetus if she wishes to have a 'natural' birth and there are no significant fetal heart rate

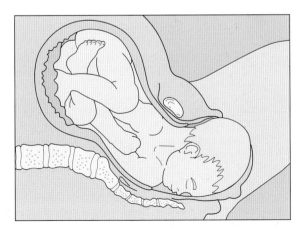

Fig. 8.10 Late second stage. The head is broaching the vulval ring – 'crowning'. The membranes have ruptured, and the perineum is stretched over the head.

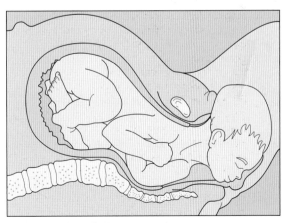

Fig. 8.11 Birth of the head. As the fetal head is pushed through the vulval ring it extends on the neck and the perineum is swept over the face. The direction of movement of the head is now upwards. The uterus has retracted to fit closely over the fetal body. The shoulders are still in the transverse diameter of the midpelvis.

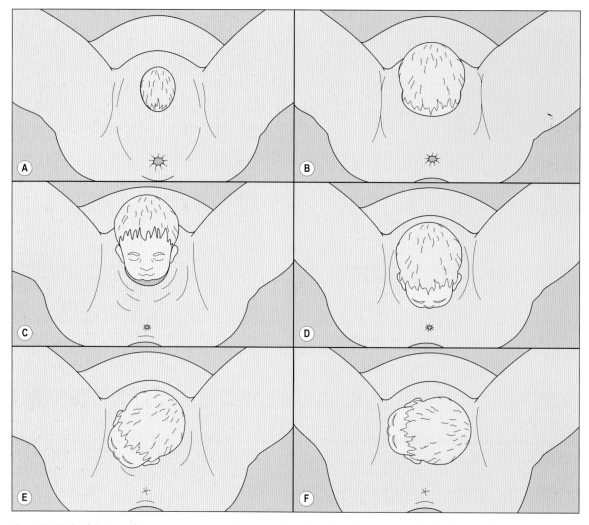

Fig. 8.12 Birth of the head. A sequence showing the progressive distension of the perineum by the head, which extends on the neck as it is born. The perineum sweeps over the forehead, face and chin. Once the head is born it drops slightly and then restitution (external rotation) occurs.

abnormalities. Once the active phase of the second stage has commenced the upper limit should be 45 minutes for a nulliparous and 30 minutes for a multiparous woman. After this time, close monitoring of the fetus is mandatory as the risk of hypoxia and acidosis increases.

BIRTH OF THE BABY

Head

As the fetal head (for this is the usual presenting part) becomes visible between the labia, the woman should be prepared for the birth. With each contraction the patient pushes and the fetal head becomes more visible, retract-

ing slightly between contractions. When the area of the visible head has increased to 5 cm, and the perineum is thin and distended, the vulva should be swabbed with chlorhexidine (1 : 1000). The medical attendant who will deliver the baby now scrubs up and puts on gloves and gown. With each contraction the fetal head is flexed by the index finger of one of the attendant's hands; the perineum is 'protected' by a pad which covers the perineum and the distended anus and is held in the attendant's other hand. In some cases the perineum tears in spite of the protection; in others a deliberate incision (an episiotomy) is made to avoid such tearing. This is discussed later.

The manoeuvres described permit the head to be born slowly, until the parietal bosses are visible (when the head is said to be 'crowned'). The mother now ceases to push with the contractions unless asked to do so by the medical attendant. Instead, she is asked to pant during each painful contraction.

To be born the fetal head now has to extend, and this is aided by the attendant's left hand keeping the head flexed and the right hand holding the perineal pad pushing the chin upwards. The forehead, nose, mouth and chin emerge and the head is born, the perineum being pressed back behind the chin. The baby's eyes are swabbed with sterile water and its head is rotated (or rotates itself) through 90°. The attendant now puts a finger inside the woman's vagina to feel whether the umbilical cord is around the baby's neck. If it is, a loop of the cord is brought down.

Shoulders

As the baby's head rotates, mucus streams from its mouth and nose. With the next contraction, the rotated head is grasped gently between the attendant's two hands, which are placed over the sides of the head, and the head is drawn posteriorly so that the anterior shoulder is released from behind the pubic bones (Fig. 8.13). Following the birth of the anterior shoulder, the baby is swept upwards in an arc to release the posterior shoulder, followed by the body and the legs (Fig. 8.14).

The mother should now be able to see and touch her baby. The baby is then laid between the mother's legs and, if necessary, its mouth and fauces are sucked clear using a suction apparatus or a soft tube and bulb. The baby is placed between the mother's legs so that it is below the level of the placenta, and its circulation will receive an

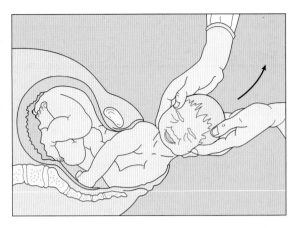

Fig. 8.14 The birth of the posterior shoulder. The accoucheur aids the birth by lifting the head gently upwards while maintaining traction. This prevents damage to the perineum.

additional 60 mL of blood as it drains from the placenta. One-third of this amount is received in the first 30 seconds after the birth and the remainder in the next 2–3 minutes. In normal cases (where the baby is not hypoxic) the attendant should not clamp, divide and tie the umbilical cord for about 2–3 minutes.

THE NEWBORN BABY

The neonate lies between its mother's legs, usually taking its first breath within seconds, and starting to cry and to move its arms and legs. It is checked for good respiratory effort, its colour and its alertness. Either an Apgar score is taken (Table 8.2) or the Basic Resuscitation Programme suggested in the UK is adopted (Fig. 8.15). Most babies establish respiration easily and quickly, but a few are born in a mild or severe hypoxic state. This problem is discussed further in Chapter 26. The baby is checked for gross malformations. It is then given to the mother for cuddling and suckling. This early mother–baby contact encourages (but is not essential for) bonding, and if the baby is put to the breast this helps to 'bring in' the milk.

Vitamin K

Most neonates develop vitamin K deficiency by the third day of life. This predisposes the baby to a bleeding diathesis (haemorrhagic disease of the newborn) caused by the depression of clotting factors II, VII, IX and X. The baby may bleed from the gastrointestinal tract, the umbilical cord, or from skin punctures. A late-onset variety of vitamin K deficiency may affect breastfed babies between 4 and 6 weeks after birth. It manifests as gastrointestinal bleeding or intracranial haemorrhage. To prevent these possible problems it is currently

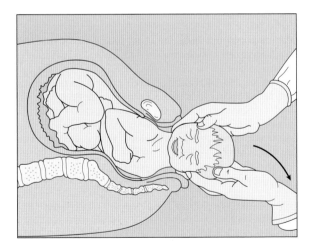

Fig. 8.13 Birth of the anterior shoulder. With the birth of the head the shoulders reach the pelvic floor and, directed by the levator 'gutter', rotate to lie in the anteroposterior diameter of the pelvic outlet. The head therefore rotates externally, or undergoes 'restitution' to its position at the onset of labour. The anterior shoulder (in this case the right one) is appearing from behind the symphysis. The birth of the shoulder is aided by downward and backward traction of the head by the accoucheur.

Table 8.2 Apgar scoring method for evaluating the infant

SIGN	0	1	2
Colour	Blue; pale	Body pink; extremities blue	Completely pink
Respiratory effort	Absent	Weak cry; hypoventilation	Good; strong cry
Muscle tone	Limp	Some flexion of extremities	Active motion; extremities well flexed
Reflex irritability (response to stimulation of sole of foot)	No response	Grimace	Cry
Heart rate	Absent	Slow (below 100)	Fast (over 100)

recommended that all newborn babies should be given phytomenadione (vitamin K_1), either 1.0 mg intramuscularly at birth or 1.0 mg orally at birth, at 3–4 days and at 6 weeks of age. The further care of the newborn infant is described in Chapter 9.

PROGRESS, MANAGEMENT AND DELIVERY OF THE PLACENTA

The third stage of labour extends from the birth of the baby to the expulsion of the placenta and membranes.

Separation of the placenta takes place through the spongy layer of the decidua basalis, as the result of uterine contractions being added to the retraction of the uterus that follows the birth of the child. The retraction of the uterus reduces the size of the placental bed to one-quarter of its size in pregnancy, with the result that the placenta buckles inwards, tearing the blood vessels of the intervillous space and causing a retroplacental haemorrhage, which further separates the placenta. The process starts as the baby is born and separation is usually complete within 5 minutes, but the placenta may be held in the uterus for longer because the membranes take longer to strip from the underlying decidua. Following the separation of the placenta, the lattice arrangements of the myometrial fibres effectively strangle the blood vessels supplying the placental bed, reducing further blood loss and encouraging the formation of fibrin plugs in their torn ends (Fig. 8.16).

Management of the third stage of labour

There are two methods of managing the third stage of labour:

- Traditional or expectant management
- Active management.

Traditional or expectant management

The placenta and membranes are allowed to separate without interference. The ulnar border of one hand is placed in the uterine fundus and the signs of placental separation are awaited. These are:

- A gush of blood
- The fundus rises in the abdomen and becomes spherical
- That part of the umbilical cord which can be seen at the vulva, lengthens
- If the fundus is lifted upwards the umbilical cord does not shorten.

Ten to twenty minutes pass before these signs appear. No attempt is made to hasten the separation – by 'fiddling' with the fundus, for example – unless haemorrhage demands action. Once the signs indicate that the placenta has been expelled from the uterus and is lying in the vagina, a uterine contraction is obtained by 'rubbing up' the uterus. The contracted uterus is pushed down towards the pelvis, so that it acts as a piston to expel the placenta and membranes from the vagina. The expelled placenta is grasped and twisted around with continuing traction to make the membranes into a twisted cord so that they are expelled intact.

Active management

As the fetal head is being born an intramuscular injection of Syntocinon 10 IU is given. The combination of oxytocin and ergometrine – Syntometrine – although widely used, is associated with a small reduction in blood loss but carries increased side-effects of nausea, vomiting and hypertension so the preferred routine prophylactic drug is Syntocinon.

The delivery of the baby following the injection is conducted slowly over 60 seconds. The umbilical cord is divided and clamped 2 minutes after the birth. The slowness is because the oxytocic effect takes about 2 minutes

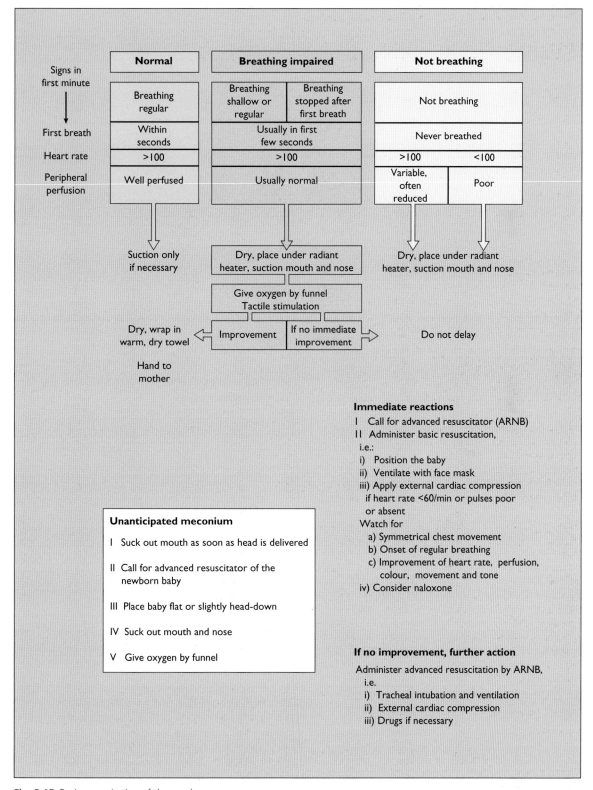

Fig. 8.15 Basic resuscitation of the newborn.

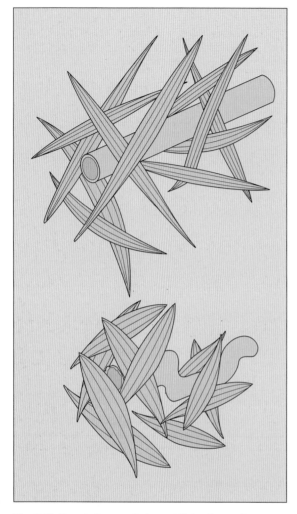

Fig. 8.16 The uterine muscle forms a 'living ligature' to occlude blood vessels.

to produce a strong uterine contraction. The attendant's left hand is placed on the uterus to detect the contraction. When it occurs, the hand is placed suprapubically and pushes the uterus upwards while the right hand grasps the umbilical cord and pulls the placenta out of the vagina in a controlled manner (Fig. 8.17). The membranes are drawn out intact by twisting them into a rope and pulling them out with a sponge forceps or the hand. In 1–2% of cases the placenta is retained, but no blood loss occurs. After a 10-minute delay another attempt is made to pull the placenta out by controlled cord traction. If this fails, manual removal is necessary (see p. 184).

The advantages of active management are that maternal blood loss is reduced by a mean of 80 mL, postpartum haemorrhage (a loss of more than 500 mL of blood) is reduced from 4% to 2% of all deliveries, there is a lower requirement for blood transfusions and the third stage of

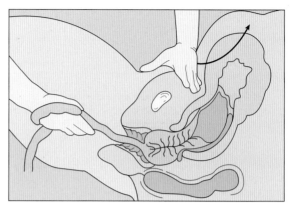

Fig. 8.17 Controlled cord traction.

labour is shortened. There is no difference in retained placenta or the need for manual removal of the placenta. The disadvantages include increased nausea and vomiting and hypertension if ergometrine, rather than oxytocin, is used. Injectable prostaglandins and oral misoprostol have been shown to be less effective than oxytocin and ergometrine for the routine management of the third stage.

Inspection of the placenta and membranes

The placenta and membranes are held up by the umbilical cord and the fetal surface is examined, attention being paid to the blood vessels to see if any run to the edge of the membranes, indicating a possible succenturiate lobe. The membranes are examined to make sure that no part remains in the uterus. The maternal surface of the placenta is examined next, any clots being washed away, so that the cotyledons can be inspected. The maternal surface is held in both hands and fitted together to make sure that no cotyledon has been left in the uterus. If any cotyledon is missing, or if most of the membranes have been left in the uterus or vagina, a doctor should explore the vagina and the uterine cavity under sterile conditions after ensuring that the woman has adequate anaesthesia.

Retained placenta

A retained placenta is one which has remained in the uterus for more than 1 hour. As a retained placenta may be associated with haemorrhage, action should be taken to remove it. The causes of a retained placenta are:

- Incarceration of a separated or partially separated placenta when, following the injection of an oxytocic drug, the closing cervix traps it.
- Uterine atony, which is accompanied by bleeding.
- A morbidly adherent placenta. In this relatively uncommon condition (1 in 1500 births)

the trophoblast has invaded the decidua and myometrium to varying degrees (placenta accreta) or has penetrated to the serosal coat (placenta percreta).

Management

If postpartum bleeding is marked, attempts should be made at once to find if the placenta has separated as described earlier, and attempts should be made to deliver it. If these measures fail it should be removed manually (see p. 184).

Should the placenta be retained for 1 hour with little bleeding the above procedures should be undertaken. A placenta accreta or percreta may resist attempts at manual removal and hysterectomy may be performed.

INSPECTION AND REPAIR OF THE GENITAL TRACT AND PERINEUM

Following the expulsion of the placenta and membranes, bleeding usually ceases. If the perineum has been torn or an episiotomy made, the tear or incision is now repaired after inspecting the vagina for damage. If a difficult forceps delivery has been made the cervix should be inspected to exclude a lateral tear.

Episiotomy

Episiotomy – a deliberate incision in the stretched perineum and vagina – was first suggested about 200 years ago, to prevent a ragged perineal tear occurring which might extend to become a third- or fourth-degree tear. The idea was that episiotomy would prevent the development of such tears and would also prevent the later development of vaginal prolapse, although the evidence for this is dubious. Routine episiotomy has major disadvantages: the woman continues to have perineal pain and discomfort for longer than one who has not had the procedure, and in addition sexual intercourse may be uncomfortable for up to 6 months afterwards.

If the episiotomy has extended to produce a third- or fourth-degree tear, unless the anal sphincter is correctly sutured the woman may develop anal or urinary incontinence.

If the accoucheur thinks that an episiotomy is required because the fetal head is overdistending the woman's perineum, they should explain what they propose to the patient. If the woman agrees to the procedure, the perineum should be infiltrated with a local anaesthetic, unless the woman has already had an epidural anaesthetic. The episiotomy incision may be midline or mediolateral (Fig. 8.18). The midline incision has the advantage that no large blood vessels are encountered and it is easier to repair. Its disadvantage is that it may extend into the rectum. If a large episiotomy is needed, for example when

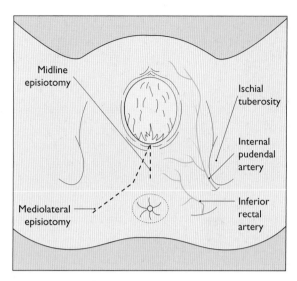

Fig. 8.18 Types of episiotomy.

a difficult midforceps delivery is anticipated, a mediolateral episiotomy is preferred.

One method of repairing an episiotomy is shown in Figure 8.19. This repair is the least painful postoperatively, particularly when 2/0 polyglycolic suture material is used.

Another method is to use continuous suture to repair the vagina and interrupted sutures for the perineal muscles and skin; a continuous subcuticular skin closure is associated with less pain and dyspareunia 3 months postpartum. The standard repair of an episiotomy is shown in Figure 8.20.

Perineal tears

Four degrees of perineal tear are recognized:

- First-degree – damage to the fourchette and vaginal mucosa, and the underlining muscles are exposed.
- Second-degree – the posterior vaginal wall and the perineal muscles are torn but the anal sphincter is intact.
- Third-degree – the anal sphincter is torn, but the rectal mucosa is intact.
- Fourth-degree – the anal canal is opened and the tear may spread to the rectum.

First-degree tears are easy to repair; one or two sutures are all that is needed. Second- and third-degree tears need more care and their repair is shown in Figure 8.20. Third- and fourth-degree tears are uncommon, occurring in less than 1% of births. They usually follow a forceps delivery in a primigravida, the birth of a baby weighing more than 4 kg, or the delivery of a fetus persistently maintaining an occipitoposterior position. Careful repair is essential, but even then half of the women have persisting anal incontinence (usually only of flatus) for about 6 months owing to poorly repaired sphincter damage, and 4% have

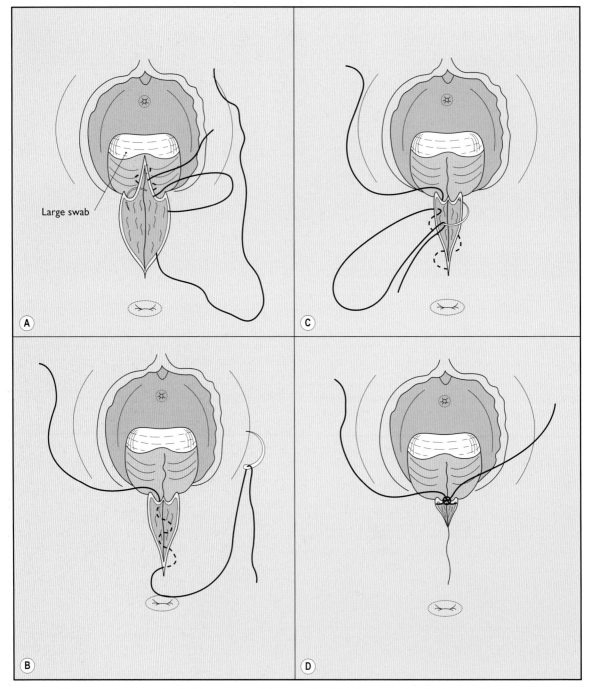

Fig. 8.19 (A) Suture of the vaginal wall. (B) The suture of the vaginal wall has been completed and the perineal muscles are being sutured. (C) The subcuticular suture of the perineal skin, starting posteriorly and finishing deep to the hymen. (D) The two strands of catgut are tied, and cut short. The knot disappears beneath the vaginal mucosa.

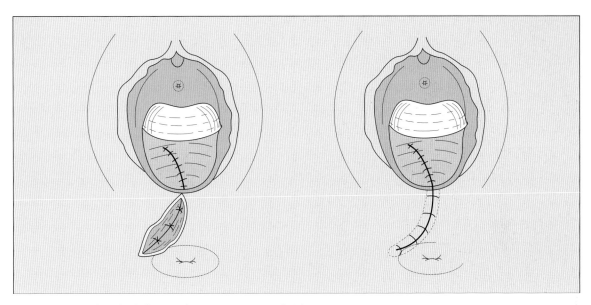

Fig. 8.20 Standard method of repair of an episiotomy or perineal tear.

faecal incontinence. Pelvic exercises may resolve the problem, but if these fail surgery may be needed. Repair of fourth-degree tears requires considerable skill, and it is essential to secure the apex of the tear otherwise a rectovaginal fistula may result. The anal sphincter retracts when torn and its exposed ends must be identified and rejoined by sutures (Fig. 8.21).

Postoperative care

The degree of postoperative pain and oedema depends on the method of delivery (forceps deliveries are followed by more oedema) and the quality of suturing. Most women need analgesics for a few days. A woman who has had the traditional interrupted sutures experiences more pain, but most patients can walk and have showers. Perineal swabbing is not usually necessary unless there is marked perineal oedema.

Episiotomies and perineal tears are not without longer-term discomfort. Twelve weeks after giving birth, 5% of women still experience some degree of pain and 15% have perineal discomfort. Sexual intercourse may be painful or uncomfortable for up to 20 weeks.

Lacerations of the lower genital tract

After a difficult delivery the vagina and the clitoral area should be inspected for lacerations. Any large laceration should be sutured. Continued bleeding in spite of a firmly contracted uterus suggests an internal laceration. The vagina and cervix should be inspected with good illumination.

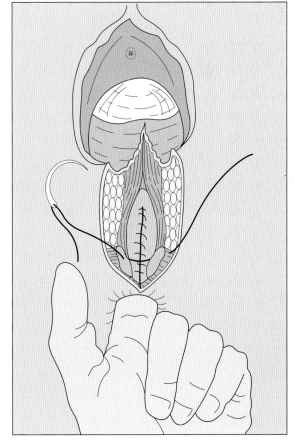

Fig. 8.21 Repair of a fourth degree tear.

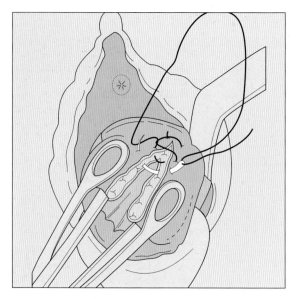

Fig. 8.22 Repair of a cervical tear.

If a lacerated cervix is found the tear is sutured, care being taken to include the apex of the tear (Fig. 8.22).

MANAGEMENT OF THE IMMEDIATE POSTDELIVERY PERIOD

The woman should remain in the delivery room for 1 hour. The medical attendants will check regularly that the uterus is contracted, that there is no excessive blood loss and that the vital signs are normal. During this time the baby will be checked thoroughly for abnormalities (see pp. 86–88), cleansed and returned to the mother to enable the parents to celebrate the birth.

Before the woman leaves the delivery room, the attendant must be sure that:

- The mother is in good general condition.
- The uterus is well contracted and contains no blood clots.
- The perineum has been properly repaired.
- The woman is not in pain from the repair.
- The woman does not have a full bladder.

PAIN RELIEF DURING LABOUR AND CHILDBIRTH

The pain of childbirth varies considerably between women. Because of this a woman has the right to know that analgesics and anaesthetics are available for her, and she can decide when she needs pain relief. This is usu-

ally more effective than if the medical attendants decide on the type of analgesia. Between 15 and 20% of women report disappointment in the pain relief they receive during their labour.

The ideal obstetric method of pain relief should:

- Do no harm to the mother or her baby
- Not prevent the patient cooperating, particularly in the second stage of labour
- Not interfere with normal uterine activity.

In early labour (the latent phase), when uterine contractions are not particularly painful, most women do not require pain relief. If the woman is very apprehensive a short-acting benzodiazepine may be given, but this is not requested by many women.

Most women seek pain relief once the active phase of the first stage begins. Several methods are available, including both drugs and non-pharmacological means.

Non-pharmacological methods

The non-pharmacological methods need to be taught during the pregnancy by a trained person, so that by the time labour begins the woman understands what she has to do. They include massage and touch, relaxation techniques, rhythmical movements, heat and cold (e.g. showers or baths), and transcutaneous electrical nerve stimulation (TENS). The effectiveness of these techniques is not clear, but some women find them very helpful in relieving pain. Water immersion during the first stage of labour reduces the use of analgesia but does not affect the duration of labour, the rate of operative delivery or neonatal outcome.

Later in the active phase, when the contractions become stronger, a woman may choose to continue with non-pharmacological methods but must be made aware that if they do not provide adequate pain relief she may obtain treatment by a pharmacological method. She must not be made to feel that she has failed if she seeks narcotics or epidural anaesthesia.

Pharmacological methods

Of the narcotics, intramuscular pethidine at a dose of 100–150 mg at intervals is chosen by many women (the opioid is effective in about 15 minutes and the effect lasts for 2–3 hours). There is some concern that if pethidine is given within 2 hours before birth the baby may have a delayed onset of breathing. If this occurs it is easily and effectively treated by injecting an opioid antagonist, for example naloxone, either into the umbilical vein or intramuscularly.

An alternative method of giving pethidine, which is available in some hospitals, is patient-controlled analgesia (PCA). Using PCA the woman controls the dose she is receiving (within limits). The method is attractive to some women, particularly after a caesarean section, but it is not widely used.

Nitrous oxide and oxygen

In most cases a 50 : 50 mixture of nitrous oxide and oxygen is given in an Entonox machine. The patient breathes the mixture during a contraction in the active phase of the first stage and during the second stage of labour. It can be used to supplement the pain relief provided by pethidine. To be effective it has to be used properly, and even if this is the case, rather less than 50% of women obtain satisfactory pain relief; 20% obtain some relief, and 30% find the method ineffective.

Epidural analgesia

Epidural anaesthesia has become increasingly popular in recent years and would be chosen by more women if the service were more readily available. In Britain, for example, the Social Services Committee has recommended strongly that Health Authorities should provide an anaesthetic service in all major obstetric units that is available within a few minutes of receiving a call. The Committee also recommends that only specifically trained doctors should give an epidural anaesthetic.

Epidural anaesthesia is the most effective way of relieving the pain of childbirth, and provides complete relief of contraction pain in 95% of labouring women. It also provides great flexibility in pain management. For example, should the delivery require forceps or vacuum extraction or be by caesarean section, epidural anaesthesia avoids possible adverse biochemical effects associated with a general anaesthetic, and can provide postoperative pain relief. The disadvantages of epidural anaesthesia are that a few women complain of dizziness or shivering, and that it may increase the duration of the second stage and lead to an increase in operative vaginal deliveries. Epidurals can cause a small rise in maternal temperature and urinary retention, requiring catheterization, is common.

Serious side-effects are uncommon. The most worrying are transient hypotension, which occurs in 20% of patients, and dural tap (in 1%), which is followed by severe headache in half of the women. If the latter occurs the injection of a small volume of the woman's blood into the dural space (blood patch) will prevent further leakage of cerebrospinal fluid and allow resolution of the headache. There is no increase in the rate of long-term back pain.

Local analgesia

Local analgesia is a choice in the relief of pain during childbirth for women who have not had an epidural anaesthetic and who require a forceps or vacuum extraction delivery; for the repair of an episiotomy or a perineal tear; and in some cases for breech delivery. Two techniques are available. These are pudendal nerve block and perineal nerve infiltration. To understand the techniques, knowledge of the nerve supply of the vulva and lower vagina is needed.

Nerve supply of the vulva

The female vulva is innervated mainly by branches of the pudendal nerve. The pudendal nerve, derived from S2, S3 and S4, leaves the pelvis medial to the sciatic nerve through the greater sciatic foramen. It then crosses the external surface of the ischial spine and re-enters the pelvis through the lesser sciatic notch and, passing along the lateral wall of the ischiorectal fossa, divides into branches that supply most of the perineum (Fig. 8.23). Further sensory branches to the skin of the perineum are derived from the ilioinguinal nerve, the pudendal branch of the posterior femoral cutaneous nerve and the genital branch of the genitofemoral nerve (Fig. 8.24).

Technique of pudendal nerve block

A 10 cm 20-gauge needle and, if available, a needle director are required. Two fingers are introduced into the vagina to palpate the ischial spine, the guide containing the needle being introduced in the groove between the index and middle finger to impinge on the spine. The guide is then directed to lie just medial to, and below, the ischial spine, and the needle is advanced 1 cm beyond the guide (if no

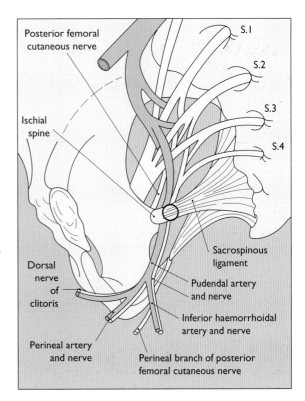

Fig. 8.23 The course of the pudendal nerve. The area in the circle that lies just medial to and below the tip of the ischial spine is the area into which the local anaesthetic is infiltrated.

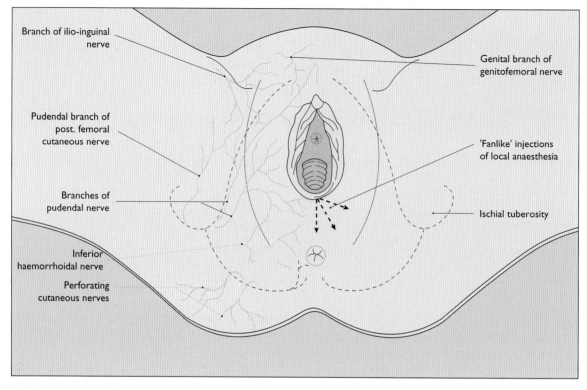

Fig. 8.24 Innervation of the perineum. On one side the nerves are shown, on the other, 'fanlike' local anaesthesia.

guide is available the needle is introduced between the fingers to the same site) and pushed through the sacrospinous ligament (Fig. 8.25); 10 mL of 0.5% lidocaine (lignocaine) are injected behind each ischial spine, and a further 10 mL are used to make a perineal infiltration. Anaesthesia should be effective within 5 minutes and it should be tested. The lower vagina and perineum become insensitive to pain. The use of pudendal nerve block is not without problems. For example, the needle may be difficult to introduce accurately in a relatively mobile patient, particularly when the fetal head is deeply engaged.

Technique of perineal nerve infiltration

Using a 7.5 cm 22-gauge needle and 20 mL of 0.5–1.0% lidocaine (lignocaine) the perineum is infiltrated in a fan-like manner, the base being the posterior fourchette at the midline. Three lines of infiltration are required, one medially as far as the anal sphincter and midway between the skin and the vaginal mucosa, and two others at 45° to block the nerves as they reach the perineum (Fig. 8.25). The analgesia is effective in about 3 minutes and lasts between 45 and 90 minutes. It should be tested by pricking the skin with a sharp needle before any procedure is begun.

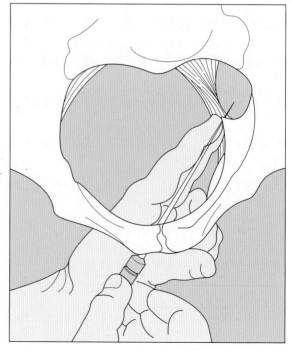

Fig. 8.25 Transvaginal pudendal nerve block.

Chapter | 9 |

The puerperium

By convention the puerperium lasts for 6 weeks from the day of the birth of the child. During this time the physiological and morphological changes that occurred during pregnancy revert to the non-pregnant state. It is also a time when the woman takes on the responsibility of caring for a dependent, demanding infant. This may cause problems, particularly if she finds it difficult to adjust to being a mother.

PHYSIOLOGICAL AND ANATOMICAL CHANGES

The endocrinological changes that occurred during pregnancy rapidly revert. Within hours of the expulsion of the placenta the levels of the placental hormones, human placental lactogen (hPL) and chorionic gonadotrophin (hCG), fall rapidly. Within 2 days hPL is undetectable in serum, and by the 10th day after birth hCG can no longer be detected. The serum levels of oestrogen and progesterone fall rapidly in the first 3 puerperal days, reaching non-pregnant levels by day 7. They remain at this level if the woman chooses to breastfeed; if she does not, oestradiol begins to rise, indicating follicular growth. In breastfeeding women human prolactin (hPr) levels rise following suckling.

The cardiovascular system reverts to the non-pregnant state during the first 2 puerperal weeks. In the first 24 hours the additional burden on the heart caused by the hypervolaemic state persists, after which time the blood and plasma volume return to the non-pregnant state. This occurs by the second puerperal week. In the first 10 days after birth the raised coagulation factors occurring during pregnancy persist, but are balanced by a rise in fibrinolytic activity.

MORPHOLOGICAL CHANGES IN THE GENITAL TRACT

Following the birth the perineum is either damaged or intact. The damage will have been repaired, but oedema of the tissues may have occurred and will persist for some days. The vaginal wall is swollen, bluish and pouting. It rapidly regains its tonicity, although it is fragile for 1 or 2 weeks.

The uterus undergoes the most marked changes. At the end of the third stage of labour the uterus is the size of a 20-week pregnancy and weighs about 1000 g. It rapidly becomes smaller, and by the end of the first puerperal week it weighs about 500 g. Its involution can be demonstrated by the fact that its size is reduced on abdominal examination by one finger's breadth a day, to the extent that on the 12th day after the birth it cannot be palpated abdominally. Its involution continues more slowly after this time, but by the end of the 6th puerperal week it is only slightly larger than it was before the pregnancy.

Concurrently with the involution of the uterus, the placental site becomes smaller. After the birth it is rapidly covered with a fibrin mesh, and thrombosis occurs in the vessels supplying it. Beneath the placental site, macrophages, lymphocytes and polymorphs form a 'barrier', which also extends throughout the endometrial cavity. Within 10 days the placental site has shrunk to a diameter of 2.5 cm, and a new growth of covering epithelium has occurred, which also covers the remainder of the uterine cavity. The superficial tissues of the uterine lining and placental site continue to be shed for 6 weeks, and form part of the lochia.

The lochia is the term used for the discharge from the genital tract that follows childbirth. For the first 3–4 days it consists of blood and remnants of trophoblastic tissue, mainly from the placental site. As the thrombosed vessels of the site become organized the character of the lochia changes. From the third to the 12th day after the birth its colour is reddish-brown, but after this time, when most of the endometrial cavity has been covered with epithelium, it changes to a yellow colour. Occasionally some of the thrombi at the end of the vessels break, releasing blood, and the lochia becomes red once more for a few days.

CONDUCT OF THE PUERPERIUM

A recently delivered woman may start walking about as soon as she wishes, go to the toilet when required, and rest when she feels tired. Some women prefer to remain in bed for the first 24 hours after the birth, and women who have had an extensive repair of a torn perineum or a large episiotomy may choose to remain in bed for longer.

A function of the medical and midwifery attendants is to make sure that the tissues are healing properly, and that the uterus is involuting normally. However, this function is less important than encouraging breastfeeding and providing information about the care of the infant when the mother goes home.

Economic pressures now dictate that most women leave hospital 1–2 days after an uncomplicated delivery and 3–5 days after a caesarean section, with supervisory care at home being provided by a combination of visiting hospital and community midwives.

Care of the puerperal woman

Regular checks are made of the temperature and pulse. The perineum is inspected each day to observe the degree of oedema (if any) and the sutures. Many women who have a damaged and repaired perineum experience considerable pain. The woman may need analgesics; perineal pain is discussed further on page 82.

The character and amount of the lochia are observed and recorded, and the height of the uterine fundus above the symphysis is checked daily.

Uterine contractions continue after childbirth. They are usually painless, but some women experience painful contractions (afterpains), especially when breast feeding. The woman may ask for analgesics.

Urinary tract problems

Micturition may be difficult in the 24 hours after childbirth because of a reflex suppression of detrusor activity caused by the pressure on the bladder base during birth. As a diuresis occurs following the birth, the woman may be uncomfortable. If she is unable to pass urine, catheterization may be required. This is more likely to occur in the puerperium rather than later, because the pregnancy-induced dilatation of the renal pelvis and ureters and the relaxation of the bladder muscle take about 3 weeks to disappear.

About 10% of puerperal women experience urinary incontinence (usually stress incontinence). In all but a few women this persists for a few weeks and then ceases. Pelvic floor exercises (see p. 311) may speed up the resolution of the problem.

Bowel problems

A few women become constipated during the puerperium. In most cases relief is spontaneous; if not, stool softeners such as oral sterculia with frangula bark granules (Normacol) or bisacodyl rectal suppositories may be prescribed.

Women who have haemorrhoids during pregnancy often complain that they are more painful in the postpartum period. One woman in 20 develops haemorrhoids for the first time during the birth, but in most cases these settle in 2 or 3 weeks.

Backache

Backache often occurs in the last quarter of pregnancy and persists after the birth, or it may occur for the first time in the puerperium. Backache affects about 25% of puerperal women, but over half of them have complained of backache before becoming pregnant. The pain can be considerable, particularly if the new mother has no help in caring for her baby. It may persist for months, but eventually settles.

CARE OF THE NEONATE

Today most hospitals have facilities for rooming-in, the baby lying in a cot close to the mother's bed, mother and baby being treated as a dyad. This has made the care of a healthy newborn infant much easier.

Checking for congenital abnormalities

A check for major abnormalities is made immediately after the birth and before the baby is given to the mother to celebrate the event. A full check is made during the baby's first day of life. The procedure is described in Box 9.1.

Box 9.1 Examination of a newborn baby

Examine the baby preferably when settled ½–1 hour after a feed. Examine gently and with warmed hands and in the mother's presence. Commence the examination with the baby clothed to accomplish as much of the examination as possible (especially steps 1–4) without disturbing the baby. Only undress the baby as required by the examination.

1. Observe the posture and any spontaneous movement; listen for audible breathing sounds.
2. Feel the anterior fontanelle.
3. Listen to the precordium for cardiac murmurs (this can be done initially through the inner garments to avoid the touch of the stethoscope on the skin – all but the softest murmurs will still be heard).
4. If the baby is still relaxed, gentle abdominal palpation is best done next, feeling especially for liver, spleen or kidney enlargement, or other tumour.
5. Commence a systematic examination commencing at the head, face and neck:
   a. Examine the head for bruising, swelling and its shape.
   b. Examine the face for abnormal features, symmetry, birthmarks.
   c. Open the mouth, examine for cleft palate, other abnormalities of palate, tongue and gums.
   d. Examine the eyes for position, strabismus, conjunctival haemorrhage or inflammation, red light reflex.
   e. Examine the neck for sternomastoid tumour, goitre, other swellings or pits, redundant skinfolds.
6. Examine the chest for shape, symmetry, signs of respiratory distress, air entry.
7. Check the umbilicus, looking for infection, hernia; check the number of vessels.
8. Examine the external genitalia; in boys check for undescended testicles, hydroceles, hernias, hypospadias; in girls check for hymenal skin tags, imperforate hymen, labial fusion. Check for imperforate anus.
9. Feel for the femoral pulses.
10. Examine the extremities and spine; observe the posture, length of limbs, range of movement; look for deformities of hands or feet – posture, size, shape and number of digits.
11. Examine the hips.
    To examine the left hip, the doctor steadies the infant's pelvis between the thumb of the left hand on the symphysis pubis and the fingers behind the sacrum. The examiner grasps the child's left thigh in the right hand and attempts to move the femoral head gently forwards and then backwards out of the acetabulum. If the head of the femur is felt to move, with or without an audible 'clunk', dislocation, or dislocability is diagnosed. If there is any doubt after the examination, real-time ultrasound is used to detect a displaced hip. In about 10% of the cases the babies' hips produce a soft 'click' rather than a 'clunk', and there is no evidence of abnormal movement of the femoral head. These babies must be examined again before discharge from hospital. If 1 month later the 'click' has changed into a 'clunk', and abnormal movement between the femoral head and the acetabulum is found, the ultrasound examination is repeated.

Care of the umbilical cord

The umbilical cord is inspected and the clamp removed, and the cord is tied and cut close to the umbilicus 24 hours after birth. The area is smeared with chlorhexidine cream, but no cord dressing or binder is used.

Weight loss

A newborn infant may be expected to lose between 5 and 10% of its birthweight during the first 4 days of life. For a healthy mature baby this causes no problems. From the fourth day the infant will be obtaining sufficient breast milk (or breast-milk substitute) to start gaining weight. No fluids other than those obtained from the breast or bottle need be given. Extra fluids should be avoided in breastfed babies as they interfere with the smooth establishment of lactation. The only reason for giving extra fluids is to counter the development of 'dehydration fever' in the baby.

Dehydration fever

Because a neonate's temperature control is not very efficient, dehydration fever may affect a few infants in the first days of life in hot, humid weather. The infant develops a high fever, looks dehydrated, and has a dry mouth and a depressed anterior fontanelle. It is vigorous and thirsty, unlike an infected infant, which is languid and febrile. Dehydration fever rarely occurs in infants who room-in and breastfeed on demand. The treatment consists of replacing the fluid and salt lost by giving oral feeds of 200 mL 1 : 5 normal saline per kg body weight per 24 hours.

The stools

In the first 2 days of life the infant's faeces are sticky and greenish-black in colour. As microorganisms invade the gut the colour of the faeces changes to yellow, with the occasional passage of greenish faeces. Breastfed babies usually defecate a soft stool which has little odour. Bottle-fed infants do not defecate as regularly and the stool, when expelled, is firmer in consistency, dark yellow, and occasionally has an offensive smell.

Jaundice

Most babies develop transient jaundice which is benign and self-limiting. A few develop more marked jaundice. If this occurs within 24 hours of birth, persists, and extends on to the infant's trunk or thighs, serum bilirubin measurements are made. A serum bilirubin reading of more than 250 mmol/L is of concern as kernicterus may occur. Advice from a paediatrician should be obtained. Treatment consists of phototherapy or, in severe cases, exchange transfusion.

Infant feeding

The establishment of maternal lactation and breastfeeding or, if the mother chooses not to breastfeed, the establishment of feeding with breast-milk substitutes, is one of the most important tasks for those caring for the infant.

LACTATION AND BREASTFEEDING

During pregnancy the breasts develop considerably. Fat is deposited around the glandular parts of the breasts. Oestrogen leads to an increase in the size and number of the ducts, and progesterone increases the number of alveoli; hPL also stimulates alveolar development and may be involved in the synthesis of casein, lactalbumin and lactoglobulin by the alveolar cells.

In spite of this activity, lactation is inhibited during pregnancy, although levels of human prolactin (hPr) rise throughout the pregnancy. The reason for this is that the high levels of oestrogen occupy binding sites on the alveoli that prevent them from responding to the lactogenic properties of hPr. In late pregnancy the breasts secrete a thickish, yellowish fluid, colostrum, which is rich in immune antibodies. The production of colostrum increases after the birth until it is replaced by breast-milk production.

As mentioned earlier, the level of oestrogen falls rapidly in the 48 hours following childbirth. This permits circulating hPr to act on the alveolar cells to initiate and maintain lactation.

Lactation is encouraged by early and frequent suckling, as this reflexly causes the pituitary gland to secrete hPr (Fig. 9.1). On the other hand, negative emotions, including the fear of failing to breastfeed, may reduce the secretion of prolactin, by promoting the release of the prolactin-inhibiting factor (dopamine) from the hypothalamus. The onset of lactation may be delayed in women who were delivered by caesarean section or following a traumatic labour and birth.

By the second or third day after the birth hPr has induced the alveolar cells to secrete milk, which is thin and bluish in colour. Initially the milk distends the alveoli and the small ducts, causing the breasts to become full, engorged and tender. Turgid veins can be seen beneath the skin, and the milk ducts can be felt as tender strings in the breast tissue. The engorgement is due to the absence of ejection of milk through the large ducts to the nipple.

Milk ejection reflex

The milk filling and distending the alveoli is unavailable to the infant until myoepithelial cells (Fig. 9.2) that surround the alveoli and smaller ducts contract in response to the milk ejection (or 'let-down') reflex. The reflex is initiated by suckling and is mediated via the hypothalamus and pituitary gland, which release oxytocin into the bloodstream (Fig. 9.3).

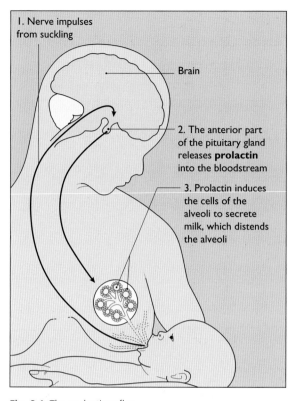

Fig. 9.1 The prolactin reflex.

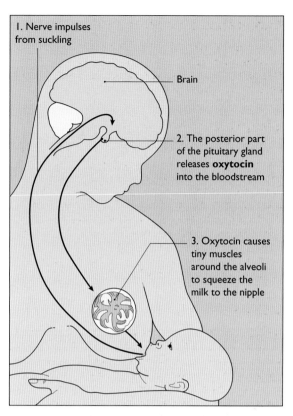

Fig. 9.3 The milk ejection reflex.

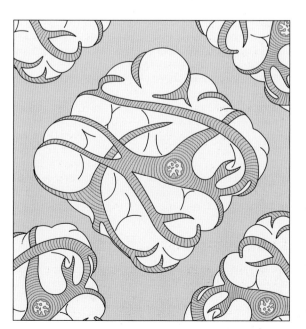

Fig. 9.2 Myoepithelial cells surrounding a partially filled villus.

The oxytocin causes contractions of the myoepithelial cells and milk is ejected from the alveoli and small ducts to flow to the large ducts and the subareolar reservoirs. Oxytocin may also inhibit the release of dopamine from the hypothalamus, further encouraging the secretion of milk.

Negative emotional and physical factors can reduce the let-down reflex, with the result that for lactation to be established the mother must be confident that she can breastfeed. The medical attendants should encourage her to be confident.

A joint statement by WHO and UNICEF summarizes the support needed for successful lactation (Box 9.2).

Nutritional needs in lactation

The energy cost of lactation is 2095 kJ/day. A woman who has been well nourished during pregnancy has fat stores of 125 700 kJ, which can be used to supply the extra energy needs of lactation. The diet of a parturient woman provides over 10 050 kJ/day and her energy needs for bodily functions and daily activity are about 8400 kJ/day, so that there is sufficient to meet the needs of lactation. However, if she is anxious she can be advised to eat an extra slice of bread with butter and cheese, which will provide the extra energy needed.

89

> **Box 9.2 Ten steps to successful breastfeeding**
>
> **Every facility providing maternity services and care for newborn infants should:**
> 1. Have a written breastfeeding policy that is routinely communicated to all healthcare staff.
> 2. Train all healthcare staff in the skills necessary to implement this policy.
> 3. Inform all pregnant women about the benefits and management of breastfeeding.
> 4. Help mothers initiate breastfeeding within a half hour of birth.
> 5. Show mothers how to breastfeed and how to maintain lactation even if they are separated from their infants.
> 6. Give newborn infants no food or drink other than breast milk unless medically indicated.
> 7. Practise rooming-in. Allow mothers and infants to stay together 24 hours a day.
> 8. Encourage breastfeeding on demand.
> 9. Give no artificial teats or pacifiers (also called dummies and soothers) to breastfeeding infants.
> 10. Foster the establishment of breastfeeding support groups and refer mothers to them on discharge from hospital or clinic.

MAINTENANCE OF LACTATION

The most effective way of maintaining lactation is regular suckling, so that both the prolactin and the milk ejection reflexes are initiated frequently, and abnormal distension of the alveoli by milk is prevented. If distension occurs, the alveoli are unable to secrete milk efficiently and at the same time suckling is avoided because of pain in the breasts. Consequently, the inhibition of the reflex that prevents the release of dopamine from the hypothalamus is lost and alveolar activity diminishes, with a further reduction of milk secretion.

Establishment of breastfeeding

The establishment of successful breastfeeding requires:

- That milk secretion occurs in the alveoli
- That the milk ejection reflex is efficient
- That the mother is motivated to breastfeed (she may need support to stay motivated).

As mentioned in Box 9.2, breastfeeding is more readily established if:

- The baby is given to the mother to caress and suckle soon after birth.
- The baby rooms-in with the mother and the staff treat them as a dyad.
- The baby is allowed to suckle frequently from birth, for a short period each time, to help 'bring the milk in'.
- Once the milk is flowing the baby is fed on demand, including at night.
- No feeds of water or of glucose water are given to the infant without the express agreement of the mother and her carers.
- The midwifery staff help the establishment of lactation by adopting a positive approach to the mother, are unhurried and supportive, and provide consistent information during the time she is establishing breastfeeding.

Technique of breastfeeding

The mother should be shown how to stroke the infant's mouth with her nipple, to induce the 'rooting' reflex in which the baby opens her or his mouth and searches for the nipple.

She then holds her breast with the nipple between her forefinger and middle finger, so that the nipple becomes more prominent and the infant is able to put its gums on the areola and not on the tender nipple itself (Fig. 9.4C).

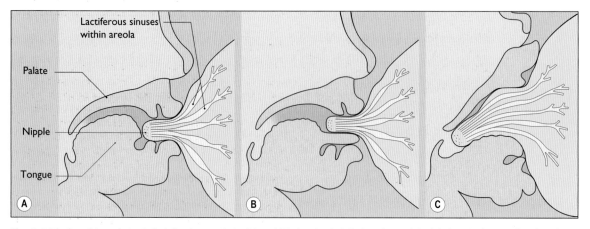

Fig. 9.4 Ideal position of nipple in infant's mouth. In (A) and (B) the nipple is being chewed; in (C) the nipple is well within the baby's mouth.

This technique enables the baby to breathe when suckling (Figs 9.5 and 9.6).

The mother is shown how to detach the infant's mouth from the nipple without causing her pain. This is done by putting her little finger into the corner of the baby's mouth to break the suction before detaching it from her nipple.

As mentioned earlier, very few babies managed in this way require additional fluids in the first 4 days of life. However, if the baby becomes clinically dehydrated, water may be given by a spoon or dropper after a feed. A feeding bottle should be avoided as it may stop the baby learning how to suck properly at the breast.

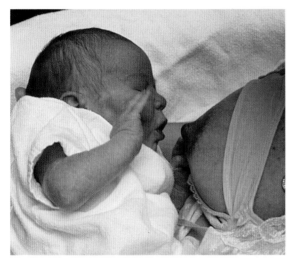

Fig. 9.5 The baby's lips are pursed awaiting attachment to the mother's breast.

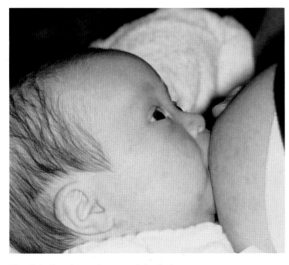

Fig. 9.6 Good attachment of the baby.

Breast engorgement

It takes a few days to adjust the supply of milk to the demand, mainly because the milk ejection reflex is not yet operating properly. During this time the breasts of some women become engorged, as described earlier. Treatment depends on the severity of the engorgement. Many nurses claim that a successful remedy consists of hot and cold towels applied alternately to the breasts, as this stimulates increased blood flow through the engorged areas. Another method is to stimulate the milk ejection reflex using an electric breast pump. Severe and painful engorgement may be reduced by prescribing small doses of bromocriptine (dopamine agonist) for 24–48 hours.

If possible the mother should continue to breastfeed in spite of the engorgement, to stimulate the milk ejection reflex.

Breast problems during lactation

Cracked nipples

Aggressive suckling by the baby may lead to cracked nipples, particularly if the nipple is not well within the infant's mouth (Fig. 9.4A and B). If the cracking is severe, the baby should not be fed from the affected breast, which should be emptied manually or by using a breast pump.

Milk stasis

This may occur early in lactation and be associated with, or follow, breast engorgement. Milk stasis is due to pressure on the main duct of a lobule by the engorged alveoli and usually settles without treatment, but may lead to non-infectious inflammation of the breast. It is thought the pressure in some of the alveoli causes seepage of milk into the surrounding breast tissues, which results in the non-infectious inflammation. Treatment of both forms, if needed, is to try to help the mother feed her baby more often and to empty the breasts manually after each feed.

Acute mastitis

Most cases of acute mastitis in the mother are caused by organisms acquired from the infant's nasopharyngeal or umbilical areas, which harbour colonies of staphylococci or streptococci that develop within a few days of birth.

Acute mastitis occurs at the end of the first week following birth. The mother develops a fever and a tender, red, firm-to-hard area is felt in one of the breasts. Treatment consists of analgesics and antibiotics. As most infections are caused by staphylococci, flucloxacillin 500 mg four times a day for 5 days is the drug of choice. If the mother is allergic to penicillin then cefalexin 500 mg or clindamycin 450 mg both four times a day for 5 days can be used. If it is not too painful, the mother should continue suckling the baby. If pus develops in the infected area, causing a breast abscess, incision of the abscess and drainage for 24 hours may be required.

Proper attention to breastfeeding reduces the chance of acute mastitis developing. The breasts should be emptied after a feed, as incomplete emptying leaves stagnant milk in the system, which may become infected. Cracked nipples should be treated, as microorganisms may invade through the cracks. Rooming-in reduces the chance of cross-infection between babies and of mastitis in the mother.

Low breast-milk supply

If insufficient amounts of breast milk are being produced to meet the baby's needs the galactagogues such as domperidone, 10 mg three times a day increasing to 20 mg three times a day after 10 days, can be tried, but only after attachment or structural impediments to suckling have been excluded. Once lactation is established the drug is withdrawn over a week. Signs of low breast-milk supply are: <6 wet nappies in 24 hours, weight gain less than 25 g per day, and finding the baby difficult to settle or lethargic.

Nipple thrush

Nipple and breast thrush is caused by overgrowth of *Candida albicans* in the nipple and ducts. It may follow antibiotic therapy and trauma to the nipple which allows the candida to enter the breast. Breastfeeding is painful and the nipple and areola appear slightly inflamed and the nipple is very tender to touch. The first line of treatment is with miconozole oral gel/cream or nystatin cream applied to the nipples, oral nystatin 500 000 units; and for the baby miconozole gel applied to its mouth until the symptoms have disappeared.

Suppression of lactation

Women who choose not to breastfeed or who stop breastfeeding may need to have lactation suppressed. Lactation will diminish and cease if the baby no longer suckles. At first the breasts become engorged but, if supported by an appropriately sized bra, will become less engorged in a few days and lactation will cease. An alternative is for the woman to be prescribed a prolactin inhibitor (dopamine receptor agonist).

Breast-milk substitutes

More than 95% of women can breastfeed if they want to, and although most women choose to breastfeed immediately after childbirth, by the sixth week of the puerperium less than 60% are still doing so.

Women who do not breastfeed choose one of the breast-milk substitutes (formula milks) available. These are based on cows' milk, modified as far as possible to have the same proportions of protein, fat, carbohydrates, minerals and vitamins as found in human milk. Provided formula milk is prepared according to the manufacturer's directions the baby will thrive, although she or he is not as well protected against infection as a breastfed infant. This is of importance in the developing countries and among poor women in all countries.

PSYCHOLOGICAL PROBLEMS IN THE PUERPERIUM

The birth of a baby places considerable stress on the mother. She has the responsibility of caring for a demanding infant, her nights are usually disturbed, and she may not feel competent or confident about her ability as a mother. It is not surprising that it takes time for her to adjust to being a mother and that she may suffer psychological disturbances.

A large number of women – probably 50% – experience a heightened state of emotional reactiveness 3–5 days after the birth and about 10% become more severely depressed. Postnatal depression is mentioned here and discussed more fully on page 187.

Postpartum blues

Why so many women develop postpartum blues is not known. Speculation about its aetiology includes hormonal imbalance (although none has been identified), reaction to the excitement of childbirth, and uncertainty by the mother about her ability to care for her dependent child. Another factor in western culture may be the expectation that a mother immediately loves her baby, when in reality mother love is a learned behaviour.

The condition leads to bursts of crying, to irritability, elation, emotional lability and, in some cases, to depression. The peak of the symptoms occurs about 3–5 days postpartum, often coinciding with the onset of lactation. Successful management consists of one of the medical or midwifery staff talking with the woman, explaining what is occurring, and if she wishes, restricting visitors. There is some evidence that postpartum blues are less likely to occur if maternal–infant bonding has occurred and if rooming-in is practised. A small proportion of women develop depression that may persist for weeks or months. It is important that all the mother's care givers actively look for the signs and symptoms during each contact with the mother in the weeks after birth. Some centres routinely use screening tools such as the Edinburgh Postnatal Depression Score to identify women at increased risk.

Adjustment to parenthood and postnatal depression (puerperal depression)

Adjustment to parenthood is difficult for most women and they can have unrealistic expectations about motherhood. On returning home after childbirth, the persistent demands of the newborn baby on energy, time and the emotions of the mother may cause considerable stress. This stress is aggravated by the nuclear family and the tendency for young people to live at some distance from their close relatives, who, in other cultures, are readily available to offer help and support. The stress becomes intensified as the mother realizes that she has the sole responsibility for a small, unpredictable infant who needs attention day and night. She may not have realized that the baby would cry so much, for so little apparent cause. Her sleep is constantly broken, and fatigue is added to her feelings of inadequacy. Her relationship with her partner also requires adjustment, and this can be emotionally disturbing, particularly if he does not do his share of parenting. As the baby occupies so much of her time, the mother finds that her day-to-day life is no longer as organized as she would wish, and feels guilty that she is not the efficient person she believed she was.

The fatigue induced by the demands of the baby, the emotional readjustment in partner relations, the guilt experienced over failing to cope as well as she expected and lack of a helpful counsellor often induces depression. In mild cases reassurance and advice and providing support for the woman are sufficient. It is also important to tell parents of local community-based help organizations that provide 24-hour home counselling and home visiting when needed. Their activities in helping women adjust to parenthood can be of great value in reducing the incidence of puerperal depression. In 10–20% of women the depression may be more severe and require medication for recovery or to prevent recurrent future depression (see p. 187).

Child abuse

Women who find difficulty in coping with their baby, or who have inappropriate or disturbed behaviour while in hospital, are more likely to abuse their baby after discharge. The prevalence of child abuse before the age of 3 years is not known exactly, but it is probable that at least six per 1000 liveborn children are abused. Mothers who have social problems, who have no supportive partner or relative, or who have marital problems are more likely to abuse their child. It is possible, by simple observation in the puerperium, to identify some vulnerable women, and this should be part of postnatal care. Preventive intervention by family doctors, paediatricians and social workers has been shown to reduce the prevalence of child neglect and abuse.

SEXUALITY AFTER CHILDBIRTH

After childbirth the demands of the new baby occupy a good deal of a mother's time. Moreover, if the mother has had a perineal tear or an episiotomy repaired – in fact if she

has needed any stitches – her perineum and vagina may be tender for several weeks or months (see p. 79). It is not unexpected that her desire for sexual intercourse is reduced. Some women who breastfeed may have a reduced libido and develop vaginal dryness, both of which are reversed when they cease breastfeeding. Intercourse is not the only way of obtaining sexual pleasure, and she may welcome touching, cuddling and stimulating her partner if he wishes. When she is ready the couple can resume intercourse. Women may consult a doctor about their lack of sexual feeling after the birth, and supportive advice is helpful.

PERINATAL BEREAVEMENT

About 12 babies in every 1000 are either stillborn or die in the first 28 days of life. These constitute perinatal deaths, and many of these babies are born preterm and are of low birthweight, and about 25% have severe congenital malformations. Parents whose baby dies in the perinatal period have grief reactions similar to those that follow the loss of any loved person. At first the mother (and often the father) feels numb and shocked. After a few days the reaction changes to a desire to understand why the baby died, or to expressions of anger or guilt about events in pregnancy or during labour. Over the next 2 or 3 months many parents are likely to review the events surrounding the baby's death, often repeatedly. More than 50% of mothers suffer from depression and anxiety, which may last for months, but in time the couple adjust, often embarking on a new pregnancy.

The severity and duration of the bereavement reaction may be reduced if the parents are given the opportunity to talk with the attending medical and midwifery staff soon after the baby's death. The talk should take place in a quiet private area, not in an open ward. Most parents want to understand what has gone wrong, and to have it explained in clear, simple language. A few become angry, blaming the staff for the child's death. The doctor or midwife should listen to the parents with sympathy and understanding and explain as clearly as possible the events surrounding the death.

In addition, the staff member should give information to the parents about the grief reaction that may be expected, and should provide reassurance that nothing the mother did, or failed to do, caused the death of the child.

Parents who wish to see their dead child (even if malformed) should be given the opportunity, so that they may mourn their loss. If they do not wish to see the child at that time, a photograph, a footprint and perhaps a lock of the child's hair should be kept with the mother's records, as later the parents may regret their decision not to have seen their child.

Before the parents see the baby they should be told how the infant will look. If there are deformities they should be described (perhaps with the aid of a photograph). The baby is presented to the parents clothed and wrapped, and when they become accustomed to him or her, the baby can be undressed by them. This procedure is often emotional, and support from a health professional may be invaluable. The parents should be told that they can spend as much time as they wish with the baby, and should be encouraged to name the child. Many parents wish to have a photograph of their dead baby. When the mother leaves hospital it is important to suggest that she makes contact with her family doctor (or health visitor), and she should be told about community-based help organizations in her area.

One woman in every five whose baby is stillborn, or who dies in the neonatal period, will suffer severe symptoms of bereavement (sleeplessness, depression and withdrawal). Women who have little or no support from husband, partner or family, who are cared for by insensitive health professionals and who lack a caring environment are more likely to be severely affected. These women in particular need help from sympathetic health professionals who listen, communicate and counsel.

There is some evidence that parents cope better, psychologically, with the next pregnancy if conception is delayed for a few months, but the decision has to be made by the couple, rather than imposed by a doctor. During the pregnancy continuity of care is important, and supportive, communicating, sympathetic health professionals help to reduce possible mothering difficulties and puerperal problems.

POSTNATAL CHECK

It is usual for the mother and her baby to be asked to return for a postnatal check 6–8 weeks after the birth. The purpose of this visit is to discuss her:

- Adjustment to parenthood
- Changes in mood or behaviour
- Need for information about child care
- Sexual relationship
- Weight change
- Contraception
- Follow-up of any complications that arose in pregnancy or during childbirth.

The doctor also examines the woman and her baby.

The maternal examination includes inspection of the perineum and vagina to ascertain that any damage has healed, to find out whether she has urinary or faecal incontinence, and to determine the muscle tone. A vaginal speculum is used to visualize the cervix and a Pap smear is taken if indicated. A bimanual examination is made to check that the uterus has involuted completely.

Follow-up examination of the newborn is made (see Box 9.1) and immunization discussed.

Chapter | **10** |

Minor complications of pregnancy

The physiological and anatomical changes that occur during pregnancy may lead to complications which, although minor in medical terms, may cause considerable distress and discomfort to many pregnant women. They are listed below in alphabetical order.

BACKACHE

Backache is common in late pregnancy and is felt over the sacroiliac joints. It is caused by relaxation of the ligaments and muscles supporting the joints, and is probably also induced by progesterone and, possibly, relaxin. It is usually worse at night and may prevent the woman from sleeping. Wearing flat-heeled shoes, avoiding heavy lifting, gentle exercise (including water-based exercise), physiotherapy and acupuncture are all beneficial.

CERVICAL EVERSION AND DISCHARGE

The high levels of oestrogen in pregnancy may increase the eversion of the endocervical columnar cells so that they appear as a red ring around the external cervical os. The cells may secrete mucus when exposed to the vagina, causing a non-infective vaginal discharge. The condition has erroneously been called a cervical erosion.

CONSTIPATION

The reduced gut motility associated with increased progesterone is aggravated in late pregnancy by the pressure of the enlarged uterus, making constipation common in pregnancy.

Treatment consists of increasing dietary fibre (for example by eating wholemeal instead of white bread) and attempting to defecate after a meal. If the constipation is causing discomfort the woman may be prescribed oral sterculia with frangula bark granules (Normacol) or the contact laxative bisacodyl.

DISPLACEMENT OF THE UTERUS

Retroversion

In 10% of women the uterus is normally retroverted; moreover, retroversion of the uterus does not hinder conception, and so when examined vaginally in the early weeks of pregnancy some women will be found to have a retroverted uterus. In nearly all cases the uterus becomes anteverted spontaneously, usually between the 9th and 11th weeks of pregnancy. Very rarely the uterus remains retroverted until after the 14th gestational week and becomes incarcerated in the cul-de-sac. If this occurs the woman complains of frequency of micturition and dysuria. If the position of the uterus is not corrected, the symptoms increase in severity and eventually there is retention of urine and an enormously distended bladder. Finally, retention of urine with overflow occurs. Examination shows a smooth, soft cystic tumour arising in the pelvis and palpable abdominally in the midline. Treatment entails inserting a catheter and decompressing the bladder slowly. When this is done the uterus usually becomes anteverted, but may need to be anteverted using the fingers by pushing up in the posterior fornix and manipulating the uterus to one side of the sacral promontory.

Uterovaginal prolapse

In multiparous women, particularly in the developing countries, uterovaginal prolapse may complicate pregnancy. In the early weeks of pregnancy the prolapse may become more prominent. As the uterus becomes an abdominal organ the pressure on the vagina is relieved to some extent, and the prolapse becomes less obvious. Occasionally a swollen, infected cervix may protrude through the vulva. The prolapse causes few problems during labour and cervical dilatation is usually rapid. Pregnancy after a vaginal repair for prolapse is considered on page 307.

DYSPNOEA

By the 15th week of pregnancy one woman in four complains of dyspnoea on exertion. The proportion increases as pregnancy advances, with the result that, by the fourth quarter of pregnancy, three-quarters of pregnant women are dyspnoeic. The condition is probably due to a lack of adaptation to progesterone-induced hyperventilation. Once pathological causes such as severe anaemia and cardiac disease are excluded, the woman can be reassured that the breathlessness will not harm her or her fetus and that no specific treatment is required.

HEARTBURN

Relaxation of the lower oesophageal sphincter permits the regurgitation of some of the stomach contents, causing irritation of the lower oesophagus. It is also possible that a similar relaxation of the pyloric sphincter permits a reflux of bile into the stomach, which may then be regurgitated into the lower oesophagus. The woman complains of heartburn, which increases as the pregnancy advances.

Treatment is difficult, but frequent small meals, avoidance of spicy food and cigarettes, and the use of antacids may relieve the discomfort. If antacids fail, floating antacids such as a sodium alginate–sodium bicarbonate mixture or the H_2 receptor antagonist ranitidine hydrochloride may give relief. If the heartburn occurs predominantly at night, the use of extra pillows to prop up the expectant mother may help.

HAEMORRHOIDS AND VARICOSE VEINS

Haemorrhoids and varicose veins of the legs, and occasionally of the vulva, become increasingly common as pregnancy advances. Haemorrhoids often become larger or may appear for the first time during childbirth. They may persist for several months after the birth and cause pain. Constipation should be avoided and topical treatment prescribed.

Varicose veins increase in size in late pregnancy. Treatment entails the woman lying or sitting with her feet up as much as possible and, if the veins are painful or disfiguring, wearing elastic stockings. The latter should be put on before the woman gets out of bed in the morning. Surgical treatment for either condition is generally contraindicated in pregnancy.

INSOMNIA

Many pregnant women find that their sleep pattern is altered. In early pregnancy they may sleep for longer than usual. In late pregnancy, because of the discomfort of the enlarged uterus, leg cramps and backache, sleep may be disturbed.

LEG CRAMPS

The cause of leg cramps is not known. They tend to occur more frequently in the second half of pregnancy, usually at night. Magnesium (lactate or citrate) 122 mg morning and

244 mg nocte reduces severe cramps in one-third of suffers compared with placebo. Calcium supplements are ineffectual. Some women obtain relief if the foot of the bed is raised about 25 cm.

MICTURITION

Frequency of micturition

Increased frequency of micturition is common in early pregnancy, when it is due to a supranormal excretion of urine by the kidney, and in the last weeks when the pressure of the fetal head causes direct irritation of the trigone.

Urinary incontinence

Urinary incontinence affects over 50% of pregnant women to some extent, and 15% complain that the leakage is troublesome. There is no specific treatment, although pelvic floor exercises may help (see Box 39.1, p. 311). Usually the leakage eases in the puerperium.

NAUSEA AND VOMITING

Nausea due to pregnancy affects over 75% of women and vomiting occurs in half of them. The symptoms usually begin in the sixth gestational week and cease by the 14th, although they may continue throughout the pregnancy. The symptoms are more common in women who have a history of unsuccessful pregnancies, or who are carrying a multiple pregnancy. One-quarter of women who have the symptoms will experience them again in a subsequent pregnancy.

The cause appears to be either the effect of the rising levels of oestrogen, or the high levels of human chorionic gonadotrophin (hCG) acting on the chemoreceptor trigger zone in the midbrain. Once the body has become habituated to the new hormonal environment, the nausea and vomiting usually cease. In addition, psychological factors may act on the emetic centre in the cerebral cortex.

Nausea and vomiting may be graded as mild, moderate or severe.

Mild

Mild nausea (and occasional vomiting) affects 45% of pregnant women and is the most common form. The nausea can occur in the morning (morning sickness), but may occur at any time of the day and can be provoked by emotional stress.

Treatment

The patient should be advised to eat frequent small meals during the day, to take fluid between (not with) meals, and to eat whatever she feels helps her nausea. If the vomiting is distressing she can be prescribed pyridoxine 50 mg 6-hourly or metoclopramide (Maxolon) 10 mg two to three times a day.

Moderate

Moderate nausea and vomiting affects 5% of all pregnant women, and 10% of all women suffering from nausea. The symptoms may occur at any time of the day or night. The patient feels miserable and may become mildly dehydrated.

Severe

This form is uncommon, affecting 1 in 1000 pregnant women. The nausea is continuous and the vomiting frequent. This is the reason for its name – hyperemesis gravidarum. The woman rapidly becomes dehydrated and ketoacidotic.

Treatment

The patient should be admitted to hospital and treatment started urgently to avoid the possibility of liver damage. An intravenous line is established and dehydration and ketosis corrected by infusing 1 L of 5% dextrose, followed by 1 L of Hartmann's solution if electrolyte disturbance is detected. The infusion should provide 3–4 L/day and is continued until hydration and electrolyte balance have been corrected. The fluid intake and output are recorded, and the urine is checked twice daily for acetone, bile, sugar and specific gravity. Plasma electrolytes are measured daily. If vomiting persists, the patient should be given metoclopramide (10 mg IV or IM) as needed. During the time that the infusion is running the patient can be given ice to suck, and oral feeding should be withheld. Corticosteroids have been used successfully in non-randomized studies. Once the vomiting has ceased the patient is treated in the same way as for the moderate form of nausea. She should remain in hospital for 2 days after the vomiting has ceased and until she has begun to gain weight.

OEDEMA

Oedema, particularly of the legs, is, in the absence of hypertension, a normal physiological adaptation to the pregnant state. The cause is water stored in the ground substance of connective tissue. In pregnancy the increased secretion of oestrogen alters the ground substance from a colloid-rich, water-poor matrix to a colloid-poor, water-rich matrix. In addition, in late pregnancy, increased mechanical obstruction to the venous return from the legs adds to leg oedema. Oedema around the ankles and lower legs is more common towards evening in hot, humid climates, and in obese women. Treatment consists of the woman sitting or lying with her legs elevated. There is no place for diuretics.

Oedema associated with a rise in blood pressure requires further investigation, particularly when the hands or face become oedematous (see Ch. 14).

PALPITATIONS, FAINTING AND HEADACHES

These symptoms are common in pregnancy and are caused by altered cardiovascular dynamics. The patient should be examined and reassured that she has no organic lesion. Auscultation of the heart may reveal a soft systolic murmur, which is due to the hypervolaemic circulation occurring during pregnancy. A murmur of this kind is not a sign of cardiac damage. Some women feel faint when lying on their back in late pregnancy because the pressure of the uterus reduces venous return to the heart (supine hypotension). Pregnant women should avoid lying flat on their backs. Headaches also appear to be due to the altered vascular dynamics.

PLACIDITY AND DROWSINESS

These symptoms are common in pregnancy and are due to the increase in circulating progesterone. This relaxation during pregnancy is enjoyed by some women, but others become frustrated by their inertia. There is no effective treatment available.

PUBIC SYMPHYSIS DIASTASIS (PELVIC OSTEOARTHROPATHY)

In a few women abnormal relaxation of the ligaments surrounding the pubic joint permits the pubic bones to move on each other when the woman walks or exerts herself. This movement may put strain on the sacroiliac joints. Pubic symphysis diastasis may occur during pregnancy or start in the puerperium. The pain may persist for the remainder of the pregnancy or for several weeks after the birth, which makes care of the neonate difficult. The patient complains of severe pubic pain, backache and sacral pain. Examination shows that the pubic joint is very tender when pressed. The diastasis can be confirmed by ultrasound or X-ray examination (Fig. 10.1). Treatment consists of bed rest on a firm mattress, with the patient nursed as far as is possible on one or other side.

PRURITUS

After exclusion of a skin rash and abnormal liver function, antihistamines can decrease the skin irritation.

SWEATING

Because of the vasodilatation and increased peripheral circulation, pregnant women 'feel the heat' and often sweat profusely, particularly in hot, humid climates. No treatment is available apart from frequent cool showers.

VAGINAL DISCHARGES

In pregnancy the quantity of normal vaginal secretions increases and many women complain of a non-irritant vaginal discharge. Vaginal infections, particularly candidiasis, are more frequent in pregnant women than in non-pregnant women. Vaginal discharges are discussed on pages 260–262.

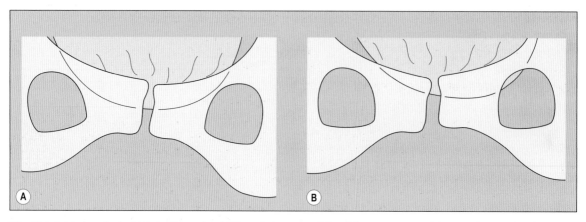

Fig. 10.1 Pelvic symphysis diastasis. The patient is 39 weeks' pregnant. The sliding movement of the symphysis is shown when (A) the patient stands on her right leg; (B) the patient stands on her left leg.

Chapter | **11** |

Miscarriage and abortion

Abortion or miscarriage is defined as the expulsion of a fetus before it reaches viability. Because of different definitions of viability in different countries, the World Health Organization (WHO) has recommended that a fetus is considered potentially viable when the gestation period has reached 22 weeks or more, or when the fetus weighs 500 g or more. As the term abortion does not differentiate between spontaneous and induced abortion the term miscarriage is widely preferred, abortion being used when the pregnancy is deliberately terminated before fetal viability. Most miscarriages occur naturally between the sixth and 10th weeks of pregnancy.

Data from several countries estimate that between 10 and 20% of clinically diagnosed pregnancies end in miscarriage. Miscarriage is more frequent among women over the age of 30 and increases further among women over the age of 35; the risk being nine times greater than for women aged 20–29. Paternal age over 40 also increases the risk, albeit not as strongly as maternal age. The risk also increases in frequency with increasing gravidity: 6% of first or second pregnancies terminate as a miscarriage; with third and subsequent pregnancies the rate increases to 16%.

AETIOLOGY OF SPONTANEOUS MISCARRIAGE

The causes of miscarriage are:
- Implantation
- Ovofetal
- Maternal.

Implantation

Implantation occurs 8–10 days after ovulation in most healthy pregnancies. The proportion ending in early loss increases when implantation is later. A refractory period after the time of uterine receptivity may provide a natural mechanism that eliminates impaired embryos. In 20% of miscarriages the trophoblast has failed to implant adequately.

In the early weeks of pregnancy (0–10 weeks) ovofetal factors account for most miscarriages; in the later weeks (11–22 weeks) maternal factors become more common (Table 11.1).

Table 11.1 Aetiological factors in 5000 abortions	
FACTOR	**PERCENTAGE**
Fetal or ovular	
Defective ovofetus	60
Defective implantation or activity of trophoblast	15
Maternal	
General disease	2
Uterine abnormalities	8
Psychosomatic	?15

Ovofetal factors

Ultrasound examination of the fetus and subsequent histological examination show that in 70% of cases the fertilized ovum has failed to develop properly or the fetus is malformed. In 40% of these cases chromosomal abnormalities are the underlying cause of the miscarriage.

Maternal factors

Systemic maternal disease (e.g. systemic lupus erythematosus), and particularly maternal infections, account for 2% of miscarriages. A further 8% are associated with uterine abnormalities, such as congenital defects, uterine myomata, particularly submucous tumours, or cervical incompetence (see p. 104). Psychosomatic causes have been suggested as leading to miscarriage, but the evidence is difficult to evaluate. Women who smoke 10 cigarettes or more per day double their risk.

MECHANISMS OF MISCARRIAGE

The immediate cause of miscarriage is the partial or complete detachment of the embryo by minute haemorrhages in the decidua. As placental function fails uterine contractions begin, and the process of miscarriage is initiated. If this occurs before the eighth week the defective embryo, covered with villi and some decidua, tends to be expelled en masse (the so-called blighted ovum), although some of the products of conception may be retained either in the cavity of the uterus or in the cervix. Uterine bleeding occurs during the expulsion process.

Between the eighth and 14th weeks the above mechanism may occur or the membranes may rupture, expelling the defective fetus but failing to expel the placenta, which may protrude through the external cervical os or remain attached to the uterine wall. This type of miscarriage may be attended by considerable haemorrhage.

Between the 14th and 22nd weeks the fetus is usually expelled followed, after an interval, by the placenta. Less commonly the placenta is retained. Usually bleeding is not severe, but pain may be considerable and resemble a miniature labour.

It is clear from this description that miscarriage is attended by uterine bleeding and pain, both of varying intensity. Although miscarriage is the cause of bleeding per vaginam in early pregnancy in over 95% of cases, less common causes, such as ectopic gestation, cervical bleeding from the everted cervical epithelium or from an endocervical polyp, hydatidiform mole, and, rarely, cervical carcinoma, must be excluded.

VARIETIES OF SPONTANEOUS MISCARRIAGE

For descriptive purposes the miscarriage is classified according to the findings when the woman is first examined, but one kind may change into another if the aborting process continues. If infection complicates the miscarriage, the term septic miscarriage is used. The various types of miscarriage are shown in Figure 11.1 and each will be considered separately later.

Threatened miscarriage

Threatened miscarriage is diagnosed when a pregnant woman develops uterine bleeding with or without painful contractions; other causes of bleeding in early pregnancy should be excluded. A vaginal examination (or vaginal speculum examination) shows that the cervix is not dilated.

A real-time pelvic ultrasound examination will clarify the diagnosis. This may show:

- A normally sized amniotic sac and a fetus whose heart is beating
- An empty amniotic sac
- A missed or incomplete miscarriage.

Only if the first finding is obtained is the diagnosis confirmed. The ultrasound finding also provides the information that the pregnancy will continue (in 98% of cases), and the patient can be reassured. If a subchorionic haematoma is detected the pregnancy should be monitored more closely, as there is a greater risk of spontaneous miscarriage, placental abruption, premature labour, intrauterine growth restriction and fetal death.

The use of ultrasound examination has meant that the treatment of threatened miscarriage has changed in recent years. It is no longer normal practice to insist that the woman remain in bed until the bleeding has ceased. However, if she feels more comfortable there, she may do

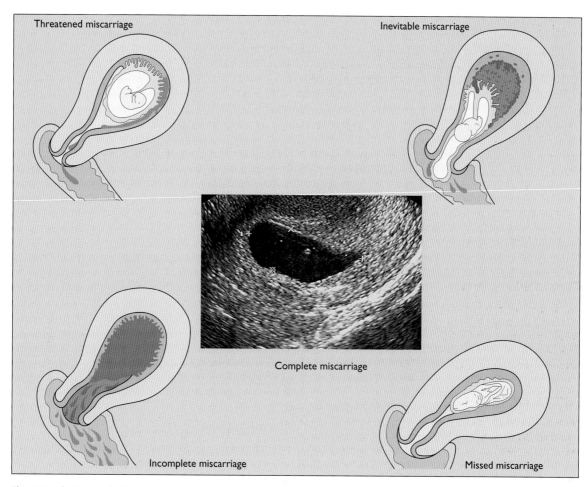

Fig. 11.1 The types of miscarriage that may be seen. In complete miscarriage the sac contains a small amount of debris.

so. Drugs, hormones (e.g. progesterone) and sedatives have no effect except as a placebo, and should be avoided.

Inevitable, incomplete and complete miscarriage

Miscarriage becomes inevitable if uterine bleeding is associated with strong uterine contractions that cause dilatation of the cervix. The woman complains of severe colicky uterine pains, and a vaginal examination shows a dilated cervical os with part of the conception sac bulging through. Inevitable miscarriage may follow signs of threatened miscarriage or, more commonly, starts without warning.

Soon after the onset of symptoms of inevitable miscarriage, the miscarriage occurs either completely, when all the products of conception are expelled, or incompletely when either the pregnancy sac or the placenta remains, distending the cervical canal. In most cases the miscarriage is incomplete. Unless the doctor has been able to inspect all the material expelled from the uterus, or has had an ultrasound examination that shows an empty uterus (or one containing less than 10 mm of tissues or blood clots), the miscarriage should be considered incomplete. This is treated by curettage; an alternative is to give misoprostol 400 µg 4-hourly for three doses or 800 µg as a single dose which will achieve a 60–80% complete evacuation of the uterus.

Treatment

A woman who is diagnosed as having an inevitable or an incomplete miscarriage and who is not in hospital should be transferred to one without delay. Before effecting the transfer, the examining doctor should give an analgesic to the patient (if required) and should make a vaginal examination. Any products of conception found protruding from the cervix should be removed by finger or sponge forceps, as leaving them may lead to vasovagal shock. If the woman is bleeding heavily an intramuscular injection of 0.5 mg ergometrine or if she is in shock intravenous ergometrine 0.25 mg, should be given.

In hospital, intervention is required unless the miscarriage is proceeding quickly and with minimal blood loss. On admission of the patient a vaginal examination is performed and any products of conception remaining in the cervix are removed by finger or sponge forceps.

If there is any doubt about the completeness of the miscarriage the patient should be taken to the operating theatre and the uterus evacuated using a sponge forceps (Fig. 11.2), followed by a careful suction curettage. Towards the end of the curettage, an injection of ergometrine 0.25 mg is given intravenously.

Follow-up

Following a complete miscarriage, or one which has been completed surgically, bleeding usually ceases within 10 days. If placental remnants have been left in the uterus the bleeding may persist beyond this time, varying in severity, and may be accompanied by uterine cramps. Examination will show a bulky uterus with a patulous os. Treatment is to perform an ultrasound, and if this shows retained products of conception, recuretting the uterus carefully. The tissue removed should be sent for histopathology, as very rarely a choriocarcinoma is present.

In a woman who is Rhesus negative, a Kleihauer test should be performed to determine the amount of fetal blood cells in the circulation, and then a prophylactic injection of 250 IU Rh D immunoglobulin should be given.

Septic miscarriage

Although less common than formerly, because of better care in hospital and fewer 'backyard' abortions, infection may complicate some spontaneous and induced abortions. In 80% of cases the infection is mild and localized to the decidua. The organisms involved are usually endogenous and are, most commonly, anaerobic streptococci, staphylococci or *Escherichia coli*. In 15% of cases the infection is severe, involving the myometrium, and may spread to involve the Fallopian tubes. If the infection spreads from the cervix it may involve the parametrium or the pelvic cellular tissues. In 5% of cases there is generalized peritonitis or vascular collapse, which is due to the release of endotoxins by *E. coli* or *Clostridium welchii* and is termed endotoxic shock.

Clinical features

In infections limited to the decidua the production of a malodorous, pink vaginal discharge is usual and the patient may develop pyrexia. In more severe, spreading infections pyrexia occurs, but its extent may not be related to the severity of the infection. Tachycardia usually develops: a pulse rate of more than 120 bpm indicates that spread has occurred beyond the uterus. Examination may show a tender lower abdomen; vaginal examination shows a boggy, tender uterus with evidence of extrauterine spread.

Investigations

A high vaginal or cervical swab is made and, if the temperature is higher than 38.4°C, a blood culture should

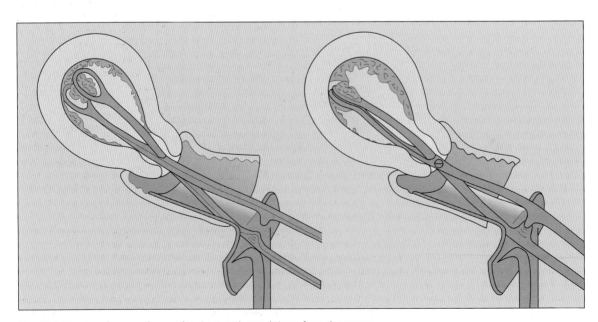

Fig. 11.2 The use of sponge forceps for clearing placental tissue from the uterus.

be taken. In severe infections serum electrolytes and coagulation studies should be undertaken.

Treatment

Antibiotics are administered at once, the precise one chosen depending on local conditions, but in general a broad-acting antibiotic and one effective against anaerobes are selected. Twelve hours after starting antibiotics, or sooner if haemorrhaging is severe and the uterus is not empty, its contents are evacuated by careful curettage. If the infection is not controlled in spite of these measures hysterectomy may be indicated.

Endotoxic shock

As already mentioned, this life-threatening condition follows 5% of septic miscarriages. Endotoxins released by *E. coli* and *Cl. welchii* are neutralized initially by phagocytes, but if this protection fails vasoconstriction of the postcapillary vessels occurs, with resulting pooling of blood, a failure of venous blood to reach the heart and a reduced cardiac output. In addition, the Gram-negative endotoxins may act directly on the blood vessels and heart, releasing substances that profoundly affect the cardiovascular system.

Clinical signs include pyrexia, rigors, hypotension, tachycardia and hypoventilation. A patient with these signs is acutely ill and should be transferred to an intensive care unit without delay.

Missed miscarriage/abortion

In a few cases of miscarriage the dead embryo or fetus and placenta are not expelled spontaneously. If the embryo dies in the early weeks it is likely to be anembryonic or blighted. In other cases a fetus forms but dies. Multiple haemorrhages may occur in the choriodecidual space, which bulge into the empty amniotic sac. This condition is called a carnaceous mole. It is thought that although the fetus has died, progesterone continues to be secreted by surviving placental tissue, which delays the expulsion of the products of conception (Fig. 11.3).

If the fetus dies at a later stage of the pregnancy, but before the 22nd gestational week, and is not expelled, it is either absorbed or mummified. The liquor amnii is absorbed and the placenta degenerates. Fetal death after the 22nd week is discussed on page 203.

Clinical aspects

With the widespread use of ultrasound a common presentation is at the time of a routine ultrasound examination when a fetal heart is not detected. Alternatively the woman may report that she has had a small amount of vaginal bleeding and this may be accompanied by the disappearance of early pregnancy symptoms (Fig. 11.3).

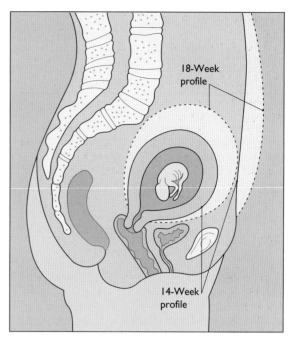

Fig. 11.3 Missed miscarriage. The duration of the pregnancy is 18 weeks but the uterus has failed to enlarge beyond the size of a 14-week gestation. Note that the abdomen is flat.

Treatment

There is no medical need to treat missed miscarriage urgently as most cases end in a spontaneous miscarriage. Information and support must be given to the parents once they become aware that the fetus has died in utero, as this can be a very traumatic experience. In most cases the woman requests an early evacuation of the uterus. Surgical evacuation when the uterine size is greater than 12–14 weeks' gestational size carries greater risk of haemorrhage and uterine and cervical damage and this must be explained. In these cases if the woman does not want to wait for spontaneous miscarriage then termination is best effected using mifepristone and misoprostol or prostaglandins, as described on page 106.

If a spontaneous miscarriage has not occurred within 28 days the pregnancy should be terminated, as coagulation defects may result.

Recurrent (habitual) miscarriage

A few women (1%) have the misfortune to miscarry successively. It has been estimated that after one miscarriage the risk of another is 20%; after two miscarriages it is 25%. If the woman has not had a previous liveborn infant after three miscarriages the chances of achieving a successful pregnancy outcome is 55–60%, but is 70% if she has

Table 11.2 Recurrent miscarriage		
POSSIBLE AETIOLOGY	**PERCENTAGE OF MISCARRIAGES OCCURRING**	
	<12 weeks	**>12 weeks**
Not known	62	35
Uterine malformations or abnormality	3	10
Cervical incompetence	3	30
Chromosome abnormality	<5	<4
?Endometrial infection	15	15
Endocrine dysfunction	3	3
Systemic disease	1	1
?Sperm factors	3	1
?Immune factors	?	1

had one or more liveborn. A woman who has three or more successive miscarriages is termed a recurrent miscarrier.

The aetiological factors in recurrent miscarriage vary depending on the population studied, but two large series, of over 100 subjects in each, offer some idea of the aetiology (Table 11.2). In Table 11.2 the causes marked with a query are speculative.

Investigation and treatment of a recurrent miscarrier

A careful medical and obstetric history may reveal systemic disease or suggest cervical incompetence. A vaginal examination may show uterine myomata or cervical incompetence, and the diagnosis can be clarified if a transvaginal ultrasound image is made. Ultrasound will also detect uterine malformations. Submucous myomata or uterine septa may be removed by abdominal surgery or under hysteroscopic vision. Cervical incompetence is discussed later.

If endometrial infection is considered a causative factor (as is the case with some specialists), endometrial tissue cultures may be made. However, it is doubtful whether toxoplasmosis, cytomegalovirus, herpes virus, rubella or listeria are causes of recurrent miscarriage.

Endocrine dysfunctions, for example polycystic ovarian disease (see p. 223), may be excluded by transvaginal ultrasound scanning and blood tests. Other endocrine disorders, such as thyroid disease and diabetes, are no longer believed to be causes of recurrent miscarriage unless they are poorly controlled.

Although it is usual to investigate both parents for chromosome abnormalities, such aberrations account for only 5% of recurrent miscarriages at the most, and no treatment is available apart from donor gametes.

Immunological causes for recurrent miscarriage have been sought. The theory is that if the two parents share several human leucocyte antigen (HLA) sites the fetus may not be able to provide a sufficient stimulus to enable the mother to produce blocking antibodies to the allogenic fetus, with the result that the fetus is aborted. However, clinical trials that entail immunizing the woman between pregnancies with paternal leucocytes, pooled donor cells or trophoblast membrane preparations to enhance her immune system, have failed to show any benefit.

A few women with an autoimmune disease, especially the antiphospholipid syndrome and systemic lupus erythematosus (SLE), have a strong blocking antibody reaction which, it is believed, may lead to recurrent miscarriage. SLE must be excluded before immunotherapy is used as SLE may be aggravated. If SLE is identified by laboratory tests, treatment with low-dose aspirin and low-dose heparin improves the live birth rate from 10% to 70%.

General measures

Women who are recurrent aborters need considerable support and care. They should be advised to stop smoking, to avoid sexual intercourse and not to travel. The results from this regimen are as good as those following the use of multivitamins, hormones (including human chorionic gonadotrophin), metallic chemicals, thyroid extract and acupuncture, all of which are advocated from time to time.

Cervical incompetence

About 20% of women who have recurrent miscarriages in the second quarter of pregnancy will be found to have cervical incompetence. The diagnosis is based on:

- A history of recurrent miscarriages occurring after the 12th week of gestation, usually starting with painless leaking of amniotic fluid.
- The easy passage of a size 9 cervical dilator through the internal os of the cervix when the woman is not pregnant, and the absence of a 'snap' on its withdrawal.
- The gradual shortening of the cervix to less than 25 mm and/or dilatation of the internal cervical os to more than 3 cm during pregnancy, as detected by ultrasound.

If cervical incompetence is diagnosed, treatment entails placing a soft unabsorbable suture (such as Mersilk 4)

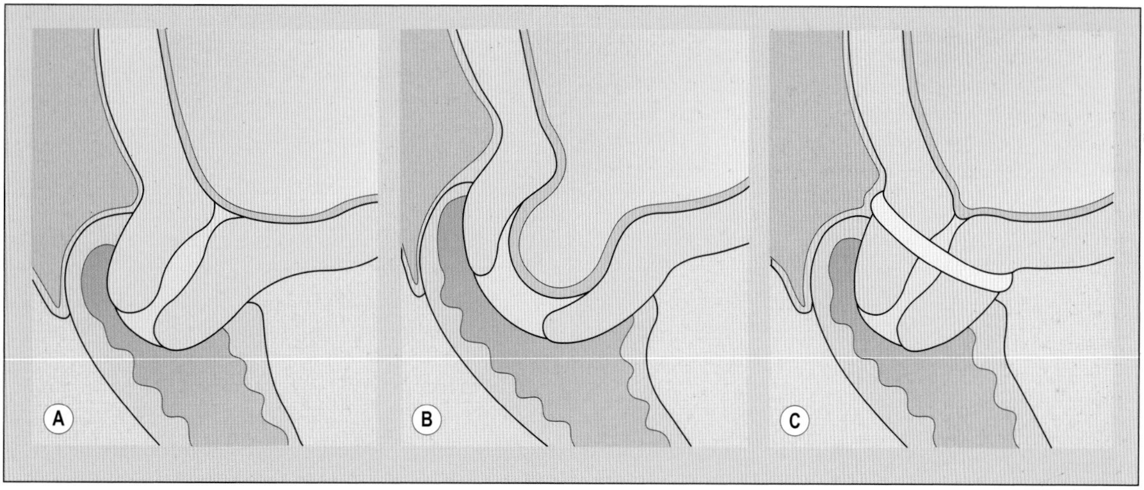

Fig. 11.4 Cervical incompetence. (A) Normal cervix at 16 weeks. (B) Incompetent cervix at 16 weeks. (C) Cerclage with an unabsorbable suture.

around the cervix at the level of the internal cervical os (Fig. 11.4). The patient may return home the same night or stay in hospital for a day, depending on the circumstances. There is no place postoperatively for the use of progesterone, uterine relaxants or narcotics. If there is doubt about the diagnosis, then surveillance with ultrasound is undertaken, cerclage being performed if there are signs of cervical shortening and/or beaking of the membranes through the internal os.

Following cervical cerclage 10% of women abort, 10% give birth prematurely, and the remainder give birth after the 36th week of pregnancy. Cervical cerclage should not be performed if the membranes have ruptured. If miscarriage or premature rupture of the membranes occurs or premature delivery becomes inevitable following cerclage, the suture must be cut. In all other cases the suture is left until about 7 days prior to term, at which time it is cut, and the woman may then be expected to give birth vaginally.

PSYCHOLOGICAL EFFECTS OF SPONTANEOUS MISCARRIAGE

For most women a spontaneous miscarriage is a distressing occurrence: over 90% express a grief reaction, which persists for a month in 20% of cases. During the period when the miscarriage threatens or is occurring many women are distressed by not knowing what the outcome will be; others are distressed by being told to rest in bed without any further explanation.

Too little information is given by many doctors (both in general and hospital practice) after a miscarriage has occurred, about the reason for the miscarriage and the outcome of a future pregnancy. Women need counselling

on these matters and need to have an opportunity to express their feelings. There are three main questions to which most women require answers:

- Why did the miscarriage occur?
- Is there anything that I did or did not do that caused the miscarriage?
- Is my next pregnancy likely to end in a miscarriage?

The doctor should provide answers sensitively and sympathetically even if the questions are not asked. This will reduce the period of grief and distress that usually follows a spontaneous miscarriage.

INDUCED ABORTION

In many countries induced (therapeutic) abortion is now legal. The exact conditions vary, but the purposes of legalizing abortion are:

- To enable women, irrespective of social or economic status, after counselling to obtain an abortion performed by a trained health professional in hygienic surroundings.
- To reduce the frequency of illegal abortions performed in unhygienic surroundings, which are often associated with high morbidity and mortality.

The main reasons for abortion are shown in Box 11.1. In most developed countries where abortion is legal, over 95% are performed for social or psychiatric reasons. It should be stressed that women rarely seek an abortion without considerable thought, and are receptive to and welcome counselling during this difficult time. It is also evident that in many cases the pregnancy could have been prevented if effective contraceptive precautions had been taken.

Box 11.1 Indications for therapeutic abortion

Social

Psychiatric
Severe neuroses, psychoses

Medical
Severe cardiac disease; heart failure
Severe chronic renal disease; renal failure
Malignant disease, especially of breast or uterine cervix

Fetal
Viral infections
Haemolytic disease
Genetic defects
Congenital defects incompatible with normal life
(e.g. anencephaly, spina bifida)

Technique of induced abortion

Abortion is safest when it is performed between the sixth and 12th gestational weeks. Only between 5 and 10% of terminations are made after the 12th week of pregnancy. Termination of the pregnancy may be surgical or medical.

The surgical approach is to evacuate the uterus using a suction curette, under local or general anaesthesia. Following curettage uterine bleeding persists for about 6 days, often being light in the first 2 days after the termination. Most gynaecologists give the woman a course of doxycycline to prevent infection.

Medical methods of termination can be used if the pregnancy is less than 9 weeks' gestation. These include the administration of a single dose of the progesterone antagonist mifepristone (200–600 mg). The mifepristone tablet is followed 36–48 hours later by a prostaglandin E_1 vaginal pessary (gemeprost) 1 mg every 6 hours for four doses. If the abortion has not started within 24 hours, gemeprost 1 mg is given 3-hourly for up to four more doses. (An alternative is oral misoprostol 200 μg repeated after 2 hours.) Bleeding usually starts during the interval between the mifepristone and the gemeprost vaginal pessary or oral misoprostol, and uterine contractions start within 4 hours of the administration of either drug. The pain may be severe and most women require narcotics. Nausea or vomiting affects one-third of patients. Bleeding persists for about 9 days, with a mean loss of 75 mL (20–400 mL). Over 98% of women abort using this regimen, but 10% require curettage for persistent heavy bleeding.

In countries where mifepristone is not available two commonly used drugs may be prescribed. Methotrexate 50 mg/m^2 body surface is given intramuscularly. This prevents folate from entering the fetal tissues, with resultant death. Misoprostol 800 μg is given intravaginally 5–7 days later, and following this 75% of women abort within 24 hours. If the abortion does not occur, the misoprostol is repeated.

After the 12th gestational week the uterus may be evacuated using the following:

- Misoprostol 100–200 μg given intravaginally every 12 hours for up to four doses
- Prostaglandin F_{2a} (Dinoprost) vaginal pessaries
- The mifepristone/gemeprost regimen mentioned earlier.

These regimens induce an abortion in 80–95% of patients and may replace dilatation of the cervix and uterine evacuation using sponge forceps and a curette, which can be a bloody and prolonged procedure.

Over 80% of women require narcotics for pain, and nausea or vomiting occurs in 30%. Following the abortion, one-third of women require evacuation of the uterus for retained products of conception.

Sequelae of induced abortion

An induced abortion performed before the 12th gestational week in a well-equipped and staffed clinic is followed by few complications. Less than 1% of women develop infection, and the mortality rate is less than 1 per 100 000 abortions. After the 12th gestational week the rate of complications rises to 3–5% and the mortality increases to 9–12 per 100 000. There is no reduction of the woman's fertility or any increase in the risk of spontaneous miscarriage, preterm birth or fetal loss in a subsequent pregnancy.

PSYCHOLOGICAL EFFECTS OF INDUCED ABORTION

Most studies have concluded that legal abortion of an unwanted pregnancy does not pose a psychological hazard for most women. Most women feel grief and guilt after a termination, but less than 10% show evidence of anxiety or depression persisting for more than a month. Most of the women adversely affected were ambivalent about having the abortion, or were pressured by parents or partner into terminating the pregnancy. This finding emphasizes that a woman seeking an abortion should be counselled before the procedure takes place, and should continue to receive support (if she chooses) during and after the operation.

Extra-uterine pregnancy/ectopic gestation

Most extra-uterine pregnancies occur in the Fallopian tubes (ectopic gestation) but, rarely, the fertilized ovum may implant onto the ovarian surface or the uterine cervix. Extremely rarely, the fertilized ovum implants onto the omentum (abdominal pregnancy).

One in 90 pregnancies is ectopic and in the United Kingdom this results in the death of 3 to 4 women each year. A combined intra-uterine and extra-uterine pregnancy is very rare and occurs 1:40 000 spontaneous pregnancies and 1 : 1000 IVF pregnancies.

AETIOLOGY

The aetiology of most cases of ectopic gestation is not known. Implantation of the fertilized ovum can only take place when the zona pellucida has partially or completely disappeared. Premature implantation could occur if the passage of the fertilized ovum along the Fallopian tube is delayed because of tubal damage following infection. Premature implantation may occur in:

- The fimbriated end of the Fallopian tube (in 17% of cases)
- The ampulla (in 55% of cases)
- The isthmus (in 25% of cases)
- The interstitial portion of the tube (in 2% of cases) (Fig. 12.1).

OUTCOME FOR THE PREGNANCY

In most cases the pregnancy terminates, in one of several ways (see below), between the sixth and 10th weeks.

Tubal abortion

This occurs in 65% of cases and is the usual outcome in fimbrial and ampullary implantation (Fig. 12.2). Repeated small haemorrhages from the invaded area of the tubal wall detach the ovum, which dies and:

- Is absorbed completely
- Is aborted completely through the tubal ostium into the peritoneal cavity
- Is aborted incompletely, with the result that the clot-covered conceptus distends the ostium
- Forms a tubal blood mole.

Tubal rupture

This occurs in 35% of cases and is more common when the implantation is in the isthmus. Whereas the rupture of the ampulla usually occurs between the sixth and

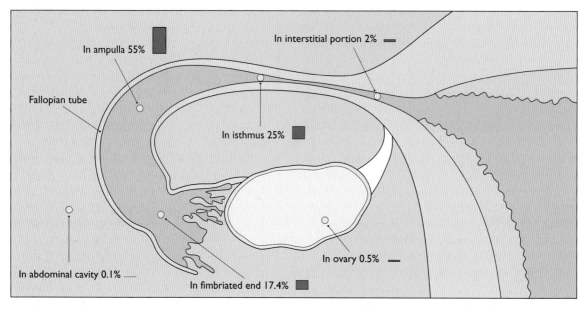

Fig. 12.1 Sites of ectopic gestation implantation, with the relative frequency of occurrence.

10th weeks, rupture of the isthmus occurs earlier, frequently at the time of the first missed period. The trophoblast burrows deeply and eventually erodes the serosal coat of the tube, the final break being sudden or gradual. Usually the ovum is extruded through the rent and bleeding continues. If the rupture is on the mesenteric side of the tube, a broad ligament haematoma will form (Fig. 12.3).

Secondary abdominal pregnancy

Very rarely the extruded ovum continues to grow, as sufficient trophoblast maintains its connection with the tubal epithelium, and later the trophoblast covering the ovisac attaches to abdominal organs. A few of these pregnancies advance to term and, in a very few, the fetus dies early and is converted into a lithopaedion.

CLINICAL ASPECTS

The possibility of an ectopic gestation should always be considered in a woman of childbearing age, especially if there is a past history of acute salpingitis. The history (Box 12.1) is of greater importance than the physical signs, as these can be equivocal. Usually there is a short period of amenorrhoea, although in 20% of cases this may not be present. The pain is lower abdominal in site, but not distinguishable from that of abortion. However, in ruptured ectopic gestation fainting usually occurs, although this may only be momentary. Vaginal bleeding follows

the pain, and may be mistaken for bleeding due to a delayed menstrual period or an abortion. The bleeding is a slightly brownish colour and continuous, and clots are rarely present (Table 12.1).

Two clinical patterns occur, and are due to the extent of the damage to the tubal wall by the invading trophoblast. The first is subacute, the second acute.

Subacute

After a short period of amenorrhoea the patient experiences some lower abdominal discomfort, which may be so mild that she considers it normal for pregnancy. Occasionally there is an attack of sharp pain and faintness, owing to an episode of intraperitoneal bleeding, and if these symptoms are marked, and particularly if the episode is followed by slight vaginal bleeding, examination may reveal tenderness in the lower abdomen; vaginal examination may show a tender fornix or a vague mass, but the signs may be insufficient to make a diagnosis. If the patient is observed, further episodes of pain are likely and the blood loss per vaginam persists until acute collapse supervenes (indicating tubal rupture or incomplete tubal abortion) or the symptoms cease (indicating complete abortion with or without a pelvic haematocele).

Acute – dramatic

Sudden collapse of the patient with little or no warning is more common when the implantation is isthmal, but is not the most frequent type of the acute clinical pattern. It is more usual for the acute rupture to supervene upon the subacute,

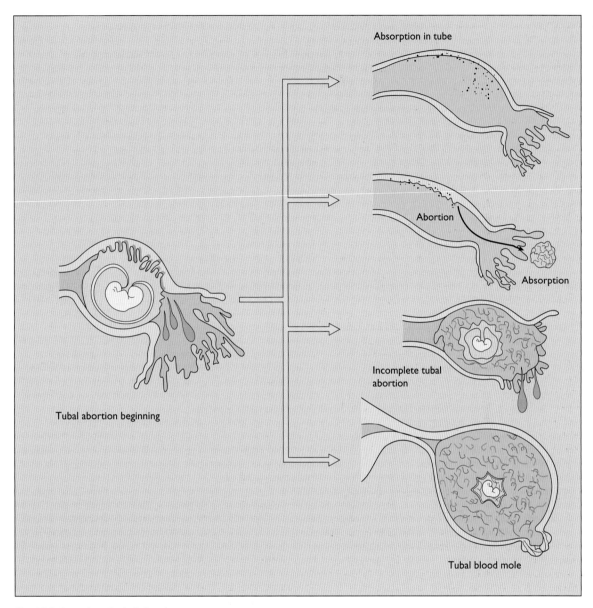

Absorption in tube

Abortion

Absorption

Incomplete tubal abortion

Tubal blood mole

Tubal abortion beginning

Fig. 12.2 Sequelae of tubal abortion.

but the mild symptoms of the latter may have been thought to be normal occurrences in pregnancy and ignored.

As the tube ruptures the patient is seized with a sudden acute lower abdominal pain, sufficiently severe to cause fainting. The associated internal haemorrhage leads to collapse, pallor, a weak, rapid pulse and a falling blood pressure. Usually the condition improves after a short time as the haemorrhage diminishes or ceases, but abdominal discomfort persists, and pain is felt in the epigastrium or is referred to the shoulder. A further episode of haemorrhage and collapse is likely, and continued bleeding can be suspected from increasing pallor and a falling haemoglobin level.

On examination the patient is shocked and the lower abdomen is tender, with some fullness and muscle guarding. Vaginal examination, which should only be carried out in hospital, shows extreme tenderness on movement of the cervix from side to side.

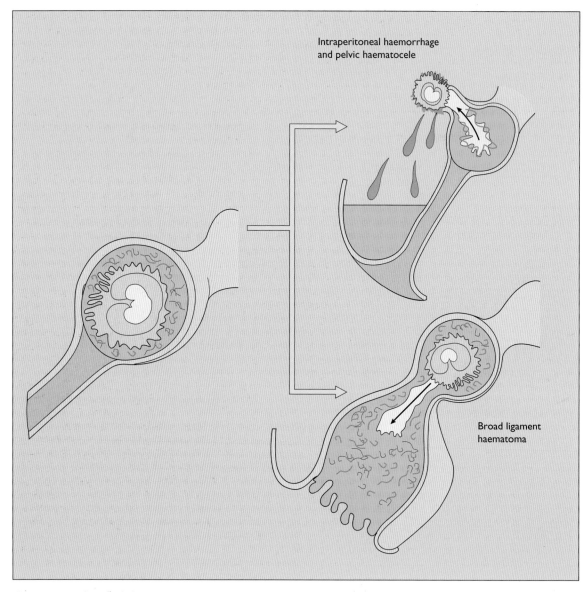

Intraperitoneal haemorrhage
and pelvic haematocele

Broad ligament
haematoma

Fig. 12.3 Sequelae of tubal rupture.

Box 12.1 **Risk factors for ectopic pregnancy**
• Previous ectopic pregnancy
• History of pelvic inflammatory disease
• Previous pelvic surgery including appendicectomy
• IVF treatment
• IUCD in situ
• Progesterone-only contraceptive pill

DIAGNOSIS

Although in acute cases the presence of internal bleeding is obvious and the diagnosis not in doubt, in subacute cases the diagnosis can be extraordinarily difficult. Laboratory tests may help, but in most instances they are not particularly informative. A radioimmunoassay for serum levels of β-human chorionic gonadotrophin (β-hCG) should be made. A negative result (<5 IU/mL) indicates

Table 12.1 Symptoms and signs in ectopic gestation

SYMPTOM/SIGN	%
Abdominal pain	90
Amenorrhoea	80
Adnexal tenderness	80
Abdominal tenderness	80
Vaginal bleeding	70
Adnexal mass	50

that the woman is not pregnant, and ectopic gestation can be excluded. If the β-hCG test is positive a pelvic ultrasound examination should be performed, preferably using a transvaginal probe. A fetal heartbeat should be detectable once the β-hCG level reaches 1500 IU. If this shows an empty uterus (Fig. 12.4), and particularly if it shows a sac and fetus in the Fallopian tube, the diagnosis is certain. and treatment should be commenced. If the ultrasound is equivocal serial measurements of β-hCG should be taken. The levels should double every 48 hours, a rise

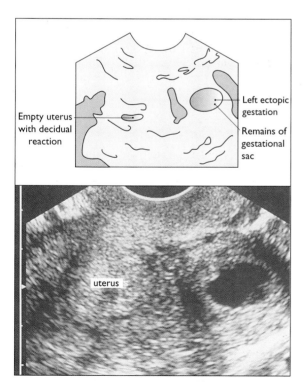

Fig. 12.4 Ectopic pregnancy.

less than 66% being suggestive of an ectopic gestation. On the other hand, if ultrasound shows an intra-uterine pregnancy, a concurrent ectopic pregnancy is extremely unlikely. Routine serum progesterone levels can help to exclude an ectopic pregnancy (>79 nmol/L) and identify a nonviable pregnancy (>15.9 nmol/L).

If ultrasound is not available, or is equivocal, the presumptive diagnosis should be confirmed by laparoscopy.

The diagnosis of suspected ectopic gestation is summarized in Figure 12.5.

TREATMENT

If an ectopic gestation is suspected the patient should be transferred to hospital without making a vaginal examination. If she is in shock, an intravenous line should be set up and transfer quickly arranged. Morphine may be given if the woman is in pain.

As mentioned, if there is any doubt about the diagnosis a pelvic ultrasound examination should be carried out to establish whether the pregnancy is intra- or extra-uterine.

Once the ectopic gestation has been diagnosed, the treatment is usually surgical or in selected cases medical. Several approaches are possible. The gynaecologist may:

- Perform a laparotomy and either excise the Fallopian tube containing the ectopic gestation, or incise the tube over the ectopic gestation and 'milk' it out.
- Insert a laparoscope to inspect the Fallopian tube and, if possible, under laparoscopic vision incise along the superior border and suck the ectopic gestation out of the tube.
- If the tube has not ruptured, the gestation sac is small on ultrasound and the hCG level is not high, the gynaecologist may inject methotrexate into the ectopic gestation so that the viable trophoblast and embryo are absorbed.
- If the woman is haemodynamically stable, the β-hCG level is <3500 IU/mL and the sac is unruptured and <3.5 cm in size, then methotrexate can be administered either as a single dose (50 mg/m² body surface area) or in four doses given on alternate days with leucovorin 7.5 mg cover on the other alternate days. Close surveillance is mandatory and the β-hCG levels are measured every 3 days for the first week, then weekly until <5 IU/mL. In addition liver function is monitored and if there is a rise in the β-hCG, abdominal pain or signs of peritoneal irritation a surgical approach is instituted. This occurs in about 7% of cases.

Following conservative surgery, or if methotrexate is used, the woman should have serum hCG measurements made weekly until negative. If the woman complains of continuing symptoms, a second-look laparoscopy may be necessary.

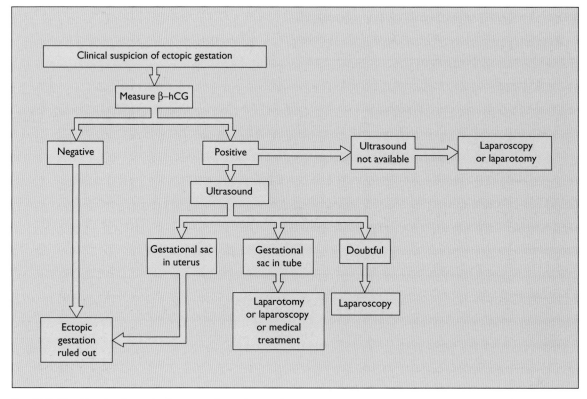

Fig. 12.5 Algorithm for diagnosis of suspected ectopic gestation.

PROGNOSIS

Less than 60% of women who have had an ectopic gestation become pregnant again. Three-quarters of these voluntarily avoid pregnancy, and one-quarter are involuntarily infertile. In a subsequent pregnancy the risk of a second ectopic gestation is 10–20%, compared to a risk of 1% in other women. Because of this, a woman who has had an ectopic gestation should be monitored carefully in the early weeks of her next pregnancy, a transvaginal ultrasound examination being made at 6–8 weeks' gestation to establish that the pregnancy is intra-uterine.

Antepartum haemorrhage

Antepartum haemorrhage is defined as significant bleeding from the birth canal occurring after the 20th week of pregnancy. The causes and proportions of cases of antepartum haemorrhage are shown in Table 13.1. In fewer than 0.05% of cases the bleeding is due to a cervical lesion, such as a cervical polyp, or rarely, a cervical carcinoma.

PLACENTA PRAEVIA

In this condition the placenta is implanted, either partially or wholly, in the lower uterine segment and lies below (praevia) the fetal presenting part. The extent of implantation may be minor, in which case vaginal birth is possible, or major, when it is not (Fig. 13.1).

Placenta praevia occurs in 0.5–2.0 % of all pregnancies, and accounts for 20% of all cases of antepartum haemorrhage. The incidence has increased between two- and threefold over the past 20 years. It is three times as common in multiparous women as in primiparae. The incidence increases with each previous caesarean section. The incidence in women who have not had a previous caesarean is 0.3%, after one is 0.8%, after two is 2.0%, and after three or more is 4.2%. The risk is also increased when a submucous fibroid is present.

The bleeding occurs when the lower uterine segment is increasing in length, and shearing forces between the trophoblast and the maternal blood sinuses occur. The first episode of bleeding occurs after the 36th gestational week in 60% of cases, between the 32nd and 36th weeks in 30%, and before the 32nd week in 10%.

Symptoms, signs and diagnosis

The bleeding is painless, causeless and recurrent. The presenting part is usually high and often not central to the pelvic brim. The diagnosis is made should an ultrasound image show that the placenta is praevia (Figs 13.2, 13.3).

If a routine ultrasound examination is made at 18 weeks the report may show that there is a low-lying placenta, but in over 85% the placenta will be normally situated by the time of delivery, as the lower uterine segment does not develop fully until late in the third trimester. A further ultrasound examination should be made at about the 34th week, or earlier if vaginal bleeding occurs.

Management

The first episode of significant bleeding usually occurs in the patient's home and is usually not heavy. The patient should be admitted to hospital and no vaginal examination made, as this may start torrential bleeding. In hospital

Table 13.1 The incidence of the causes of antepartum haemorrhage

	INCIDENCE (%)
Placenta praevia	0.5
Placental abruption	
Mild or indeterminate	3.0
Moderate grade	0.8
Severe grade	0.2
Cervical bleeding	0.05

the patient's vital signs are checked, the amount of blood loss assessed and blood cross-matched. Heavy blood loss may require transfusion. The abdomen is palpated gently to determine the gestational age of the fetus, and its presentation and position. An ultrasound examination is made soon after admission, to confirm the diagnosis. Further management depends on the severity of the bleeding and the gestational age of the fetus.

In cases of severe bleeding, urgent treatment to deliver the baby (and the placenta) is required, irrespective of the gestational age of the fetus. If the bleeding is less severe, expectant treatment is appropriate if the fetal gestational age is less than 36 weeks. As the bleeding tends to recur, serum should be held in the blood bank in case an urgent transfusion is required and the safest option for the woman is to remain in hospital. In selected cases where there is no further bleeding for 4–7 days and the woman can readily return to hospital if she has further bleeding then she may be allowed to rest at home. An episode of severe bleeding may lead to urgent delivery, but in most cases the pregnancy can continue until term (37 or more weeks). All but the most minor degrees of placenta praevia will require delivery by caesarean section. Blood should be cross-matched and readily available during delivery and the immediate puerperium.

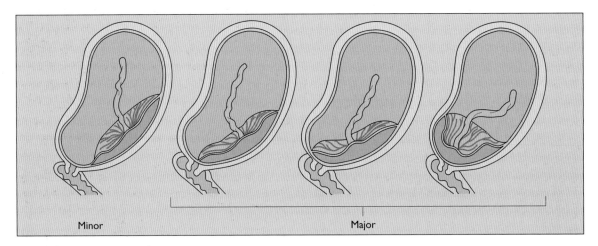

Minor   Major

Fig. 13.1 Degrees of placenta praevia.

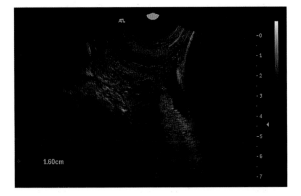

Fig. 13.2 Grade 2 placenta praevia reaching 1.6 cm from internal os.

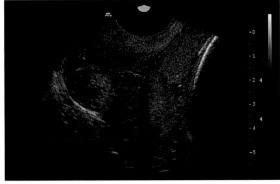

Fig. 13.3 Vaginal scan showing grade 4 placenta praevia covering internal os.

Complications

Episodes of heavy bleeding may occur at any time, during which the fetus may die from hypoxia. Following the birth, postpartum haemorrhage may occur because the trophoblast has invaded the poorly supported veins of the lower uterine segment. In most cases the haemorrhage ceases after the administration of oxytocics, but occasionally the bleeding cannot be staunched. Compression of the placental bed by an intrauterine balloon catheter may control the bleeding, otherwise caesarean hysterectomy is required.

The perinatal mortality is less than 50 per 1000 and primarily due to prematurity. The maternal mortality is low, provided the case is managed by an experienced obstetrician and no vaginal examination is performed before admission to hospital.

PLACENTA ACCRETA

Morbid adherence of the placenta occurs in 1/1500 to 1/2500 pregnancies and the incidence is reported to be increasing. One likely reason is the rising caesarean section rate. If the placenta implants over a uterine scar from a previous caesarean section, the trophoblast can penetrate through the scarred decidua and myometrium, becoming morbidly adherent. Unless the area of adherence is small, conservative management is not usually possible and the woman will require immediate caesarean hysterectomy to preserve her life. The haemorrhage is frequently accompanied by disseminated intravascular coagulopathy, and this should be anticipated in any woman who has had a previous caesarean section and has an anterior low-lying placenta. The risk of placenta praevia or accreta rises from 4% if there has not been a previous caesarean section to 14% after one, 35% after two, and 50% after three.

PLACENTAL ABRUPTION (ACCIDENTAL HAEMORRHAGE)

The term 'accidental haemorrhage' derives from an observation made in 1775 that in placenta praevia haemorrhage is inevitable, whereas in the other group of antepartum haemorrhage it is due to some 'accidental' circumstance. About 4% of pregnant women have a placental abruption, which can be subdivided into three groups. In the first the bleeding is slight, and when the placenta is examined after the birth no retroplacental bleeding can be observed. This group is classified as antepartum haemorrhage of unknown aetiology. It accounts for 75% of cases of accidental haemorrhage.

In the second and third groups there is evidence of retroplacental bleeding. The amount of blood lost to the circulation may be moderate or severe. These two groups are classified as abruptio placentae. Abruptio placentae accounts for 25% of cases of accidental haemorrhage. In four-fifths of cases of abruptio placentae the amount of blood lost to the circulation is moderate (<1500 mL), and in one-fifth the blood loss is severe (>1500 mL).

Aetiology and pathology of abruptio placentae

The aetiology is obscure, the only relevant associations being multiparity, cigarette smoking, cocaine use, multiple pregnancy, and polyhydramnios. Hypertensive diseases in pregnancy are associated with abruptio placentae in about 15% of cases, but it is not clear whether the hypertension is an aetiological factor. Occasionally it can result from direct trauma to the maternal abdomen or by compression of the uterus onto the sacral promontory during deceleration in a motor vehicle accident.

The cause of the retroplacental bleeding is damage to the walls of the maternal venous sinuses supplying the placental bed. The bleeding spreads and causes detachment of the placenta to varying degrees. The blood then trickles down between the uterine decidua and the amniotic sac to appear in the vagina and vulva (revealed haemorrhage), or is retained behind the placenta (concealed haemorrhage). In a few cases of severe bleeding the blood is forced by intrauterine pressure between the myometrial fibres towards the serosal layer of the uterus. If the amount of blood is large, the uterus has the appearance of a bruised, oedematous organ, described as apoplexie utéroplacentaire, or couvelaire uterus. This is a rare occurrence in today's obstetric practice.

In severe cases of abruptio placentae shock may result from the distraction and separation of the myometrial fibres. Another complication is the release into the circulation of thromboplastins from the damaged vessels, which cause widespread intravascular coagulation. The microthrombi are dissolved by fibrinogens, mainly plasmin, with the release of fibrin degradation products and the possible development of consumptive coagulopathy. In severe cases some microthrombi escape lysis and are deposited in the endothelium of the vessels supplying the glomeruli of the kidneys. This may lead to tubular necrosis and oliguria or anuria.

Signs, symptoms and treatment of antepartum haemorrhage

The symptomatology is related to the degree of bleeding and the extent of placental detachment (Table 13.2).

Slight haemorrhage

The amount of blood lost is less than 500 mL and there is no disturbance of the maternal or fetal condition. An ultrasound examination shows that the placenta is not lying in

Table 13.2 Comparison of the clinical picture in the various grades of accidental haemorrhage

	SEVERITY OF BLEEDING		
	Mild	Moderate	Severe
Pulse	No change	Raised	Raised
Blood pressure	No change	Lowered	Lowered
Shock	None	Often	Always
Oliguria	Rare	Occasionally	Common
Hypofibrinogenaemia	Rare	Occasionally	Common
Uterus	Normal	Tender	Tender and tense
Fetus	Alive	Usually dead	Dead
Blood loss (litres)	<1	1–3	3–6

the lower uterine segment and no retroplacental clots can be seen. If the patient has been admitted to hospital she may go home once the bleeding ceases or, if the pregnancy has advanced to 37 weeks, she may choose to have labour induced by amniotomy, provided that the condition of the cervix warrants this.

Abruptio placentae: moderate placental detachment and haemorrhage

Usually at least one-quarter of the placenta has become detached and more than 1000 mL of blood have been lost to the circulation. The woman complains of abdominal pain and the uterus is tender because blood has infiltrated between its muscle fibres. The patient may be shocked, with a high pulse rate, but paradoxically in 5% of cases the pulse rate is within the normal range until delivery, at which time it rises precipitously. The fetus is hypoxic and may show abnormal heart rate patterns on a cardiotocogram.

Abruptio placentae: severe placental detachment and haemorrhage

In cases of severe placental detachment at least 1500 mL of blood have been lost to the circulation. The woman is usually in shock; her uterus is firm to hard and very tender. The fetus is almost always dead. As pre-eclampsia is associated with only about one-third of cases, the blood pressure may be in the normal range in spite of the shock. Most coagulopathies occur in this group.

Management of abruptio placentae

Management consists of restoring the blood lost, prevention of coagulopathy and monitoring urinary output:

- At least 1500 mL of blood should be transfused in cases of moderate detachment, and 2500 mL in cases classified as severe detachment. The first 500 mL are transfused rapidly. Rapid blood transfusion prevents renal 'shutdown' and anuria. The central venous pressure is monitored and the remainder of the transfusion adjusted accordingly. The blood loss and the height of the fundus are monitored.
- Venous blood is examined 2-hourly for evidence of coagulopathy and, if present, this is treated. Adequate rapid transfusion and amniotomy or caesarean section usually prevent it from occurring.
- Urine output is measured 2-hourly. Oliguria may occur, but diuresis follows the birth provided that sufficient blood has been transfused.
- If the fetus is alive the decision has to be made whether to perform a caesarean section or the artificial rupture of the amniotic membranes (ARM). If the latter is chosen the circulating blood volume must first be restored. The fetal heart is monitored, and if the fetal CTG shows non-reassuring patterns a caesarean section is performed; however, it is imperative that first the mother is adequately resuscitated. If there are ominous CTG abnormalities the long-term prognosis for the baby is poor.

Maternal and fetal loss

Maternal mortality depends on the speed and adequacy of treatment. Today, few women should die from abruptio placentae. Fetal mortality depends on the degree of placental separation.

Chapter | **14** |

Hypertensive diseases in pregnancy

Between 5 and 8% of pregnancies are complicated by hypertensive diseases. These are gestational hypertension, pre-eclampsia, chronic hypertension, essential and secondary and superimposed pre-eclampsia.

CLASSIFICATION

Gestational hypertension

Gestational hypertension is classified as hypertension that arises after 20 weeks' gestation without any of the other features of pre-eclampsia and resolves within 3 months of delivery.

Pre-eclampsia

Pre-eclampsia is a multisystem disorder; hypertension is usually the first manifestation, followed by proteinuria. The clinical diagnosis of pre-eclampsia requires the onset after 20 weeks' gestation of hypertension and one or more of:

- Proteinuria – >300 mg/24 h or urine protein/creatinine ratio >30 mg/mmol
- Renal insufficiency – serum/plasma creatinine >0.09 mmol/L or oliguria
- Liver disease – raised serum transaminases and/or severe epigastric/right upper quadrant pain
- Neurological problems – convulsions (eclampsia); hyperreflexia with clonus; severe headaches with hyperreflexia; persistent visual disturbances (scotomata)
- Haematological disturbances – thrombocytopenia; disseminated intravascular coagulation; haemolysis
- Fetal growth restriction.

The hypertension of pre-eclampsia returns to normal within 3 months of delivery.

Chronic hypertension

- **Essential hypertension**: blood pressure ≥140 mmHg systolic and/or ≥90 mmHg diastolic (K5) prior to conception or in the first half of pregnancy without an apparent underlying cause.
- **Secondary hypertension**: hypertension associated with renal, renovascular and endocrine disorders and aortic coarctation.

Pre-eclampsia superimposed on chronic hypertension

This is diagnosed when one or more of the systemic features of pre-eclampsia develops after 20 weeks, i.e. in addition to a rise in blood pressure and/or a sudden increase in protein excretion.

GESTATIONAL HYPERTENSION

Pregnancies complicated by gestational hypertension have a good prognosis. The blood pressure should be carefully monitored and this can normally be done in a Day Assessment Unit or with ambulatory home blood pressure monitoring. Careful surveillance should be maintained to exclude the development of pre-eclampsia.

If the blood pressure exceeds 140/90 then antihypertensive therapy, as detailed in Table 14.1, is commenced, with the objective of maintaining the systolic pressure between 110 and 140 mmHg and the diastolic between 80 and 90 mmHg.

Table 14.1 Summary of the management of pregnancy-induced hypertension

CLASSIFICATION	OBSERVATIONS	TREATMENT
Gestational hypertension	Report rise in blood pressure or excessive weight gain to obstetrician	Assess in day assessment unit or ambulatory blood pressure monitoring at home
Moderate pre-eclampsia	In hospital: Four-hourly recording of the blood pressure Twice-daily urine testing for protein Regular observation of the patient's condition, including fluid intake and output Bed rest, but toilet privileges allowed	Admit to hospital Sedation (if indicated) Methyldopa (starting) 250 mg two to three time daily increasing to max. 3 g daily Labetalol (starting) 100 mg twice daily or atenolol (starting) 100 mg in evening or oxprenolol (starting) 20 mg three times daily or methyldopa (starting) 250 mg three times daily Nifedipine 10–20 mg twice daily to max. 40 mg b.d.
Severe pre-eclampsia	Two-hourly blood pressure recording for 6 hours, then 4-hourly Urine testing for protein twice daily Fluid intake and output recorded Careful observation of the patient for the signs of imminent eclampsia Complete bed rest for 24 hours, thereafter possible toilet privileges	Admit to hospital Depending on the severity of the illness give: a. Magnesium sulphate (see p. 121). b. Hydralazine – start 5–10 mg IV slowly, repeat 20–30 min. Continue infusion 50–300 μg/min, rate to keep BP around 140/90
Imminent eclampsia	The patient requires careful systematic observation as eclampsia is a possible outcome The blood pressure requires frequent estimation, at intervals determined by the obstetrician Fluid intake and urinary output must be measured meticulously, and the urine tested quantitatively for protein	Magnesium sulphate (see p. 121). Hydralazine intravenously Caesarean section

PRE-ECLAMPSIA

Pathogenesis

The aetiology of pre-eclampsia is not known, but there is evidence that the disorder has a genetic basis as the daughters and sisters of women who had pre-eclampsia are at increased risk. Late in the first trimester the secondary invasion of maternal spiral arteries by trophoblasts is impaired, so that they remain high-resistance vessels, which consequently leads to impairment of placental function. As pregnancy advances, placental hypoxic changes induce proliferation of cytotrophoblasts and thickening of the trophoblastic basement membrane, which may affect the metabolic function of the placenta. Normally the endothelial cells secrete vasodilator substances (including nitric oxide). Damaged cells secrete less vasodilators. In consequence, endothelial cells of the placenta secrete less vasodilator prostacyclin and the platelets more thromboxane, leading to generalized vasoconstriction and decreased aldosterone secretion. The results of these changes are maternal hypertension, a 50% reduction in placental perfusion, and a reduced maternal plasma volume. If the vasospasm persists trophoblastic epithelial cell injury may occur, and trophoblast fragments are then carried to the lungs, where they are destroyed, releasing thromboplastins. In turn, thromboplastins cause intravascular coagulation and deposition of fibrin in the glomeruli of the kidneys (glomerular endotheliosis), which reduces the glomerular filtration rate and indirectly increases vasoconstriction. In advanced, severe cases fibrin deposits occur in vessels of the central nervous system, leading to convulsions.

Prevention

Prophylactic aspirin therapy given to women at high risk of developing pre-eclampsia (essential hypertension, type 1 diabetes, previous severe pre-eclampsia) results in a modest reduction (OR 0.87; 95% CI 0.79–0.96). Calcium supplementation in at-risk women is associated with a 50% reduction in gestational hypertension and pre-eclampsia. Antioxidant therapy (vitamins C and E) has not been shown to be effective for prevention of pre-eclampsia.

Management

The management of pre-eclampsia is shown in Table 14.1. The basic principles of maternal treatment are to control the blood pressure and to prevent convulsions.

For the fetus the aim of treatment is to permit continued growth until it is sufficiently mature to survive outside the uterus, or until the risk of intra-uterine death is estimated to be greater than that of extra-uterine death. The duration of treatment depends on:

- The severity of pre-eclampsia
- The duration of the pregnancy
- The patient's response to treatment.

There is no cure for pre-eclampsia except to terminate the pregnancy and deliver the fetus and placenta. The treatment is merely to buy time so that the fetus becomes more mature in the uterus.

Pre-eclampsia diagnosed before week 32 of pregnancy

Before the 32nd week of pregnancy the objective is to keep the fetus in utero until the 35th week or longer. Fetal wellbeing is monitored by daily fetal movement counts, or 3 cardiotocograph examinations per week (see p. 153). Two sinister signs are slow fetal growth detected by serial ultrasound examinations, and abnormal Doppler umbilical blood flow measurements.

Platelet counts are made at intervals in cases of severe pre-eclampsia. In most cases a reduced platelet count returns to normal after the birth, but a few patients who have severe pre-eclampsia complain of upper abdominal pain, nausea or vomiting. If the platelet count is less than 100 000 the woman may have the HELLP syndrome (haemolysis, elevated liver enzymes, low platelets). Treatment consists of correcting the thrombocytopenia and delivering the fetus; systemic high-dose corticosteroids can shorten the recovery phase.

If the pre-eclampsia worsens the pregnancy must be terminated, usually by caesarean section.

Pre-eclampsia diagnosed between the 32nd and 35th weeks of pregnancy

Pre-eclampsia diagnosed between the 32nd and 35th weeks is managed in the same way as before the 32nd week, but should delivery of the fetus be indicated the choice is caesarean section or induction of labour.

Pre-eclampsia diagnosed after the 35th week of pregnancy

Pre-eclampsia diagnosed after the 35th week of pregnancy should be controlled rapidly and labour induced or a caesarean section performed, depending on the condition of the fetus and the state of the cervix.

Women with pre-eclampsia should not be allowed to exceed full term, as the risk of intra-uterine death increases after term.

Care after birth

The woman needs to have close monitoring of her blood pressure until it resolves. If the blood pressure remains high antihypertensive agents should be continued. Proteinuria often persists for longer and is of little consequence. One-third of the women will have non-proteinuric hypertension in a subsequent pregnancy, but the rate of recurrence of severe pre-eclampsia is less than 5%.

If severe pre-eclampsia presents before 34 weeks' gestation a careful search for an underlying medical disorder, such as renal disease, should be made.

ECLAMPSIA

The purpose of treating hypertensive disorders in pregnancy is to prevent eclampsia. The word arises from the Greek for 'like a flash of lightning', and this is how the disease may occur.

Eclampsia is characterized by convulsions and coma, which usually occur in patients who have severe pre-eclampsia or imminent eclampsia, and in patients in whom gestational proteinuria has been superimposed on chronic hypertension. In 10–30% of women there are no warning signs, the fits occurring 'like a flash of lightning'. With better antenatal care and early recognition and treatment of pre-eclampsia and chronic hypertension, the incidence of eclampsia has fallen. In developed countries eclampsia occurs in 1 : 2000 pregnant women, but in the developing countries the incidence is higher.

Pathophysiology

The changes that occur in severe pre-eclampsia are more marked in eclampsia: vasospasm is intense, with tissue hypoxia; the glomerular filtration rate is further reduced and urinary output falls; intracellular water retention impedes cellular metabolism and cerebral oedema may occur; blood viscosity increases, platelet levels fall and coagulation defects arise.

Clinical picture

The convulsion is preceded by a disorientation stage during which the woman becomes restless, twitches, and develops spasmodic respiration. Within a minute she passes into the tonic stage of the convulsion: her back arches, her hands clench, she grimaces, her breathing ceases and she becomes cyanosed. In this stage she may bite her tongue. She then passes into the clonic stage of the convulsion, when her body jerks uncontrollably, frothy saliva may fill her mouth and her breathing

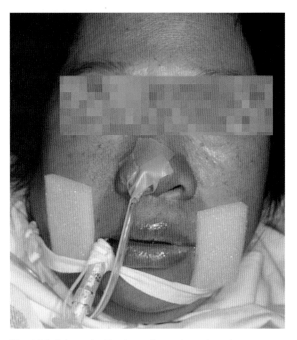

Fig. 14.1 Eclampsia. The face of an eclamptic patient.

becomes stertorous. Finally, she becomes comatose (Fig. 14.1). The coma may persist for an hour or longer, or recurrent convulsions may occur.

The convulsions occur in late pregnancy in 40% of cases, intrapartum in 30%, and a few hours after the birth in 30%.

Management of eclampsia

The aims of treatment are:

- To control the fits by relieving the generalized vascular spasm and decreasing the sensitivity of the brain to stimuli
- To reduce the blood pressure to prevent cerebral haemorrhage
- To deliver the fetus.

Midwifery care

The quality of the midwifery care of an eclamptic patient is crucial. The patient is nursed on her side, with her head and shoulders raised, and a catheter is inserted into her bladder. The attending midwives must:

- Detect any changes presaging a second convulsion
- Prevent the woman injuring herself during a convulsion
- Provide continuous oxygen
- Keep the mouth and fauces clear of any saliva by suction
- Monitor vital signs and urinary output.

Medical and drug treatment

Drug treatment - magnesium sulphate

Magnesium reduces the risk of recurrent seizures by relieving vasospasm and inducing cerebral vascular dilatation. It increases the release of prostacyclin, improving uterine blood flow, inhibits platelet activation and protects endothelial cells from injury.

Magnesium sulphate may be given intravenously or by deep intramuscular injection (Box 14.1). The intravenous route is preferred, as intramuscular injections are painful and are followed, in 5% of cases, by deep abscess formation.

The regimen is as follows:

- Loading dose when the eclamptic patient is first seen: $MgSO_4$ 4 g IV over 10–15 minutes, followed by $MgSO_4$ 1 g/h (as an infusion of $MgSO_4$ 5 g in 500 mL of normal saline).
- Continuing treatment: rate of infusion to provide 1 g/h until 24 hours have passed since the last seizure, or the woman has given birth.
- Magnesium is excreted by the kidneys and is a smooth muscle relaxant. It is important that tendon reflexes, respiratory rate (>16/min) and urine output (>25 mL/h) are monitored to detect magnesium toxicity. If this occurs the management is:
  - Respiratory arrest: intubate, ventilate, and stop the $MgSO_4$ infusion. Give 1 g calcium gluconate IV (the antidote to magnesium toxicity)
  - Respiratory depression: give oxygen by mask, calcium gluconate 1 g IV, and maintain a clear airway
  - Absent patellar reflexes: if respiration is normal, stop the $MgSO_4$ infusion until reflexes return. If respiration is depressed, treat for this condition
  - Poor urinary output (<100 mL in 4 hours): if there are no other signs of magnesium toxicity, reduce the rate of the IV infusion to 0.5 g/h and monitor fluid balance.

Antibiotics should be prescribed.

If cardiac failure occurs, furosemide (frusemide) 20 mg may be given intravenously, but because of the hypovolaemia it should be used with care.

Box 14.1 **Magnesium sulphate treatment for eclampsia**

Loading dose

$MgSO_4$ 4 g intravenously over 5 to 15 minutes

Maintenance dose

$MgSO_4$ 1 g per hour in solution of 5 g in 500 mL normal saline

---

Medical treatment

Once good control of the blood pressure and the convulsions has been obtained the pregnancy should be terminated. Depending on the period of the gestation, the health (alive or dead) of the fetus and its presentation, and on the condition of the cervix, delivery may be effected by caesarean section or labour may be induced using prostaglandins or by amniotomy. In most cases of eclampsia the induction of labour is followed rapidly by the birth of the infant. As postpartum haemorrhage may occur, prophylactic intravenous Syntocinon should be given on the birth of the infant. The patient should continue to be monitored at least for the first 4 days of the puerperium.

Prognosis in pre-eclampsia and eclampsia

In developing countries it is estimated that 50 000 maternal deaths annually are due to pre-eclampsia. Today few women in the developed countries should die from severe pre-eclampsia or from eclampsia. Most deaths are from cerebral haemorrhage or cardiac failure.

CHRONIC HYPERTENSION

Most women with chronic hypertension have been diagnosed before pregnancy; a few are found to be hypertensive at the first antenatal visit. In the absence of a secondary cause for hypertension (for example renal artery stenosis or phaeochromocytoma), a raised blood pressure (>140/90 mmHg) which persists and is present before pregnancy or detected before the 20th gestational week, is diagnostic of essential hypertension. It is important to remember that the small physiological fall in blood pressure in the first half of pregnancy may be exaggerated in women who have chronic hypertension, and some cases may be missed.

Essential hypertension complicates 1–3% of pregnancies and is more frequent in women over the age of 35.

Pathophysiology

The generalized vasospasm of essential hypertension is counterbalanced by an increased stroke volume and heart rate, which maintains an adequate blood flow to most organs with the exception of the uterus. Although uterine blood flow is increased in normal pregnancy the increase is less in women who have essential hypertension, and the higher the blood pressure the less the increase. This may reduce fetal growth and increase perinatal loss.

Pregnancy affects the course of essential hypertension. In 60% of affected women a rise in blood pressure occurs, and in 30% significant proteinuria (>300 mg/L)

is detected. The changes usually occur after the 30th week of pregnancy. Essential hypertension with super-imposed proteinuria is indistinguishable from severe pre-eclampsia.

Treatment

The aims of treatment are:

- To obtain and to maintain as good a blood supply to the uterus as possible
- To control the level of the blood pressure and prevent the superimposition of proteinuria
- To terminate the pregnancy if the patient's condition deteriorates markedly, or if the fetus fails to grow adequately in the last quarter of pregnancy.

Maintenance of uterine blood supply

Usually the woman is instructed to rest more to improve the uterine blood supply.

Control of the hypertension

Most patients will be taking an antihypertensive drug and a physician should be consulted to confirm that the drug is required and that it is safe to be given during pregnancy. Diuretics should be avoided as these agents reduce plasma volume and uteroplacental blood flow. Most experience has been obtained using methyldopa, but it appears that β-blockers such as atenolol and labetalol, and calcium-channel blockers (e.g. nifedipine) are safe. Angiotensin-converting enzyme (ACE) inhibitors should be avoided because of their potential teratogenicity.

Avoidance of problems

The woman should be seen more frequently during the antenatal period, the frequency depending on the severity of the hypertension. Her lifestyle should be checked, and if she is obese a reduction diet should be prescribed. If the fetus shows signs of growth restriction, biophysical tests for fetal wellbeing should be started (Ch. 20), and if conditions deteriorate induction of labour should be discussed with the patient. It is safer for the fetus to be born earlier rather than later, and the patient should not become postdate as the risk of perinatal loss increases.

RENAL DISEASE IN PREGNANCY

Less than 0.2% of pregnant women, and less than 5% of women with hypertension in pregnancy, have renal disease. In most cases the diagnosis is known beforehand, but routine examination of a midstream specimen of urine (which is made to detect asymptomatic bacteriuria) may occasionally detect an affected woman. Most affected women have no impairment of renal function, which is tracked by periodic serum creatinine measurements. If the level rises to more than 0.18 mmol/L and there is evidence of poor fetal growth, either renal dialysis or induction of labour should be performed after consultation with a renal physician.

Women with a renal transplant have a 90% likelihood of a successful pregnancy outcome providing that the woman's renal function has been stable for 2 years before conception, that she is normotensive or her hypertension is well controlled and she has minimal proteinuria. Close monitoring of both renal and fetoplacental function is required and delivery by caesarean section needs only to be performed for obstetric indications.

Chapter | 15 |

Cardiovascular, respiratory, haematological, neurological and gastrointestinal disorders in pregnancy

CARDIOVASCULAR COMPLICATIONS IN PREGNANCY

It will be recalled that pregnancy places an increased strain on the heart because of the increased rate and stroke volume. The burden on the heart reaches its maximum at about the 28th week and continues into the puerperium. If a pregnant woman has heart disease, the increased strain may affect her wellbeing.

At present, in the developed countries between 0.2 and 0.5% of pregnant women have heart disease. In 30% of cases a woman has mitral valve disease; in 20% ventricular septal defect; in 15%, atrial septal defect; in 15%, aortic stenosis; and in the remainder, other defects.

Diagnosis

In most cases the diagnosis has been established before the pregnancy, but the doctor should auscultate the woman's heart at the first antenatal visit. Any suspicious signs, particularly a diastolic or loud systolic murmur, should lead to referral to a cardiologist.

Management in pregnancy

The initial assessment of the pregnant woman should be made in conjunction with a cardiologist, after which the medical management of the pregnancy can be carried out by the attending doctor, the patient being reviewed by the cardiologist at intervals. The aims of management are:

- To avoid those factors that predispose to heart failure
- Should failure occur, to treat it vigorously.

Factors that predispose to heart failure include anaemia, infections (particularly urinary tract infections) and the development of hypertension. If any of these are found, treatment should be started.

The woman's cooperation, and that of her family, should be obtained. Her daily activities should be evaluated and changes suggested if this is appropriate.

The patient should be seen at intervals of no more than 2 weeks up to the 28th week of pregnancy, and thereafter weekly by a doctor (if it causes less stress on the woman, it could be her GP in collaboration with the obstetrician and the cardiologist). At each visit cardiac function is assessed by inquiring about breathlessness on exertion, or if she has a cough or orthopnoea. Her lungs are auscultated to detect rales.

Many cardiologists place pregnant women in categories suggested by the New York Heart Association, and the management is planned according to this. Initially most pregnant women are in class 1 or 2, but during pregnancy in 15–55% some degree of cardiac decompensation occurs.

Class 1

The patient has no symptoms, although signs of cardiac damage are present. She can undertake all physical activities. In this class, no additional treatment is needed.

Class 2

The woman is comfortable at rest, but ordinary physical exertion usually causes fatigue, palpitations and, occasionally, dyspnoea. Most patients in this class do not require treatment, but if the woman's social conditions are unfavourable or if signs of a deterioration in cardiac reserve occur, she should be admitted to hospital.

Class 3

Less than ordinary physical exertion causes dyspnoea and fatigue, although the patient is comfortable when resting. Most women in this class should be admitted to hospital for rest, but home conditions and responsibilities have to be assessed and help provided if needed.

Class 4

Women in this class are seriously ill. The patient is breathless even when resting. Hospital admission is mandatory.

Heart failure

Should the woman develop heart failure the principles of treatment are no different from those of non-pregnant women. Digoxin is given to control the heart rate and increase the time for blood flow into the left ventricle. Diuretics (such as furosemide) are given when pulmonary oedema is present. There is no consensus as to whether women who are not in cardiac failure should be given prophylactic digoxin, but most experts agree that if the woman is at risk of atrial fibrillation or has mitral heart disease and an enlarged left atrium, digoxin is indicated.

Management during childbirth

Most women who have heart disease have an easy, spontaneous labour and there is no indication for inducing labour on account of the cardiac condition. During labour the patient should be nursed either on her side or well propped up, as compression of the aorta in the supine position may cause marked hypotension. The woman's fluid balance and her pulse rate should be checked at intervals. If the woman requires anaesthesia, an epidural blockade is the preferred choice as it decreases sympathetic activity, and reduces both oxygen consumption and variations in cardiac output.

Delay in the second stage of labour should be rectified by the use of forceps or vacuum extractor, but there is no need for prophylactic instrumental delivery. The third stage is conducted in the same way as in non-cardiac patients, and active management using Syntocinon is safe, unless the woman is in heart failure. The accoucheur should always bear in mind that in general, women with cardiac disease tolerate postpartum haemorrhage poorly.

The risks and management of specific cardiac conditions are summarized in Table 15.1.

The puerperium

The burden on the heart continues into the puerperium. For the first 24–48 hours the patient must be constantly observed for signs of decompensation. She should then be closely monitored for the first few days, and additional support should be made available when she returns home.

Prognosis for mother and baby and for future pregnancies

The prognosis for the mother is dependent on the underlying aetiology. With good antenatal care the risk to the mother or fetus if the disease is mild is not usually increased during the current pregnancy. Women with significant impairment of cardiac function should be dissuaded from further pregnancies until the condition of the heart has been assessed and further treatment, including surgery, discussed.

Table 15.1 Management of specific cardiac conditions

CONDITION	PREGNANCY RISKS	MANAGEMENT
Atrial septal defect	Rarely causes problems	Nil specific after exclusion of other secondary complications
Ventricular septal defect	Small defects rarely cause problems	Avoid hypertension, endocarditis prophylaxis
Patent ductus arteriosus	Small shunts rarely problematic	Exclude pulmonary hypertension
Coarctation of aorta	Corrected, few problems; uncorrected, maternal mortality (15%)	Prevent hypertension, use epidural in labour
Primary pulmonary hypertension	Maternal mortality of 50%	Offer termination Anticoagulation, O_2 therapy, epidural in labour Assisted vaginal delivery
Eisenmenger's syndrome	Maternal mortality 30%, termination mortality 10%	As for pulmonary hypertension
Fallot's tetralogy	Good outcome if corrected Uncorrected – increased, risk miscarriage, IUGR, prematurity	Avoid hypotension which can cause shunt reversal, assisted vaginal delivery
Mitral stenosis	Uncorrected – IUGR and prematurity, maternal mortality 5–15%	Control heart rate with β-blockers, use epidural, assisted delivery not mandatory, endocarditis prophylaxis
Aortic stenosis	Endocarditis. Severe – IUGR, maternal mortality 5–15%	Avoid hypo- and hypervolaemia, endocarditis prophylaxis
Prosthetic heart valves	Pregnancy accelerates need for replacement, thromboembolism	Careful anticoagulation throughout pregnancy
Marfan syndrome	Aortic root involvement – maternal mortality up to 50% Autosomal dominant so 50% fetuses affected	β-Blockers, serial echocardiography, avoid hypertension, epidural and assisted vaginal delivery

VENOUS THROMBOEMBOLISM IN PREGNANCY

Venous thromboembolism (VTE) affects between 50 and 60 pregnant or postpartum women per 100 000, with a mortality rate of 1 per 100 000 maternities. It is highest in women aged over 39, the mortality rate being 1 per 3300. The prevalence of VTE is equally distributed throughout pregnancy, but the day-by-day risk is greatest in the immediate puerperium. The major risk factors include caesarean section, obesity, prolonged immobility, pre-eclampsia, current infection, previous VTE and familial thrombophilia.

Treatment of a pulmonary embolus during pregnancy consists of unfractionated heparin (UH), initially intravenously (40 000 U/day by continuous infusion in normal saline) to obtain a concentration of 0.6–1.0 U/mL. Once full heparinization has been obtained for 3–7 days, the infusion may be replaced by calcium heparin given subcutaneously. A deep vein thrombosis (DVT) is treated either with UH if delivery or surgery is imminent, or low molecular weight heparin (LWMH) given subcutaneously. UH is substituted for LMWH 24–36 hours prior to delivery. UH is suspended once labour is established or 6 hours before surgery, and recommenced 2–6 hours after vaginal or caesarean delivery. If the woman has a high risk of VTE antenatally (includes recurrent VTE, previous idiopathic VTE or previous VTE and a strong family history of VTE) she may be given LMWH prophylaxis throughout pregnancy and for 6 weeks postpartum (see also postpartum thromboembolism, p. 186).

ANTIPHOSPHOLIPID SYNDROME

Antiphospholipid syndrome (APS) is associated with early-onset pre-eclampsia, intrauterine fetal growth restriction, preterm birth, miscarriage, fetal death and venous thromboembolism. Diagnosis requires at least one of the clinical criteria and one of the laboratory criteria (see Box 15.1). Women who have suffered from clinical complications should be screened and referred for specialist evaluation.

Because of the high-risk nature of the pregnancy, women with APS should be managed by a specialist team and require close surveillance during pregnancy. Low-dose aspirin and heparin has been shown to reduce the risk of pregnancy loss (RR 0.48; 95% CI 0.33–0.68).

RESPIRATORY CONDITIONS

Asthma

The effect of pregnancy on asthma is variable, but most asthmatic women experience fewer attacks. Well-controlled asthma has no effect on the course of pregnancy, labour or the birthweight of the infant; suboptimal treatment is associated with growth restriction, premature birth and increased perinatal mortality. Treatment is no different from that of a non-pregnant asthmatic woman. Regional anaesthesia is preferable to general anaesthesia if the woman requires an operative delivery.

Pulmonary tuberculosis

Although the prevalence of pulmonary tuberculosis in most developed countries is low, it appears to be increasing with increased movement of populations. Over 8 million new cases are being reported per annum.

A patient diagnosed with active tuberculosis in the first half of pregnancy should be treated with isoniazid and ethambutol. After the 20th week rifampicin may be used.

Box 15.1 Criteria for diagnosis of antiphospholipid syndrome

Clinical	Laboratory*
Recurrent early pregnancy loss	Lupus anticoagulant
Fetal death	Anticardiolipin
Preterm birth <34 weeks for	antibodies
pre-eclampsia or fetal growth	Anti-β_2 glycoprotein
restriction	IgG or IgM
Thrombosis	
Venous	
Arterial including stroke	
Autoimmune thrombocytopenia	

*moderate to high levels

The management of labour does not differ from that for a non-infected woman. If the mother's sputum shows acid-fast bacilli, after the birth the baby should be separated from her, vaccinated with bacille Calmette–Guérin (BCG) and remain separate for about 6 weeks. If the mother's sputum has no acid-fast bacilli the baby should be vaccinated with BCG and may remain with her and be breastfed if the mother wishes it.

ANAEMIA IN PREGNANCY

Anaemia, the most common haematological abnormality encountered during pregnancy, remains an important cause of adverse maternal–fetal outcome worldwide. Iron deficiency and acute blood loss are the leading causes of maternal anaemia. All pregnant women should have a blood sample tested for the presence of anaemia at the first antenatal visit.

During pregnancy, the plasma volume begins to increase by the sixth week of gestation, peaking at around 30 weeks, with a total extra volume of 1.2–1.3 litres by term. The red cell mass also slowly increases, but proportionately less than the plasma volume. This results in reference values for haemoglobin in pregnancy being lower than in age-matched non-pregnant females and is sometimes referred to as the 'physiologic anaemia of pregnancy'. A haemoglobin less than 110 g/L in first trimester and less than 100 g/L in late second or third trimester should be considered as anaemia and investigated further.

Iron requirements during pregnancy increase in response to fetal growth and development and the increase in maternal red cell mass. Total iron requirements in normal pregnancy have been estimated as approximately 1300 mg/day. Iron is absorbed predominantly through the proximal small intestine and is highly regulated. Iron absorption is increased in iron deficiency and in pregnancy.

Iron deficiency

Worldwide, iron deficiency remains a significant cause of maternal anaemia. A serum ferritin less than 15 µg/L indicates body iron depletion and values <12 µg/L are associated with iron deficiency. In iron deficiency the mean red cell volume (MCV) and mean red cell haemoglobin (MCH) are usually reduced. Inadequate dietary iron intake and gastrointestinal blood loss (hookworm infestation) are the commonest causes of iron deficiency. Prevalence rates for iron deficiency are increased amongst women from lower socioeconomic groups, teenage mothers, those eating predominantly vegetarian or vegan diets, and women with closely spaced pregnancies.

Treatment of iron deficiency and routine iron supplementation

Pregnant women with iron deficiency anaemia should be treated with oral iron. Oral iron replacement containing

30–60 mg elemental iron is usually used. Women who are unable to take oral iron or in those with malabsorption (coeliac disease), intravenous iron can be considered. Blood transfusion for the treatment of iron deficiency anaemia should be avoided unless there is active bleeding or cardiovascular compromise.

Routine iron supplementation is known to decrease the prevalence of maternal anaemia at delivery. However, it is unclear whether routine iron supplementation provided to well-nourished women who are not anaemic affects perinatal outcome. Among fertile women including those from higher socioeconomic groups, a significant proportion have depleted iron stores or iron stores which are inadequate to meet the needs of pregnancy. When available, decisions regarding an individual woman's iron supplementation during pregnancy should take into account her baseline haemoglobin and ferritin results.

Folate and vitamin B$_{12}$

Folate (also called folic acid) is a B-group vitamin. Folate requirements are increased in pregnancy. Body stores of folate may be rapidly exhausted and generally last less than 3 weeks. Red cell folate (RCF) is a more accurate measure of folate status than serum folate. Routine measurement of RCF is not required but should be considered if there is an increased MCV, prolonged hyperemesis/poor oral intake in pregnancy or gastrointestinal pathology (coeliac disease, Crohn's disease, gastric bypass).

Routine supplementation with folate (0.4–0.5 mg) is recommended for all women prior to conception and for the first trimester to reduce the incidence of neural tube defect. Higher doses of folate (4 mg/day) throughout pregnancy are required in folate deficiency and in women with increased folate requirements (for example those with chronic haemolysis or beta thalassaemia minor).

Vitamin B$_{12}$ is essential for infant neurodevelopment. Undiagnosed maternal vitamin B$_{12}$ deficiency may result in irreversible neurological damage to the breastfed infant. Although maternal vitamin B$_{12}$ deficiency is uncommon, the majority of women with deficient B$_{12}$ levels are asymptomatic. Routine measurement of vitamin B$_{12}$ is not required; however, serum vitamin B$_{12}$ levels should be checked in the following circumstances: the complete blood count is suggestive of megaloblastic anaemia (increased MCV, hypersegmented neutrophils); vegetarian or vegan diet; gastrointestinal pathology (coeliac disease, Crohn's disease, gastric banding/bypass); family history of vitamin B$_{12}$ deficiency or pernicious anaemia.

Acute blood loss

Haemorrhage remains a leading preventable cause of maternal mortality particularly in the developing world. Deaths from haemorrhage would be dramatically reduced if all pregnant women could access a skilled birth attendant at the time of childbirth, and have access to quality emergency obstetric care including a safe blood supply.

THALASSAEMIA AND HAEMOGLOBINOPATHIES

The haemoglobinopathies (thalassaemia and sickle cell disease) (Box 15.2) are inherited disorders of haemoglobin. They are autosomal recessive defects, and characterized by reduced production of one or more of the chains of globin that make up haemoglobin. Carriers (who have only one affected globin locus) remain healthy throughout life. People who are homozygous or doubly heterozygous have haemoglobin disorders of varying clinical severity.

Ethnic populations at increased risk for thalassaemia or sickle cell disorders include those from Africa, the Mediterranean region, the Middle East, South East Asia including the subcontinent, Western Pacific region, Caribbean and South American countries.

In α-thalassaemias the α chains accumulate and eventually precipitate, causing severe anaemia (thalassaemia major, or Cooley's anaemia). The β-thalassaemias may be either heterozygous, when they are symptomless, or homozygous, when they produce severe anaemia.

Thalassaemia in a woman who is anaemic in pregnancy can generally be excluded if the MCV is greater than 80 fL. An MCV of less than 80 fL indicates that haemoglobin electrophoresis should be performed. An HbA$_2$ greater than 3.5 indicates a β-thalassaemia trait. Because a significant number of women with α-thalassaemia and other rarer haemoglobinopathies have normal red cell indices, routine haemoglobin electrophoresis should be offered to all previously unscreened pregnant women from communities at greater risk because of ethnicity.

A pregnant woman carrying the thalassaemia trait has a 30% chance of becoming anaemic and a similar chance of developing urinary tract infection. Thalassaemia major in the fetus can be detected in the first quarter of pregnancy by chorionic villus sampling. If the test is positive, termination of the pregnancy is an option for the parents.

In sickle cell anaemia a defective gene on the chromosome responsible for haemoglobin synthesis leads to the

---

Box 15.2 The thalassaemias

Homozygous β-thalassaemia

Homozygous haemoglobin S (sickle cell disease)

Homozygous haemoglobin Lepore

Bart's hydrops (four-gene deletion α-thalassaemia)

Haemoglobin H disease hydrops (2 α gene deletion plus point mutation)

Haemoglobin E/β-thalassaemia

Haemoglobin Lepore/β-thalassaemia

Haemoglobin S/β-thalassaemia

Haemoglobin C/β-thalassaemia

Haemoglobin O Arab/β-thalassaemia

Haemoglobin S/C or S/D disease

production of abnormal haemoglobin and an erythrocyte life of less than 15 days. The episodes of erythrocyte destruction may cause severe haemolytic anaemia and bone pains, because of infarction of the vessels supplying the bones.

All pregnant women suspected of carrying an abnormal haemoglobin should be given folate (15 mg daily) routinely, and have frequent haemoglobin estimations. If the haemoglobin level falls below 60 g/L a direct or an exchange transfusion should be made. Infections, especially of the urinary tract, should be treated and prophylactic antibiotics given during childbirth and the puerperium. If a bone pain crisis occurs heparin should be given and the haemoglobin measured every 2 hours; a fall of more than 2 g indicates the need for an exchange transfusion.

Issues for antenatal care include:

- Accurate diagnosis of women with thalassaemia minor in order to avoid confusion with iron deficiency since the MCV and MCH are reduced in both conditions
- Antenatal screening to identify carriers and offer them partner screening to facilitate informed choices about reproduction
- Neonatal screening programmes aim to identify infants with sickle cell disease (SCD) in order to commence early prophylactic penicillin and comprehensive care.

Antenatal or preconceptual screening

Carrier screening should be offered to a woman if she and/or her partner are identified as belonging to an ethnic population whose members are at higher risk of being carriers.

Screening consists of a complete blood count, as well as haemoglobin electrophoresis or high performance liquid chromatography (HPLC). This investigation should include measurement of HbA_2 and HbF and a serum ferritin (to exclude iron deficiency) should be performed simultaneously.

If a woman's screening is abnormal, then screening of her partner should be performed.

If both partners are found to be carriers of thalassaemia or an Hb variant, they should be referred for genetic counselling. Prenatal diagnosis may be offered to couples at risk for having a fetus with a clinically significant thalassaemia or haemoglobinopathy. Screening programmes should aim to identify couples at risk for having a child with Bart's hydrops fetalis (four-gene deletion alpha thalassaemia), beta thalassaemia major (homozygous β-thalassaemia, β/E-thalassaemia) and sickle cell disease (HbSS, HbSC, S/β-thalassaemia).

Pregnancy care in women with serious haemoglobin disorders

Women with homozygous or doubly heterozygous haemoglobin disorders require special attention during pregnancy. Women with SCD have higher rates of spontaneous miscarriage, preterm birth, fetal growth restriction and perinatal morbidity and mortality. Infections and sickling crises are more common during pregnancy. Reproductive failure is common in women with beta thalassaemia major because of endocrine damage resulting from iron overload. In well-chelated patients, pregnancies occur. Cardiac complications may occur during pregnancy from iron-related cardiac damage.

RED CELL ALLOIMMUNIZATION

Pathophysiology

During pregnancy, fetal cells may cross the placenta and enter the maternal circulation, exposing the mother to 'foreign' paternally acquired red cell antigens. This fetomaternal haemorrhage (FMH) is most likely to occur at delivery (60% of pregnancies) but may also occur spontaneously during pregnancy and in association with threatened or complete miscarriage, after trauma or placental abruption, with termination of pregnancy and after invasive procedures such as amniocentesis, chorionic villous sampling (CVS), external cephalic version (ECV) and curettage. Exposure to 'foreign' red cell antigens may also occur through blood transfusion.

Exposure to foreign red cell antigens may result in the development of alloantibody. Development of antibody depends on a number of factors including the potency or antigenicity of the antigen, the dose of antigen to which the mother is exposed, the responsiveness of her immune system and ABO compatibility between the mother and fetus. Rh D is the most immunogenic of the red cell antigens. A single pregnancy with an Rh D positive, ABO compatible fetus initiates immunization in about 1 in 6 Rh D negative women.

Antibodies of the immunoglobulin G (IgG) class are actively transported from mother to fetus, commencing in the second trimester and increasing exponentially towards term. Haemolytic disease (HDN) occurs when the fetal red cell life-span is shortened by the action of a specific antibody derived from the mother and transferred across the placenta. Antibody-coated red cells are removed from the circulation by the fetal liver and spleen resulting in anaemia. This increased breakdown of haemoglobin results in increased pigment in the amniotic fluid.

In mild cases of HDN, the fetus may be born with minimal or no clinical affects and postnatal observation may be all that is required. The direct antiglobulin test (DAT) on cord blood is positive reflecting the presence of maternally-derived IgG on the infant's red cells. In some cases hyperbilirubinaemia may develop requiring phototherapy or sometimes exchange transfusion for the prevention of bilirubin encephalopathy.

In severe cases, there may be early onset of fetal anaemia. The fetal response to anaemia results in increased haemopoiesis in the liver and spleen resulting in enlargement of these organs. As anaemia progresses, decompensation occurs with development or cardiac compromise, ascites, pleural effusions and polyhydramnios (immune hydrops fetalis). Without treatment this condition may result in fetal death.

Investigations

The presence of red cell antibodies in maternal blood may be detected by an indirect antiglobulin test (IAT). A routine ABO and Rh D blood group and antibody screen (IAT) should be performed at the first antenatal visit. If a clinically significant red cell antibody is detected, levels should be monitored periodically through pregnancy by either titration or measurement.

Antigens that stimulate antibodies known to cause clinically significant haemolytic disease are shown in Box 15.3.

The aim of surveillance during pregnancy is to ensure that the fetus does not develop life-threatening anaemia. Antibody titration or quantitation give an indirect measure of the likelihood of fetal anaemia, as severe fetal disease is unlikely at low antibody levels such as a titre below 1 in 16. At antibody titres above these levels, fetal monitoring through ultrasound is usually performed. Fetal haemoglobin concentration may be measured from a sample collected at cordocentesis (fetal blood sampling). As this

is an invasive procedure associated with significant risk to the fetus (1–2% chance of fetal loss), it is usually only performed when there is a high likelihood of moderate to severe anaemia requiring fetal transfusion.

Indirect methods of screening for moderate to severe fetal anaemia are available. Spectrophotometric examination of amniotic fluid is performed to identify the presence of bilirubin. A sample is collected at amniocentesis and bilirubin is measured as a change in optical density at 450 nanometres (OD 450) (Fig. 15.1). The OD 450 level is then interpreted using a curve (Liley, Queenan or Robertson) that predicts the degree of anaemia based on the amount of haemolysis at a given gestation (Fig. 15.2). Depending on the gestational age at which the OD 450 reaches a critical level, either delivery or cordocentesis (fetal blood sampling) with intrauterine transfusion can be arranged. The OD 450 is most widely used in Rh D alloimmunized pregnancies and may underestimate the degree of anaemia in Kell immunization. In Kell immunization both haemolysis and suppression of red cell production contribute to anaemia.

Non-invasive screening for moderate to severe fetal anaemia is now widely used. Measurement of the peak systolic velocity in the middle cerebral artery and interpretation of the result using gestation-specific charts allows prediction of fetuses at risk of moderate to severe anaemia. In the same way as with amniocentesis, if the middle cerebral artery Doppler is above 1.5 multiples of the median (MoM), either delivery or cordocentesis and intrauterine transfusion can be performed, depending on gestation.

The infant

At birth, the infant is examined to determine the degree of fetal haemolysis, taking particular account of hepatosplenomegaly, ascites, and pleural effusions. The outlook for severely hydropic infants is guarded. A blood sample

---

Box 15.3 Antigens that stimulate antibodies that can cause significant haemolytic disease of the newborn (HDN)

Rhesus antigens	Kell antigen	Kidd antigens	Duffy antigens
D	K	JKa	Fya
C		Jkb	Fyb
c			
E			
e			

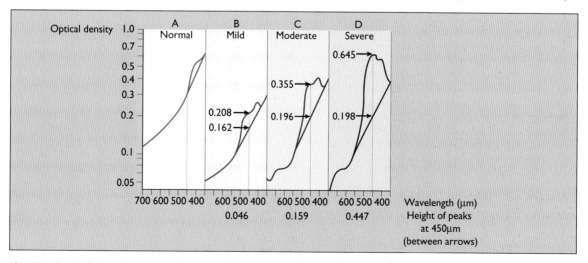

Fig. 15.1 Spectral absorption curves of amniotic fluid in (from left) normal late pregnancy; mild, moderate and severe haemolytic disease.

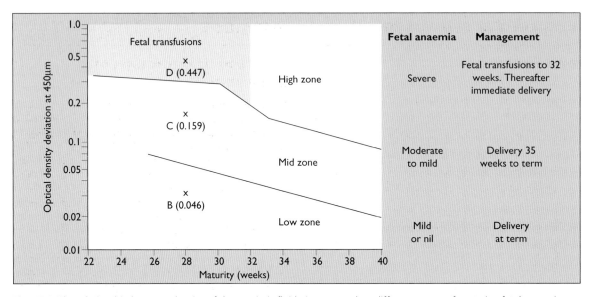

Fig. 15.2 The relationship between the size of the amniotic fluid pigment peak at different stages of maturity, fetal anaemia and management. (The peak figures from Fig. 15.1 B, C and D are charted.)

is collected to determine haemoglobin concentration, the serum bilirubin, ABO and Rh D blood group and direct antiglobulin test (DAT or Coombs' test).

Careful follow-up of the infant for development of jaundice is essential. In adults and older children development of jaundice is usually first seen in the sclera. The sclera are difficult to see in a newborn infant due to the eyelids which may be swollen or closed. Jaundice may be detected in the skin but is usually not visible until the bilirubin exceeds 100–120 µmol/L and may be difficult to detect in darker-skinned infants.

High levels of unconjugated bilirubin may be toxic to the brain, and can cause the disease called kernicterus. The acute signs of kernicterus include lethargy, poor feeding, temperature instability, hypertonia leading to arching of the head, neck and back (opisthotonus), spasticity and seizures. Death or severe neurological disability may follow. The risk of developing kernicterus increases with increasing unconjugated bilirubin (concentrations greater than 340 µmol/L are considered unsafe), decreasing gestation, asphyxia, acidosis, hypoxia, hypothermia, meningitis, sepsis and decreased albumin binding.

Therapies to manage jaundice include adequate hydration, phototherapy, and exchange transfusion. Exchange transfusion is undertaken to prevent kernicterus. The rate of rise as well as the actual bilirubin level must be taken into account. The red cells used for exchange transfusion must be ABO compatible with the infant and negative for the relevant antigen to which the maternal antibody is directed.

Prevention of Rh D alloimmunization

Since the 1960s there has been considerable success in preventing Rh D immunization in Rh D negative women.

Rh D immunization mainly affects Caucasian women where up to 15% of the population are Rh D negative. Lower rates of Rh D negative women are seen in African, Asian and Middle Eastern populations.

The principle of prevention is passive immunization. Rh D negative women are given an injection of anti-D antibody at a time when fetal cells may be present in the circulation. The injected anti-D antibody binds to any fetal Rh D positive red blood cells present in the circulation and allows them to be cleared by the maternal liver and spleen before an immune response can occur. For anti-D antibody to be effective, it must be given at the right time and in the right amount.

Anti-D is given to Rh D negative women in the following circumstances during pregnancy:

- Threatened or spontaneous miscarriage, invasive procedures (amniocentesis or chorionic villous sampling), trauma, placental abruption, termination of pregnancy, curettage
- Routinely antenatally at 28 and 34 weeks' gestation
- Routinely at delivery if the infant is Rh D positive.

The dose of anti-D must be sufficient to remove all fetal cells from the maternal circulation. The Kleihauer–Betke test which identifies fetal cells in maternal blood is used to determine the volume of FMH and should be used to assess whether additional doses of anti-D are required for sensitizing events in the second and third trimesters and postnatally. Anti-D should be administered as close to the sensitizing event as possible and within 72 hours. It may still have an effect if given up to 9–10 days after the event.

NEUROLOGICAL DISORDERS

Epilepsy

Epilepsy is a common disorder and a third of women with epilepsy will suffer increased convulsions during pregnancy, owing to stress and decreased biological availability of their anticonvulsant therapy because of decreased absorption and increased hepatic and renal clearance. There is some controversy about the teratogenic effects of the commonly used anticonvulsants, with reports of a two- to threefold increase in malformations. There is evidence of similar malformations (particularly facial dysmorphism, hypoplastic fingernails and shortened phalanges) in women with epilepsy who have not taken drugs. Carbamazepine is considered to be the safest drug, although it has been associated with a small increase in the risk of spina bifida, and so additional prophylactic folate therapy is important.

During pregnancy drug levels should be monitored regularly and dosages adjusted accordingly. Most women with epilepsy labour normally, caesarean section being reserved for those with frequent stress-associated seizures. After delivery the drug dose may need to be reduced. Breastfeeding is not contraindicated despite the drugs crossing into the breast milk.

Headaches

Most pregnant women report headaches, most commonly because of tension or migraine. Tension headaches can be treated with paracetamol if necessary. Migrainous headaches tend to be worse in the first and second trimesters. β-Blockers are effective, as are tricyclic antidepressants; ergot derivatives are contraindicated because of their vasoconstrictor and direct effects on the uterus. Persistent headaches, especially with atypical features, should be carefully investigated to exclude other serious causes. CT or MRI scans of the head can be safely performed in pregnancy.

Bell's palsy

Paralysis of the facial nerve occurs three times more frequently in late pregnancy and the puerperium than in non-pregnant women. Prednisolone (1 mg/kg daily) is commonly used and most recover completely within 6 weeks.

Carpal tunnel syndrome

This is a common complaint caused by pressure on the median nerve as it passes through the carpal tunnel. Night wrist splints are usually effective, and it usually resolves early in the puerperium. Surgical decompression is rarely required.

GASTROINTESTINAL DISORDERS

Intrahepatic cholestasis of pregnancy (ICP)

ICP occurs most commonly in the third trimester and is characterized by generalized pruritus which is most severe on the palms and soles, elevated serum bile acids and usually the transaminases are elevated. The diagnosis is made after exclusion of other hepatic disorders. The condition resolves rapidly after delivery. The incidence varies among ethnic groups; 1% Caucasians, 5% Hispanics and 10% reported in Chile. There is debatably an association with late fetal death, meconium staining of the liquor, and postpartum haemorrhage. There is a small increase in premature births.

Treatment is with ursodeoxycholic acid 10–25 mg/kg divided into two doses daily although this does not have a marked effect on pruritus. Because of the reported association with late fetal death it is common practice to deliver the woman by 37–38 weeks'.

Inflammatory bowel disease

Severe active Crohn's disease and ulcerative colitis can cause infertility and if active in early pregnancy will double the rate of miscarriage. Later in pregnancy active disease is associated with premature birth. The rate of relapse of inflammatory bowel disease is not influenced by pregnancy. Because of potential malabsorption a higher dose (4 mg) of folic acid for neural tube defect should be prescribed, anaemia managed and a specialist dietitian consulted to prevent malnutrition. The woman's usual medication can be given as there are no clear contraindications to steroid and sulfasalazine therapy in pregnancy. If the woman requires a caesarean section for obstetric indications, previous abdominal surgery can make access to the lower uterine segment difficult.

Appendicitis

Acute appendicitis coincidentally complicates 1 in 1500 pregnancies. The diagnosis in pregnancy is hampered as the classical symptoms of nausea, vomiting and anorexia are common occurrences of pregnancy and the upward displacement of the ileocaecal junction by the enlarging uterus, can distort the localization of the abdominal pain. If diagnosis is delayed and peritonitis and perforation occur fetal loss can be as high as 40% and maternal death can result. Therefore a high index of suspicion in the presence of unresolving abdominal pain is vital. MRI has been shown to be the most reliable imaging modality with a high sensitivity for identifying acute appendicitis. As the pregnancy advances the abdominal incision needs to be made higher so a right paramedian incision will give the best access in the second and third trimesters. Postoperatively careful observation should be kept for signs of preterm labour.

Chapter 16

Endocrine disorders in pregnancy

DIABETES MELLITUS

During pregnancy the placenta secretes substances that have an anti-insulin action, including human placental lactogen (hPL), progesterone, human chorionic gonadotrophin (hCG), cortisol and cytokines including TNFα. If the maternal β islet cells are unable to produce the additional insulin required to counteract this effect, the woman will develop hyperglycaemia (gestational diabetes). The incidence of glucose intolerance during pregnancy reflects the background prevalence of type 2 diabetes and impaired glucose tolerance. In some communities this reaches 10% or more using the current criteria.

As maternal glucose, but not insulin, can readily cross the placenta, the fetal pancreas will secrete additional insulin if there is maternal hyperglycaemia. This fetal hyperinsulinaemia can result in macrosomia, polycythaemia, impaired lung maturation, neonatal hypoglycaemia, jaundice, hypocalcaemia and hypomagnesaemia. Offspring may develop glucose intolerance in childhood and they are more prone to adult obesity.

Maternal hyperglycaemia, at the time of conception and during embryogenesis, can cause major fetal abnormalities (neural tube defects, cardiac abnormalities, skeletal abnormalities) and increase the risk of miscarriage.

Detection of gestational diabetes

Routine screening of all pregnant women for hyperglycaemia should no longer be considered controversial as two large RCTs have both shown benefit from treating gestational diabetes and the results from the Hyperglycaemia and Adverse Pregnancy Outcome study (HAPO) are being used to define the diagnostic criteria that predict an adverse perinatal outcome. The two currently most widely used criteria are detailed in Table 16.1.

Women who are more likely to develop gestational diabetes are those who have a previous history of gestational diabetes; who suffered an intra-uterine death late in pregnancy; who have a close family member or members who are diabetic; who are from an ethnic group with a high prevalence of type 2 diabetes; who are older than 30 years, who have persistent glycosuria, or where there is

Table 16.1 The diagnosis of gestational diabetes

	ORAL GLUCOSE LOAD (g)	PLASMA GLUCOSE LEVEL (mmol/L)			
		Fasting	1 hour	2 hour	3 hour
Glucose challenge test (non-fasting)*	75		8.0		
	50		7.8		
Glucose tolerance test GTT (fasting)†	100	5.0	9.2	7.9	7.1
	(O'Sullivan and Mahan criteria)		(2 or more values exceeded)		
	75	<7.0	≥7.8–11.1		
	(WHO Criteria)				

*If the plasma glucose exceeds these values GTT should be done. †If fasting ≥7.0 or 2 hour ≥11.1 then classified WHO diabetes

fetal macrosomia should be tested early in pregnancy, ideally before they conceive. If the test is negative they should be retested at the beginning of the third trimester when all women should be screened.

Management of diabetes

Pre-pregnancy advice

Ideally, women who are known to be diabetic and women who have had gestational diabetes should be seen before they become pregnant. This consultation offers the opportunity to explain to the woman the reasons for meticulously maintaining her blood glucose at normal levels before conception, and to ensure dietary advice has included taking folic acid to reduce the risk of neural tube defects. Each woman needs to be assessed for the presence of any complications associated with diabetes, such as diabetic retinopathy and nephropathy. Women who are taking oral hypoglycaemic agents should preferably be changed to insulin therapy.

Pregnancy

In pregnancy the key principles of management include:

- A multidisciplinary team, including an endocrinologist, a diabetic educator, a dietitian, a neonatologist and obstetrician, is desirable for management.
- Euglycaemia should be maintained throughout, with fasting blood glucose less than 5.0 mmol/L and if measured 1 hour after eating less than 8 mmol/L and 2 hours after eating less than 7 mmol/L.
- Ultrasound examination in the first 12 weeks of pregnancy provides accurate dating of the pregnancy, and ultrasound between 18 and 20 weeks of pregnancy allows exclusion of any major malformations and, around 34 weeks of pregnancy, permits assessment of fetal growth. Ultrasound scans may be performed more often if there is any suspicion of abnormal fetal growth.

- Fetal wellbeing is monitored with fetal movement counts, Doppler umbilical blood flow and cardiotocography (see Ch. 20 for management of high-risk pregnancy).
- Optimal time for delivery is different for each case and is determined by the presence or absence of complications.
- The woman should be delivered in a hospital with neonatal facilities and facilities for performing an urgent caesarean section.

Maternal complications

Women with diabetes are more prone to pre-eclampsia (especially if there are any microvascular complications), urinary tract infections, polyhydramnios and candida vaginitis. Diabetic ketoacidosis must be avoided as it may cause fetal death. The incidence of the complications (Table 16.2) depends largely on the quality of the care and blood glucose control of the diabetic woman before and during pregnancy.

Management of gestational diabetes

Many women with gestational diabetes can maintain euglycaemia by diet and exercise alone, but up to 60% may need insulin therapy. The same principles of management are used for women with diabetes prior to pregnancy. Fetal and maternal complications are less frequent in gestational diabetes and the risk of congenital abnormalities is not increased, as diabetes does not arise in early pregnancy. Oral hypoglycaemic agents, although not currently the treatment of choice, have been successfully used to achieve euglycaemia, especially in women who are unable or unwilling to use insulin.

Timing of delivery

Most diabetic women whose diabetes is well controlled will be able to continue their pregnancy to full term.

Table 16.2 The effects of diabetes mellitus on pregnancy	
CONDITION	**RISK (PERCENTAGE OF WOMEN AFFECTED)**
Pre-eclampsia	10–20
Polyhydramnios	20–25
Bacteriuria	7–10
Congenital malformations	6
Perinatal mortality	20–100 per 1000

If metabolic control has been inadequate and polyhydramnios or fetal macrosomia is present, delivery by 38 weeks is indicated.

Management of labour

Labour can be induced in the usual way, and the fetus monitored as for any high-risk pregnancy. Blood glucose levels need to be monitored at frequent intervals and, if necessary, an infusion of short-acting insulin can be given. The fetus should be monitored throughout labour. During vaginal delivery shoulder dystocia should be anticipated.

The risk of shoulder dystocia is 14% if the birthweight is between 4000 and 4500 g (twice that for the offspring of non-diabetic women) and 52% for birthweights greater than 4500 g (three times greater); consequently, elective caesarean section is recommended if the estimated fetal weight is more than 4000 g. A caesarean section may be performed if there is significant macrosomia or non-reassuring fetal status, or if labour fails to progress satisfactorily. Uncomplicated diabetes is not an indication for operative delivery.

As maternal insulin requirements quickly return to prepregnancy levels after delivery, monitoring of blood glucose levels is important.

The newborn baby

Following delivery the baby (Fig. 16.1) should be carefully assessed by a neonatologist. Early feeding with oral glucose if necessary is important to minimize the risk of neonatal hypoglycaemia. The blood glucose levels should be monitored before each feed for the following 2 days. If hypoglycaemia persists the baby may require enteral feeding or intravenous glucose or glucagon.

Babies of diabetic mothers who had difficulty controlling their blood glucose during pregnancy are likely to have poor temperature control, to feed slowly, and to be jaundiced, hypocalcaemic and hypomagnesaemic. If these babies are born before term they are more likely

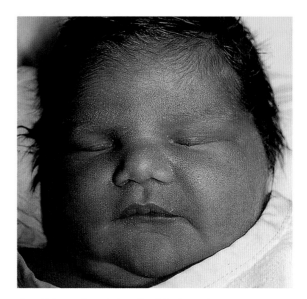

Fig. 16.1 Newborn baby of a diabetic mother.

to develop the respiratory distress syndrome because there is delayed resorption of lung fluid, which causes transient tachypnoea in the newborn baby.

Later in life these babies are at risk of developing abnormal glucose tolerance and obesity, particularly if the mother's diabetic control has been suboptimal.

Follow-up of women who have had gestational diabetes

Follow-up is important as up to 50% of women with gestational diabetes may develop overt diabetes, usually type 2, and if this is detected early there is an opportunity to minimize the development of the complications of diabetes. Regular testing for hyperglycaemia should be performed, at least every 2 years if the GTT is normal and they are of child-bearing age, thereafter every 3 years, and every year if there is impaired fasting or impaired glucose tolerance.

At these follow-up visits women who have had gestational diabetes can be encouraged to follow a diet appropriate for a diabetic, avoiding refined carbohydrates and ensuring adequate dietary fibre. Because of the risk of developing diabetes they should be advised to take the following measures:

- Avoid becoming overweight or obese
- Take regular exercise
- Avoid cigarette smoking
- Be checked annually for hypertension.

These women should also be reminded that they have a 50% chance of developing gestational diabetes in a future pregnancy. If the woman is intending to become pregnant again, testing for hyperglycaemia immediately before conception is recommended. Otherwise, testing should be done as soon as possible in early pregnancy.

THYROID DISEASE

Autoimmune hyperthyroidism (Graves' disease)

Autoimmune hyperthyroidism (Graves' disease) may precede pregnancy or may arise in pregnancy because of the hypermetabolic state of the mother. Untreated hyperthyroidism carries an increased risk of premature delivery (10–25%), growth restriction and fetal death (8–15%). In pregnancy, treatment with propylthiouracil (starting with 100 mg 8-hourly and titrating according to thyroid-stimulating hormone (TSH) and T_4 levels and clinical symptoms) is preferred as it inhibits thyroxine synthesis and the peripheral conversion of T_4 to T_3. It does cross the placenta, and so consequently the objective is to maintain the free T_4 index in the normal range so that the fetus does not become hypothyroid. Ultrasound examination of the fetus is used to assess fetal heart rate, goitre and growth particularly if the mother remains hyperthyroid. Labour is usually uneventful and a thyroid storm is rarely seen in pregnancy. About 10% of neonates become thyrotoxic in the neonatal period because of the transplacental passage of thyroid-stimulating immunoglobulins. Affected babies can be identified during pregnancy by measuring the level of maternal TSH receptor antibody in the last trimester.

Parenchymatous (colloid) goitre

Although the mother's thyroid gland enlarges in pregnancy, it is uncommon for it to cause symptoms. The cause of the goitre is partly due to decreased absorption of iodine in the first half of pregnancy. A pregnant woman should take iodized table salt to prevent the fetus developing colloid goitre.

Hypothyroidism

The most common causes of hypothyroidism in women in the reproductive age group are Hashimoto's thyroiditis, surgery (thyroidectomy) and radiotherapy for thyroid carcinoma. Also at risk are women with other autoimmune diseases such as type 1 diabetes. Inadequately treated hypothyroidism increases the risk of infertility, pre-eclampsia, growth restriction, premature birth, placental abruption and fetal death. In early pregnancy an increased need for thyroxine occurs that is associated with a rise in T_3 and T_4, which plateaus at about the 30th week. In women with hypothyroidism this rise cannot occur, and these women need more thyroxine than when not pregnant. The preferred replacement is the pure T_4 preparation levothyroxine. The extra quantity needed can be estimated from the serum thyroid-stimulating hormone (TSH, or thyrotrophin) level, a fall indicating a need for more thyroxine, above the average daily dose of 100 μg, as required. The compliance of the patient should be ensured, as insufficient thyroxine may increase maternal and fetal morbidity.

PITUITARY DISEASE

Prolactin-secreting adenomas

Women with known macroadenomas should be treated with surgery or radiation before becoming pregnant, as up to 33% develop symptoms during pregnancy (headaches, visual field defects) if untreated. Microadenomas rarely (5%) cause symptoms, and if enlargement is detected this can be treated with bromocriptine. There are no particular complications associated with labour, and breastfeeding is not contraindicated.

Diabetes insipidus

This disorder is rarely encountered in pregnancy and the treatment is synthetic vasopressin (DDAVP) administered intranasally. Oxytocin release is independent of vasopressin secretion, and thus labour and lactation are not usually affected by the condition.

ADRENAL DISEASE

Cushing syndrome

Women with untreated Cushing syndrome are usually infertile owing to the inhibition of gonadotrophin release by the excess androgen secretion. Pregnancies in women with treated Cushing syndrome are complicated by an increased risk of preterm delivery and hypertension (both up to 66%) and perinatal deaths (7%). These complications appear to be more common with adrenal adenomas than with hyperplasia. Non-suppressible tumours may need to be treated surgically, and this is associated with an improved pregnancy outcome.

Addison disease

In treated women the pregnancy is usually uneventful, replacement therapy is given with cortisone acetate and fludrocortisone acetate, and additional doses are required during the stress of labour and delivery.

Phaeochromocytoma

This may present in pregnancy as a hypertensive crisis or as severe pre-eclampsia. Diagnosis is made by detecting elevated catecholamines in a 24-hour urine collection. If detected before 24 weeks surgical excision is usually performed; after this time, phenoxybenzamine is used to achieve stabilization, with delivery by caesarean section when fetal maturity is assured, to avoid the excessive catecholamine release associated with labour.

Chapter 17

Infections during pregnancy

With the exception of poliomyelitis, pregnancy does not alter a woman's resistance to infection. The severity of any infection, however, correlates positively with its effect on the fetus. For example, the more severe the infection and the earlier in pregnancy it occurs, the greater is the risk of miscarriage or of intra-uterine death of the fetus.

Infections have an indirect and a direct effect on the fetus. The indirect effect operates by reducing the oxygenation of the placental blood, and by altering the nutrient exchange through the placenta. The direct effect depends on the ability of the invading organism to penetrate the placenta and infect the fetus. Viruses, being smaller than bacteria, are able to do this more easily. At first, the virus multiplies in the trophoblast and subsequently invades the fetus. Most viral infections do not affect the fetus unless the mother's infection is very severe. Three exceptions to this are rubella, cytomegalovirus and herpes simplex infections. These infections may cause congenital defects. The clinical effects of infections are microcephaly, congenital heart disease, eye damage (such as cataract), deafness, hepatosplenomegaly (with jaundice), purpura and, later in childhood, mental handicap.

As maternal antibodies cross the placenta they offer the fetus a degree of immunity, except in the case of a primary infection. The fetus becomes immunologically competent from about the 14th week of gestation, but the efficacy of this protection is low until the second half of pregnancy.

URINARY TRACT INFECTION

Urinary tract infection is the most disturbing of the bacterial infections. It occurs because the urinary tract dilates owing to the relaxation of the muscles of the ureter and the bladder in pregnancy, with consequent urinary stasis.

Asymptomatic bacteriuria

The prevalence of asymptomatic bacteriuria (defined as more than 100 000 bacteria per mL of urine) in pregnancy is 6%, similar to that in non-pregnant sexually active women; 30% of pregnant women who have asymptomatic bacteriuria will develop symptomatic urinary tract infection. Unless the infection is treated these women have an increased risk of delivering a low-birthweight baby, delivering prematurely and having postpartum endometritis.

Because of this risk, pregnant women should be screened for asymptomatic bacteriuria in early pregnancy. A midstream specimen of urine is sent to a laboratory for culture. In 85% of cases *Escherichia coli* is isolated, and in the remainder a variety of microorganisms are found. As the procedure is costly, other procedures, such as dip slides covered with a culture medium and reagent strips, have been developed and are reliable screening methods.

Treatment of asymptomatic bacteriuria consists of prescribing amoxicillin 500 mg/clavulanic acid 125 mg or cefalexin 2 g as a single dose or in appropriate doses for 5–7 days. Seven days after the woman has finished the antibiotics, a midstream specimen of urine is re-examined. If the asymptomatic bacteriuria has not been eliminated, a longer course of antibiotics is prescribed. Regular follow-up urine cultures must be made, and recurrences treated.

Pyelonephritis

As mentioned above, about 30% of women who have untreated bacteriuria will develop pyelonephritis during pregnancy, as will 1% of women who do not have the condition. Pyelonephritis can cause premature rupture of the membranes and perinatal death

The infection occurs when bacteria, growing in the stagnant urine, spread from the bladder to the ureter and then to the renal pelvis. Haematogenous infection is very uncommon. Pyelonephritis usually begins after the 20th week of pregnancy. In mild cases the woman complains of tiredness and urinary frequency, and occasionally dysuria. More severe infections start suddenly, with chills and rigors, fever, and pain over one or both renal areas. The patient may rapidly become dehydrated. The diagnosis is confirmed by examining a midstream specimen of urine, having excluded other causes of abdominal pain such as acute appendicitis and abruptio placentae.

Treatment consists of correcting the dehydration and prescribing appropriate antibiotics, having tested for bacterial sensitivity. In most cases, a cephalosporin or amoxicillin is appropriate initial treatment. As some women with pyelonephritis are nauseated, the antibiotic may have to be given intravenously. Follow-up examinations of a midstream urine culture at 2-week intervals for the remainder of the pregnancy should be instituted. Some authorities recommend prophylactic antibiotics for the duration of the pregnancy.

VAGINAL INFECTIONS

Vaginal infections during pregnancy due to *Candida* spp., *Trichomonas* and bacterial vaginosis are discussed on pages 260–262. The diagnosis and treatment are the same as in pregnancy.

BACTERIAL INFECTIONS

Group B streptococcus

Colonies of group B streptococci (GBS) are harboured in the lower vagina and/or rectum of 18–27% of pregnant women.

If group B streptococcal infection is present during labour the bacteria may colonize the neonate. Over half of babies born through an infected vagina are colonized, and 2–5% of them develop early onset GBS neonatal sepsis. The mortality rate for premature affected infants is 25–30%, for those at term 2–8%, and neurological sequelae for the survivors of 15–30%.

Up to 80% of cases of early-onset disease are associated with obstetric risk factors: preterm delivery, prolonged rupture of membranes for more than 18 hours, maternal fever >38° during labour. Treatment of known carriers or those at high risk with penicillin during active labour reduces both neonatal and maternal morbidity.

Two approaches to selecting those for treatment are widely used: one treats on risk factors alone, the other takes a low vaginal and a rectal swab at 36 weeks' and then treats those with positive isolates. Both regimens have been shown to be effective. See Box 17.1.

Box 17.1 **Strategies to prevent early-onset group B streptococcus (GBS) neonatal sepsis**

A. Screen all women between 35–37 weeks with low vaginal and anorectal swab

If positive or previous baby with early onset GBS or GBS bacteriuria during index pregnancy:

- Give 1.2 g IV benzylpenicillin when in labour or ruptured membranes followed by 600 mg IV 4-hourly until delivered
- If allergic to penicillin give clindamycin 600 mg IV 8-hourly or erythromycin 500 mg 6-hourly

B. Treat if positive risk factor(s)

- Premature labour before 37 weeks
- Previous early onset GBS disease
- When anticipate membranes will have been ruptured >18 hours before delivery
- Intrapartum fever ≥38.0°C
- GBS bacteriuria during pregnancy

Gonorrhoea

Depending on the population studied, between 1 and 6% of pregnant women are found to have gonorrhoea on culture studies using the Thayer–Martin medium. Many have no symptoms. In symptomatic gonorrhoea the woman complains of dysuria and a vaginal discharge which occurs within 5 days of sexual intercourse. If the symptoms suggest gonorrhoea, or if the woman's sexual behaviour suggests that she may have gonorrhoea, cervical and urethral swabs should be taken and inoculated directly on to preheated plates of culture medium. In addition, vaginal swabs should be made for other vaginal infective organisms. The management of gonococcal infection is discussed on page 264.

Syphilis

The importance of syphilitic infection in pregnancy is that treponemes are able to penetrate the placenta after the 15th week of pregnancy and infect the fetus, resulting in congenital syphilis in 20–50% and perinatal death in 20–30%. If the fetus survives the initial infection, by the time of the birth it is in the second stage of syphilis.

For this reason every pregnant woman should be offered screening for syphilis using a reagin test (either the VDRL or the rapid plasma reagin (RPR) test), although the incidence of syphilis in most areas is less than 0.1%. The test should be made at the first antenatal visit and, in regions with a high prevalence, repeated at the 30th week of pregnancy. False positives may occur, and so a woman who has had a positive screening test is investigated using a procedure that detects specific antitreponemal antibodies in her serum (e.g. the *Treponema pallidum* haemagglutination test, TPHA; the fluorescent treponemal antibody test, FTA-ABS; or the *T. pallidum* immobilization test, TPI).

The treatment is that described on page 259 for non-pregnant women. Follow-up serological tests are made monthly for 3 months, every 2 months for the next 6 months, and every 3 months for the next year.

As the signs of syphilis in a neonate are often equivocal and the serology is inaccurate, the infant of a woman who has been diagnosed as having syphilis while pregnant, and who has not had a complete course of treatment and follow-up, should be given a full course of antibiotic treatment (aqueous procaine benzylpenicillin 50 000 U/kg body weight daily for 10 days).

OTHER INFECTION

Toxoplasmosis

Toxoplasma gondii infects 2–10 pregnant women per 1000. In 90% there are no clinical signs. Infections acquired in pregnancy may lead to a miscarriage or congenital infection of the fetus, one fetus in four being affected. The risk of fetal disease is highest in the first trimester; most neonates infected in the third trimester are asymptomatic with delayed sequelae, including developmental delays. The eyes and the central nervous system may be severely damaged.

Screening tests for toxoplasma are available but are not cost-effective. If chosen they are best carried out before pregnancy, and seronegative women should be retested in each of the quarters of pregnancy.

Preventive measures taken by a pregnant woman are more cost-effective:

- A pregnant woman should avoid touching cat faeces.
- She should avoid touching her eyes or mouth while handling raw meat, wash her hands after handling it, and should only eat well-cooked meat.
- The woman should wash vegetables and fruit thoroughly before eating them and, if a gardener, should wear gloves.

A proven infection may be treated with pyrimethamine plus sulfadiazine, with supplementary folic acid to counteract their antifolate activity.

VIRAL INFECTIONS

Seven viral infections need some discussion.

Rubella

Rubella infection is widespread. By the age of 19 more than 85% of people have been infected, and nine out of 10 of those infected have lifelong immunity.

Should rubella occur in a non-immune woman in the first 14 weeks of pregnancy, viraemia and infection of the fetus are almost certain, and more than 40% of the infected fetuses will be damaged by the virus. The virus invades actively dividing cells and alters the genome. Infection in weeks 4–12 of pregnancy affects the lenses of the eyes (causing cataract) or the ears (causing deafness). Infection between the fifth and 12th weeks damages the chambers of the heart. As well as causing damage to specific organs, rubella infection may cause widespread cellular damage, leading to fetal growth restriction, thrombocytopenia, hepatosplenomegaly and vasculitis and, in particular, renal artery stenosis.

These problems could be avoided if all women were immunized against rubella between the ages of 11 and 13 using a live attenuated strain of the virus (the RA 27/3 strain). Programmes to accomplish this have been developed in many countries.

A woman should be tested for rubella antibodies either when she decides to become pregnant or at the first pregnancy visit. If this test is positive the woman is immune to rubella. A non-immune woman who is not pregnant may be offered vaccination but should avoid pregnancy for

3 months. If a pregnant woman is inadvertently vaccinated the risk of the baby being infected is extremely small: no cases of congenital rubella syndrome have been reported in these circumstances.

A problem arises when a pregnant non-immune woman develops a rubelliform rash (as in half of women the rash is not due to rubella), or if the woman has been in contact with a case of rubella. A serological test should be made as soon as possible, preferably within 15 days of the appearance of the rash or the contact. If the rubella IgG is positive the woman may be reassured that her baby is in no danger of being infected. If it is negative then a second test measuring the IgM levels should be taken 21 days later. If the woman seroconverts, the problems of congenital infection should be discussed with her and a therapeutic abortion is an option she may wish to consider.

Genital herpes

A general discussion on herpes simplex virus (HSV) can be found on this page. In pregnancy HSV may cross the placental barrier to infect the fetus, and is more likely to be found in primary than in recurrent infections. Overall the risk is low, only one fetus per 11 000 live births being infected. The transmission risk is greater during childbirth, particularly if the mother has her first attack (40–50% risk), compared with a risk of <5% for a recurrent infection.

These findings suggest that:

- A woman with a history of genital herpes need have no anxiety that her baby will be infected and may expect to be delivered vaginally, unless a recurrence of the infection or a new infection occurs during the pregnancy.
- If a first infection or a recurrence of genital herpes occurs during the pregnancy, but has healed by the time labour starts, the woman may give birth vaginally.
- If herpetic lesions are present when the membranes rupture or labour starts, a caesarean section should be performed to avoid the risk that the baby will acquire a herpetic infection during the passage through the birth canal.

The strategy of taking endocervical swabs for viral culture every 2 weeks from the 34th week of pregnancy can be abandoned, as positive HSV-infected swabs do not predict the risk of the infant being exposed to herpes infection during birth. The infant only needs treatment with aciclovir if it is clinically ill or has positive viral cultures. Severe neonatal HSV infection carries a 30% risk of neonatal death and neurological damage occurs in 40% of the survivors.

Hepatitis B

Less than 0.5% of women in the developed nations are hepatitis B carriers but, in contrast, up to 30% of migrants from parts of Africa and east and southeast Asia have hepatitis B surface antigen (HBsAg) in their blood and are potentially infectious to healthcare workers, who may be infected by contact with blood and other body secretions. Many units now screen all pregnant women for hepatitis B. Precautions are taken when caring for such women in childbirth, and most hospitals have developed appropriate protocols.

It is also known that the hepatitis B virus is readily transmitted to the baby, probably during the birth. Babies at particularly high risk are those whose mothers have HBcAg as well as HBsAg in their blood. If not treated, many of the babies will develop hepatocellular carcinoma in adulthood. This can be avoided to a large extent if babies at high risk are given hepatitis B immunoglobulin together with hepatitis B vaccine 10 µg at birth, and two further injections of the vaccine at the ages of 1 and 6 months. Many centres offer hepatitis B vaccination to all children.

Hepatitis C

Hepatitis C infection is usually contracted from needle sharing (50–70% of IV drug users are hepatitis C positive), from contaminated blood transfusions or from contaminated instruments, e.g. tattooing or body piercing. In Australia the prevalence of hepatitis C is 13/1000. The risk of vertical transmission to the fetus is 3–7%, but if associated with HIV infection and a high viral load can reach 25%.

Currently there are no effective management strategies to reduce transmission, including caesarean section and the avoidance of breastfeeding. Fetal scalp electrode application and fetal scalp blood sampling should be avoided. The antiviral agents (interferon and ribavirin) used to treat hepatitis C in the non-pregnant are teratogenic. If identified, women should be referred for specialist assessment and treatment after delivery, and the baby followed up so that it can also be treated if its HCV RNA serology stays positive after 12–18 months.

Cytomegalovirus infection (CMV)

Over half of all pregnant women show serological evidence of previous CMV infection. One per cent of women may become infected with CMV during pregnancy, most of whom are asymptomatic. The infection is associated with an increased perinatal mortality, and 3–7% of the infants have congenital abnormalities.

Screening has proved to be of no value – there is no vaccine available.

Human immunodeficiency virus infection (HIV)

Although in western countries most cases of HIV infection occur in homosexual or bisexual men, intravenous drug users who share needles are increasingly being infected, as are some heterosexual men and women who do not abuse drugs. In sub-Saharan Africa and south and southeast Asia many heterosexual women and men are HIV positive and the numbers are increasing. Infected women who become pregnant have a 30% risk of transmitting the virus to the fetus, and all infected fetuses will be antibody positive and develop AIDS. There is a strong argument that screening for HIV infection should be offered to all pregnant women, particularly as the use of antiretroviral drugs antenatally and intrapartum, delivery by caesarean section and bottle feeding can significantly reduce the risk of vertical transmission of the disease to 2%.

HIV infection has no adverse effect on pregnancy, nor has the pregnancy any adverse effect on the progress of HIV infection. As the HIV infects the amniotic fluid as well as the women's blood, full infectious disease control precautions should be taken by attendant medical staff during labour and childbirth. Delivery by caesarean section reduces the risk of transmission to the baby by 50%; vaginal delivery may be considered if the viral load is <1000 copies per mL. Coexisting STIs, chorioamnionitis and ruptured membranes for more than 4 hours quadruple the risk for the baby. If vaginal delivery is undertaken then invasive procedures such as fetal scalp electrodes, scalp blood sampling and episiotomies should be avoided, the baby should be washed as soon as possible, and given AZT (azathioprine) within 8 hours of delivery and for the next 6 weeks. In communities where access to triple therapy is limited a single dose of nevirapine 200 mg at the onset of labour reduces the vertical transmission. The decision on whether or not to breastfeed will depend on the risk of other infections due to suboptimal hygiene in the preparation of formula feeds.

Chickenpox (varicella)

Varicella infection is common, over 80% of pregnant women testing positive for IgG antibodies to the varicella zoster virus (VZV). Primary infection can result in serious complications for both mother and baby, because during pregnancy the maternal immune system is less efficient. Pneumonia occurs in 10% of women and can result in death. If the infection occurs in the first trimester, 0.4% and in the second trimester 2% of the fetuses are infected, and the viral vesicles can cause a wide spectrum of abnormalities, including limb hypoplasia, microcephaly, cortical atrophy, cataracts, psychomotor retardation, convulsions and intrauterine growth restriction. If the maternal infection becomes apparent 7 days before or 7 days after delivery, the baby is at risk of developing disseminated varicella infection, as maternal antibody production will not yet be adequate.

If there is doubt about the diagnosis or previous history of infection, maternal blood should be taken for anti-VZV, IgG and IgM antibodies. If there is a high risk of maternal or fetal complications, the mother should be given 12.5 units per kg of VZV immunoglobulin (VZIG)

intramuscularly within 96 hours of exposure. For severe maternal infection, aciclovir 10–15 mg/kg should be given every 8 hours. An infected infant may be given VZIG and aciclovir.

Many communities offer varicella zoster vaccination, and this should be considered for women who are seronegative before they conceive.

INFECTIONS IN THE TROPICS

Helminth infestations – hookworm disease

Endemic infections by helminths are almost universal among rural dwellers in the tropics and subtropics, and the most serious of these is hookworm disease. Two types of hookworm are found, *Ancylostoma duodenale* and *Necator americanus*. In the gut the worms attach to the villi by suckers, and feed on blood obtained from the villi; after passing through their bodies this blood is excreted into the lumen of the bowel. The blood loss due to hookworm is related closely to the hookworm load, and varies from 2 to 90 mL/day. Hookworm infestation is a cause of iron deficiency anaemia, and this is particularly serious in pregnancy. Treatment consists of eliminating the worms by administering bephenium hydroxynaphthoate (Alcopar) in a dose of 5 g daily for 3 days, and treating the anaemia with iron.

Malaria

Exacerbation of malaria, or relapse in a partially immune woman, is particularly common during pregnancy, and each attack may precipitate abortion or the onset of premature labour. The fetus is protected by the placenta in most cases, although large numbers of immobilized parasites may be found in the placenta, particularly if the infection is by *Plasmodium falciparum*. Occasionally, in non-immune patients, congenital transmission of malaria occurs.

Pregnant women travelling to an area where malaria is endemic should take prophylactic antimalarial drugs. If the strains of *P. falciparum* in the area are chloroquine resistant, problems arise. The alternative drugs, Fansidar and Maloprim, affect folic acid synthesis and may induce a fatal Stevens–Johnson syndrome. They should be avoided. If the risk of chloroquine resistance is low, chloroquine and proguanil should be given. If the risk of chloroquine resistance is high, a pregnant woman should postpone her visit until she has given birth.

Any pregnant woman developing a high fever in a malarial area should be suspected of having the infection, and if this is confirmed by finding parasites in a thick blood film, treatment is given with chloroquine 600 mg (base) initially, followed 8 hours later by 300 mg, and 300 mg daily for the next 3 days.

Diseases of the placenta and membranes

ABNORMAL PLACENTATION

The shape of the definitive placenta is determined at the time the placenta forms, the variations found (Fig. 18.1) mostly having no clinical significance.

The umbilical cord may enter the placenta at its midpoint, may join it at an edge (marginal insertion of the cord), or the umbilical vessels may run some distance along the membranes (velamentous insertion of the cord). Should the vessels run across the cervix they may be compressed by the fetal head during labour, or bleed causing fetal anaemia. In some cases the placenta is smaller than the chorionic plate and the trophoblast invades the decidua laterally more deeply, giving a ridged appearance on the placental surface (placenta circumvallata). In most cases this has no clinical significance, but occasionally may be found in women who have antepartum or intrapartum haemorrhage. In other cases the placenta has an accessory lobe separated by membranes from the main placenta (placenta succenturiata).

In a few cases the trophoblastic invasion is not regulated by maternal immune defences and the myometrium is invaded, causing placenta accreta, increta or percreta. Haemangiomata occur in 1% of placentae. In most cases they are small and of no clinical significance, but larger haemangiomata may be associated with polyhydramnios, antepartum haemorrhage or preterm labour.

GESTATIONAL TROPHOBLASTIC DISEASE

Gestational trophoblastic disease is uncommon affecting 1/750 pregnancies of women of non-Asian ethnicity but 1/380 of those from Asia. It is potentially lethal, but with treatment a 98% cure rate is attainable. The disease occurs in two forms (Box 18.1).

Hydatidiform mole

The tumour may have completely or partially replaced the placenta (Fig. 18.2). In the complete form, hydropic swelling and vesicle formation is associated with trophoblastic proliferation and a paucity or absence of blood vessels within the villi (Fig. 18.3). No fetus can be found. Five per cent of complete moles undergo malignant change.

In the partial form a fetus is present but areas of the placenta show the changes described for the complete mole. Partial moles become malignant less frequently (0.05%).

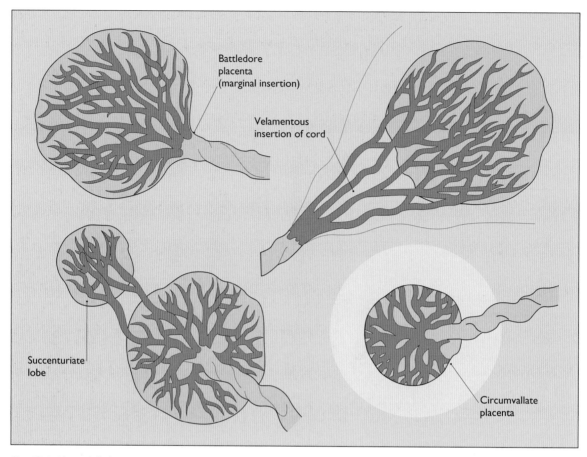

Fig. 18.1 Abnormal placentation.

Malignant trophoblastic disease

The tumour may be confined to the uterus (invasive mole) or spread via the bloodstream to distant organs (choriocarcinoma).

In the invasive mole the trophoblast-covered villi penetrate the myometrial fibres and may extend to other organs, the appearance of the villi remaining that of the benign tumour.

Box 18.1 **Classification of trophoblastic neoplasms**

Benign trophoblastic disease (hydatidiform mole)

Complete hydatidiform mole
Partial hydatidiform mole
Hydropic degeneration of the trophoblast

Persistent trophoblastic disease (often malignant)

Apparently confined to the uterus (invasive mole)
Usually with extra-uterine spread (choriocarcinoma)

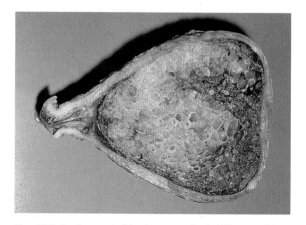

Fig. 18.2 Benign trophoblastic tumour (hydatidiform mole): gross specimen. Note the grape-like masses.

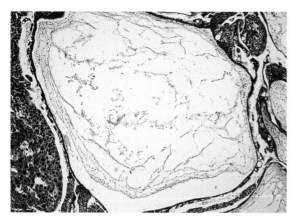

Fig. 18.3 Microphotograph of a benign trophoblastic tumour (hydatidiform mole), showing the distended villi and irregular trophoblastic proliferation.

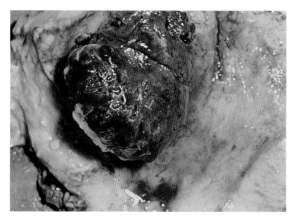

Fig. 18.4 Choriocarcinoma.

In choriocarcinoma (Fig. 18.4) the tumour is characterized by sheets of trophoblastic cells, both syncytio- and cytotrophoblasts, with few or no villi formed.

Aetiology

Gestational trophoblastic disease is caused by a genetic disorder in which a spermatozoon enters an ovum that has lost its nucleus, or in which two sperms enter the ovum. In over 90% of complete moles only paternal genes are found, and in 10% the mole is heterozygous. In contrast, partial moles usually have a triploid chromosomal constitution, with two sets of paternal haploid genes and one set of maternal haploid genes.

The development of gestational trophoblastic tumours is thought to be due to a defective maternal immune response to the invasion by the trophoblast. In consequence, the villi become distended with nutrients. The primitive vasculature within each villus does not form

properly, with the result that the embryo starves, dies and is absorbed, whereas the trophoblast continues to thrive and, in certain circumstances, invades the maternal tissues.

The increased syncytiotrophoblast activity leads to an increased production of human chorionic gonadotrophin (hCG), chorionic thyrotrophin and progesterone. A fall in oestradiol secretion occurs, as oestradiol synthesis requires enzymes from the fetus, which does not exist. The raised hCG levels may induce the development of theca lutein cysts of the ovary.

Diagnosis of benign gestational trophoblastic disease

The first sign is bleeding per vaginam, which tends to persist. The bleeding may be followed fairly soon by uterine contractions and the expulsion of grape-like material. In other cases the tumour grows without symptoms. During this time examination will show the following features:

- The uterus is usually larger than expected from the gestational dates and is 'doughy' to the touch.
- Fetal heart sounds cannot be heard.
- Ultrasonic scanning shows a distinct speckled appearance (Fig. 18.5).
- If serum hCG is measured it is found to be unexpectedly high (Fig. 18.6).

Treatment

If the patient is admitted expelling the tumour, no immediate treatment is needed unless the expulsion slows down, at which time a digital evacuation of the uterus is carried out. Blood is obtained for possible transfusion, as the expulsion is often accompanied by marked blood loss.

If the diagnosis is reached before the expulsion of any vesicles, the uterus may be evacuated using a suction curette. The administration of prostaglandins or oxytocics

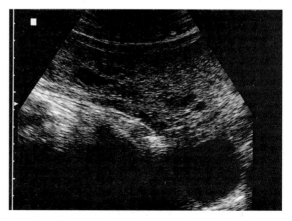

Fig. 18.5 Twin gestation at 16 weeks with a hydatidiform mole on the right and a fetus and normal placenta on the left.

143

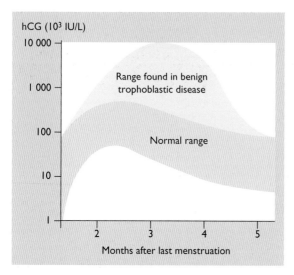

Fig. 18.6 Chorionic gonadotrophin excretion in trophoblastic disease. The normal range is shown in pink; levels found in trophoblastic disease are shown in the blue area.

to induce contractions should be avoided as these may lead to the intravascular dissemination of trophoblast. Gentle curettage may be performed later to remove any residual trophoblast. Some authorities give a single course of chemotherapy if they think that the woman presents with increased risk factors. If bleeding persists for more than 21 days a further curettage may be indicated.

Women over the age of 40, or women who have completed their family, may prefer to have a hysterectomy, to avoid potential malignancy.

Follow-up

Follow-up is important as the disease persists in between 5 and 10% of cases, often developing a malignant form. Follow-up is primarily by serial β-hCG assays as outlined in Box 18.2 and Figure 18.7. Many countries have a molar register so compliance with follow-up can be monitored.

Malignant gestational trophoblastic disease

Malignancy follows a complete mole in 15% of cases and 0.5% after a partial mole. It follows a spontaneous abortion in 1 in 5000 cases, and a viable pregnancy in 1 in 50 000 cases.

Women who have had a benign gestational trophoblastic tumour are at greater risk of developing a malignancy if the woman:

- Is over the age of 40
- Secretes large amounts of β-hCG (>100 000 IU/mL)
- Has theca lutein cyst(s) more than 6 cm in diameter.

> ### Box 18.2 Follow-up of benign trophoblastic disease using a specific radioimmunoassay
>
> 1. Radioimmunoassay of serum β-hCG at 7–10-day intervals. If the level falls serially no drug treatment is needed. Complete disappearance of β-hCG takes 12–14 weeks on average.
> 2. When β-hCG level has been normal for 3 consecutive weeks, test monthly for 6 months.
> 3. If the assay shows normal β-hCG levels for 6 consecutive months, follow-up can be discontinued.
> 4. During the follow-up period pregnancy should be avoided. Oral contraceptives may be prescribed.
> 5. If the serum β-hCG level plateaus for more than 3 consecutive weeks, or rises, or if metastases are detected, treat with methotrexate or actinomycin D.

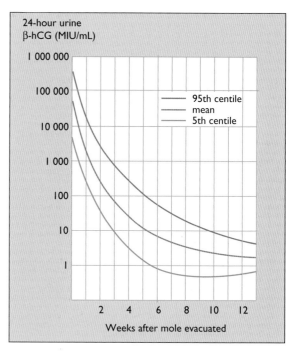

Fig. 18.7 Hormone follow-up of benign trophoblastic disease (mean and 95% confidence limits).

Malignant gestational trophoblastic disease is best managed at special centres, where meticulous follow-up is conducted. Treatment is by chemotherapy (Table 18.1) and follow-up is shown in Box 18.3.

Following a molar pregnancy and after their β-hCG have returned to normal, women should be offered contraceptive therapy and advised not to conceive for a further 6 months. The risk of a further mole in a subsequent pregnancy is 1 in 55.

Table 18.1 Chemotherapy in malignant trophoblastic disease

	NON-METASTATIC mg/kg IM	METASTATIC mg/kg IM
Initial course		
Methotrexate at 48-hour intervals for 4 doses	1	1.5
Folic acid (citrovorum factor) on alternate days, 24 hours after the injection of methotrexate	0.1	0.15
Subsequent courses 1. If response, i.e. a fall in the β-hCG level <20%, repeat the regimen 2. Without response, increase methotrexate by 0.5 mg/kg and folic acid by 0.05 mg/kg 3. If no response after two consecutive courses change to actinomycin D 4. If no response to actinomycin D after two courses change to three chemotherapeutic drugs used in combination. Currently etoposide + methotrexate + cyclophosphamide (or vincristine) are recommended		
Laboratory tests Full blood count, platelet count, SGOT (serum glutamic oxaloacetic transaminase) on day 1 (before starting therapy) and days 3, 5, 7, 11, 15, 18, 21		

Box 18.3 **Principles of the management of malignant trophoblastic disease**

1. During treatment the serum levels of the β-hCG are assayed each week.
2. Provided that the β-hCG level continues to fall after a course of chemotherapy, withhold further courses.
3. When the β-hCG level is normal for 3 consecutive weeks, assay each month for 6 months.
4. If the β-hCG level remains normal for 12 months, discontinue follow-up. Patients should avoid pregnancy throughout this period.
5. Repeat the course of chemotherapy if the β-hCG level plateaus for more than 3 consecutive weeks, or rises, or if new metastases are detected.
6. If the β-hCG level plateaus after 3 consecutive courses of chemotherapeutic agent, or if it rises during a course, change to another chemotherapeutic regimen.

ABNORMALITIES OF THE AMNIOTIC FLUID

Amniotic fluid is secreted into the amniotic sac by the amniotic cells, which lie over the placenta. The fluid is 99% water and increases in quantity during pregnancy. In the amniotic sac it is swallowed by the fetus. Most of the swallowed fluid is absorbed by the fetal intestinal villi and enters the fetal circulation. From the circulation most is exchanged in the placenta, but some is returned to the amniotic sac by transudation through the fetal skin. In the last quarter of pregnancy fetal urination adds to the amniotic fluid.

Polyhydramnios

Polyhydramnios is caused by increased secretion of amniotic fluid because of a large placenta, or by a fetal malformation that prevents the fetus swallowing the fluid or prevents the absorption of the fluid through the fetal intestinal villi. Examples of the former are multiple pregnancy and diabetes and, of the latter, anencephaly, spina bifida, and atresia of the upper gastrointestinal tract.

The fluid may accumulate rapidly (acute polyhydramnios), which causes considerable distress to the mother. She may develop dyspnoea, tachycardia, vomiting and severe abdominal pain. It is most frequently associated with monochorionic twins. Treatment consists of removing amniotic fluid by amniocentesis, repeated if necessary. Laser ablation of the communicating vessels on the surface of the placenta is effective therapy when there is evidence of twin to twin transfusion. The slow accumulation of amniotic fluid is more commonly found (chronic polyhydramnios). Symptoms similar to those of acute polyhydramnios may be experienced by the expectant mother, and examination shows a distended uterus from which a fluid thrill can be obtained. Ultrasound scanning will confirm the diagnosis and identify the presence of either a multiple pregnancy or a fetal abnormality (in most cases).

Treatment

A patient who has a minor degree of polyhydramnios may be relieved by sedation at night. If the symptoms become worse between 30 and 35 weeks of pregnancy, an amniocentesis using a spinal needle to remove no more than 500 mL at any one time (to reduce the onset of preterm labour) may be performed, although half the women go into labour as a result. After the 35th week labour may be induced by vaginal amniocentesis if the symptoms become worse, or if a gross fetal malformation is present. The liquor should be released slowly to prevent cord prolapse. Postpartum haemorrhage is likely and prophylactic oxytocin should be given.

The baby or babies should be examined carefully to detect fetal malformations, including oesophageal and duodenal atresia.

Oligohydramnios

Oligohydramnios is caused by defective liquor-secreting cells or, in late pregnancy, by renal tract malformations that prevent fetal urination; it also occurs in postdatism and following rupture of the membranes. If oligohydramnios occurs early in pregnancy abortion is usual. Should the pregnancy continue, amniotic bands may develop which may damage the fetus. Later in pregnancy, oligohydramnios may cause pulmonary hypoplasia pressure deformities, such as wry neck, altered shape of the skull or club foot, and the fetal skin is dry and leathery. If oligohydramnios is suspected a detailed ultrasound should be undertaken.

In labour the lack of amniotic fluid may lead to umbilical compression and fetal distress. Some obstetricians try to prevent this complication by the transcervical infusion of saline into the amniotic sac.

ABNORMALITIES OF THE UMBILICAL CORD

A normal umbilical cord is 45–60 cm long, but extremes of 2 cm and 200 cm have been recorded. The umbilical cord usually contains one vein and two arteries set in Wharton's jelly. In 1% of cords only one artery is formed, and this may be associated with congenital malformations. Long cords have no clinical significance unless they form a coil, or coils, around the fetal neck. A cord of normal length may be shortened by coiling around the fetus. During childbirth the cord may be pulled tight as the fetus descends, reducing the oxygen supply and, occasionally, causing fetal death. Knots, either true or false, may occur in the umbilical cord. True knots may lead to a reduced fetal circulation. False knots are accumulations of Wharton's jelly and have no clinical significance.

Chapter | **19** |

Variations in the duration of pregnancy

The duration of human pregnancy averages 260 days from conception and 280 ± 14 days from the first day of the last menstrual period. In 7–13% (Australia and USA respectively) of pregnancies the duration of pregnancy is curtailed and a preterm birth (less than 36 completed weeks) occurs. In 7% of cases the pregnancy is prolonged, defined as gestation more than 41 completed weeks (i.e. 41 weeks and 6 days).

PREMATURE OR PRETERM BIRTH

There are some problems inherent in defining preterm birth as one that occurs before the 36th completed week of pregnancy. This is because the survival of the neonate depends not only on the duration of the pregnancy, but also on the baby's birthweight.

Studies of preterm births show that premature birth may be associated with low social class, young maternal age, eating disorders leading to a low body weight (body mass index <19), fetal abnormalities, multiple pregnancy and smoking. Preterm births may also be associated with medical complications, such as a history of abortion or stillbirth, uterine bleeding in pregnancy (threatened abortion, abruptio placentae and placenta praevia), hypertensive disorders and anaemia.

Bacterial vaginosis (see p. 262) has been implicated, which has been associated with an increase in preterm birth two to three times that of women who do not have bacterial vaginosis (15–20% compared with 6%). A Cochrane review of antibiotic therapy to eradicate bacterial vaginosis showed that it was effective in reducing the incidence of preterm birth, but only in women with a previous history of spontaneous premature delivery (RR 0.37). Progesterone as a depot intramuscular injection or as pessaries reduces the recurrence of preterm birth by 35%. Treatment with metronidazole actually increases the rate of preterm birth. It should also be noted that a large number of preterm births follow a spontaneous rupture of the membranes from unknown causes (Table 19.1).

Prevention of preterm birth

Ceasing smoking is an effective way of preventing preterm birth, leading to a reduction of 16% in preterm birth and 19% reduction in low birthweight. Increased contact with health professionals to provide better social support (France), the prophylactic use of tocolytic agents such as terbutaline (Germany), uterine activity monitoring at home or in hospital (USA) or bed rest in early pregnancy have been tried and have not been shown to be effective.

Regular antenatal examinations will detect medical conditions complicating pregnancy at an early stage of their development, but it is uncertain if this will reduce the incidence of preterm birth. Cervical cerclage increases the duration of pregnancy in women who have a diagnosis of incompetent cervix, but not in other cases.

Table 19.1 Causes of curtailment of pregnancy and prematurity

CAUSE	PERCENTAGE
No cause found (including premature rupture of the membrane)	35–45
Hypertensive disorders	18–30
Multiple pregnancy	12–18
Maternal disease	5–15
Abruptio placentae	5–7
Placenta praevia	3–4
Fetal malformations	1–2

PRETERM LABOUR

The diagnosis of preterm labour must be made carefully or women who are having mild contractions, which do not cause cervical dilatation, will be included. The criteria for diagnosis are:

- The gestational period is less than 36 completed weeks.
- Uterine contractions, preferably recorded on a tocograph, occur every 5–10 minutes, last for at least 30 seconds and persist for at least 60 minutes.
- The cervix is more than 2.5 cm dilated and more than 75% effaced.

Using these criteria, two-thirds of women presenting with presumed preterm labour will not be in labour. They need reassurance, not drug treatment.

A confirmatory test is to measure fetal fibronectin, which in cases of preterm labour is released into cervical and vaginal secretions. A negative test means that it is very unlikely that the woman will deliver within 7 days (negative predictive value approaches 100%). A positive test can occur in association with coitus, vaginal infection and examination. Its specificity is low and positive predictive value is 35–50%. Its main benefit is to reduce the need to transfer women in possible preterm labour to tertiary units and/or to commence tocolytic therapy.

If the criteria are met, the woman is in preterm labour. If the pregnancy is less than 35 completed weeks' gestation and the woman is not in a facility with a neonatal intensive care unit, she should have uterine contractions suppressed and be transferred as soon as possible to such a facility. If she has access to neonatal intensive care the choice is to attempt to suppress uterine activity or to permit labour to proceed. In some third-level hospitals women who start preterm labour at or after the 34th week of gestation are permitted to

proceed, as the premature infant can be competently cared for with no increase in perinatal mortality.

The greatest challenge is the management of a woman whose labour starts when the gestation period is less than 34 completed weeks.

Management of preterm labour of less than 34 completed weeks

The major risk to the fetus is pulmonary immaturity. The principal objective of management is to enhance surfactant production in the fetal lungs to prevent hyaline membrane disease. The usefulness of bed rest to prevent premature rupture of membranes is uncertain. To be effective corticosteroids, two doses of 11.4 mg betamethasone 24 hours apart, must be given to the mother more than 24 hours and less than 10 days before birth. The corticosteroids also reduce the chance of intraventricular haemorrhage in these infants. After 34 weeks' gestation this treatment is no longer necessary, as lung maturation is adequate. The common practice of repeating the corticosteroids 7–10 days later if delivery has not occurred has been questioned, as a number of animal studies have reported effects associated with changes in the development of the central nervous system, pancreatic function and growth restriction. The most recent randomized control trial of one further course of betamethasone reported a reduction in neonatal morbidity without any apparent increased risk.

Once labour is established, tocolytic therapy can be administered (Table 19.2) to postpone delivery for at least 24 hours to allow steroid-induced lung maturation to occur. This time can also permit the mother to be transferred to a hospital with neonatal intensive care facilities.

The current tocolytic drug of choice is the calcium-channel blocker nifedipine, which has been shown in a Cochrane analysis of 12 random controlled trials (RCTs) to be superior to the β mimetics, reducing the number of women delivering within 7 days (RR 0.76). In addition there were significantly fewer neonatal complications, including necrotizing enterocolitis, respiratory distress syndrome, intraventricular haemorrhage and jaundice. Of major importance is that few women taking nifedipine had to stop treatment because of side-effects. Other drugs such as nitric oxide donors – nitroglycerin or magnesium sulphate – have not been shown to be effective tocolytic agents. There is insufficient evidence to recommend continuation of any oral therapy after successful inhibition of uterine contractions.

Before starting tocolytic therapy, the following conditions should apply:

- The pregnancy is less than 35 weeks.
- There has been confirmation of preterm labour.
- The cervix is less than 5 cm dilated.
- There is no evidence of abruptio placentae.
- There is no evidence of chorioamnionitis.
- The fetus is alive and no potentially lethal malformations have been detected by ultrasound.

Table 19.2 Tocolytic drugs in the management of preterm labour

DRUG	DOSE	SIDE-EFFECTS
Calcium-channel blocker		
Nifedipine	10 mg orally; repeated 20 min later if contractions persist (max. 40 mg in first hour). If contractions cease, 20 mg by mouth 4–6-hourly	Substantially less than with beta agonists. Principal side-effect: headache; others: hypotension, nausea, palpitation
Beta agonists		
Salbutamol	Infused at 4 µg/min, increasing by 4 µg/min every 20 min until uterine contractions suppressed; dose maintained for 6 hours and then reduced. Oral salbutamol started 8 mg 6-hourly for 5 days	Tachycardia, palpitations, apprehension, anxiety. Increase in cardiac output. Pressure in the chest
Ritodrine	Infused at 50 µg/min increased by 50 µg every 10 min until the contractions cease. Maximum dose 350 µg/min. Run for 24 hours then oral ritodrine 10–20 mg 2–6-hourly	Hypokalaemia. Pulmonary oedema and myocardial ischaemia in 5%. Fluid retention in all women

Note: Calcium-channel blockers and beta agonists are relatively ineffective if the cervical dilatation is >5 cm.

These exclusions mean that fewer than 15% of women in preterm labour should receive tocolytic drugs.

The membranes should be kept intact for as long as possible, and when they rupture a vaginal examination is carried out to exclude a prolapsed cord. If labour starts either it may be allowed to proceed, or a caesarean section may be performed. If there is a delay when the infant's head is in the pelvic outlet, a forceps delivery may be appropriate.

The place of caesarean section in the management of preterm labour is controversial. Most obstetricians believe that if labour starts when the pregnancy is 26–31 weeks' gestation, caesarean section should be performed if:

- The fetus does not present cephalically.
- There is associated antepartum haemorrhage.
- The labour fails to progress normally.
- Fetal distress develops.

Although there can be little disagreement about these indications, the routine use of caesarean section to deliver babies weighing less than 1500 g is debatable; current evidence shows it increases maternal morbidity, but is insufficient to determine if there is a benefit to the neonate.

PRELABOUR RUPTURE OF THE MEMBRANES (PROM)

Prelabour (premature) rupture of the membranes may lead to the onset of preterm labour, with or without other causal factors. In most cases the baby is born within 7 days of the rupture; 50% within 2–4 hours, 80–90% by 7 days. Rupture of the membranes after the 35th week is of less clinical significance, and if labour does not start quickly it may be induced by the use of Syntocinon (see p. 190),

depending on the state of the cervix. A woman whose cervix is 'not favourable' (see p. 189), may prefer to delay induction for 48–72 hours in the anticipation that, during this time, the cervix will ripen and induction will be easier and more successful.

A multicentre study of 5000 women with prelabour rupture of the membranes, whose gestation was greater than 37 weeks, showed that there was no increase in the caesarean section rate or in infection whether or not induction, using oxytocics, or expectant treatment was chosen. The mother should be informed of the choices and her wishes accepted. Routine antibiotic therapy has been shown to reduce maternal infection, but to have no significant beneficial effects on the neonate. If the woman is a carrier of group B streptococcus she must be informed that there is an increased risk of neonatal morbidity.

The real problem occurs when the membranes rupture between the 26th and 35th weeks (preterm premature rupture of membranes PPROM), as the longer the birth is delayed the more mature the baby becomes. Against this is the risk of ascending intra-uterine infection occurring. The woman should be admitted to or transferred to a hospital with a neonatal intensive care level nursery. A high vaginal swab is also taken for bacteriological examination.

Regular assessments of maternal temperature and pulse are made to detect intra-uterine infection, and observations are made to see if the amniotic fluid continues to leak. An ultrasound examination may be carried out to determine whether oligohydramnios has occurred.

The use of prophylactic tocolytics has been suggested, but studies show them to be of little value. Prophylactic corticosteroids should be given, as the risk that they will increase the chance of intra-uterine infection is less than their beneficial effect on fetal lung maturation.

Prophylactic erythromycin should be given to the mother, as four trials have shown a significant reduction in the number of babies born within 48 hours, and a reduction in neonatal infection and the need for oxygen therapy. The use of Augmentin was associated with an increased incidence of necrotizing enterocolitis and therefore it should not be used.

If antibiotics are not given and the mother develops signs of intra-uterine infection (chorioamnionitis), such as tachycardia, fever (higher than 38°C), leucocytosis and an offensive vaginal discharge, antibiotics should be prescribed and delivery expedited. In most cases the infection is polybacterial, with anaerobes and group B streptococci predominating. Antibiotics are chosen that take these findings into account.

If labour does not start within 48 hours the patient may ambulate, and provided her home conditions are suitable and she lives near the hospital, may go home. At home she should rest as much as possible, avoid sexual intercourse, and return to hospital if she develops a fever or an offensive vaginal discharge.

FETAL MATURITY

As more women attend for antenatal care early in pregnancy and with the increasing use of ultrasound, the degree of maturity of the fetus is generally known to within 2 weeks. In a few cases the woman does not seek medical attention until the third trimester, at which time the estimation of fetal maturity is less exact. In a mature fetus, hyaline membrane disease is unlikely to develop. Even if it does, neonatologists today have effective treatments. If there is then a need to determine the lung maturity this can be done by measuring the lecithin/sphingomyelin (L/S) ratios. As pregnancy advances the L/S ratio increases (Figs 19.1 and 19.2).

POST-TERM PREGNANCY

Historically in 10% of cases the pregnancy lasted for more than 42 weeks; accurate dating of pregnancy by ultrasound and a policy of offering induction after 41 weeks and 3 days in many centres has resulted in only 1–2% of pregnancies proceeding past 42 weeks'. In some cases there may be a genetic cause for postdatism, but for most the aetiology is not known.

The risk of a post-term pregnancy is that the perinatal mortality rate increases, being doubled at 42 weeks' and 6 times at 43 weeks' compared with 39–40 weeks'. At least

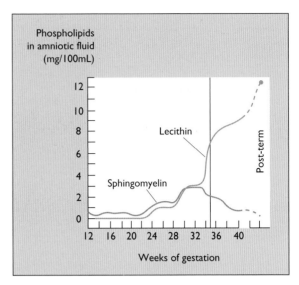

Fig. 19.1 Changes in the concentration of lecithin and sphingomyelin in amniotic fluid.

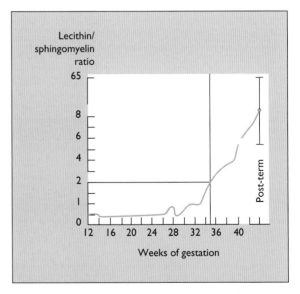

Fig. 19.2 Mean lecithin and sphingomyelin ratios during normal gestation.

one-third of the increased mortality is due to the death of a malformed fetus.

Management

If the woman is an older primigravida, has a history of infertility or has pre-eclampsia, diabetes mellitus or other pregnancy complications, the pregnancy should be terminated before it becomes post-term. In other cases three options are available and they should be discussed with the patient and her partner. These are the induction of labour, to continue with the pregnancy, or to perform an elective caesarean section. The induction of labour at 10 days post-term has been shown to be associated with lower rates of caesarean section and reduced neonatal morbidity and perinatal mortality.

If the option of continuing with the pregnancy in the expectation that labour will commence spontaneously is chosen, the welfare of the fetus must be monitored. The mother records fetal movements daily, non-stress cardiotocography is performed twice weekly, and ultrasound examinations are made to measure the volume of the amniotic fluid. An amniotic fluid index of less than 5 is considered abnormal. Umbilical blood flow may also be measured. Abnormalities in these tests (see Ch. 20) may indicate the need for induction of labour or caesarean section.

Chapter 20

The at-risk fetus

The birthweight of an infant depends on its genetic growth potential, which may be restricted or enhanced by the growth support provided by the mother, the functional integrity of the placenta and the ability of the fetus to use the nutrients provided.

Most fetuses grow normally throughout pregnancy (see Fig. 6.13, p. 46). Some fetuses are genetically programmed to have a low growth potential. They are healthy, but small at birth. Some have a genetic defect which reduces their growth potential and causes slow intra-uterine growth, which may not become apparent until some time in the second half of pregnancy. Some fetuses grow normally initially, but in the last trimester of pregnancy their growth is restricted by alterations in uteroplacental function. This has led to the use of the descriptive term placental dysfunction or placental insufficiency.

Within genetically set limits, the actual fetal growth depends on:

- An adequate supply of nutrients (especially glucose) and oxygen from the mother
- An adequate placental transfer of nutrients, which depends on a good blood supply reaching the placenta
- A good fetal circulation
- Functioning fetal pancreatic β cells, as insulin is one of the main regulators of fetal growth, provided that nutrients are available.

Of all these factors, an adequate blood supply reaching the placenta so that exchange of nutrients across the placenta can take place seems the most important.

With this background the identified causes of fetal growth restriction can be defined (Table 20.1). The degree to which these causes affect fetal growth depends on the amount of placental functioning reserve, and so not all women having these complications will give birth to a growth-restricted fetus.

A growth-restricted fetus is more likely to develop metabolic disturbances, such as acidosis, hypoglycaemia and erythroblastosis. If the disturbances are severe the fetus may die in utero. Less severe disturbances tend to become worse during labour, causing clinical or monitor-detected fetal distress, or the baby may be born with signs of severe hypoxia. Thus the fetus in an affected pregnancy is at greater risk of dying in utero or, if born alive, of needing resuscitation and possibly of being brain damaged (cerebral palsy). The pregnancy is high risk. Not all high-risk pregnancies have a growth-restricted fetus, but many do.

Table 20.1 Aetiological factors in fetal growth restriction (placental dysfunction)

	PERCENTAGE
Maternal causes	
Hypertensive disorders	60
Prolonged pregnancy	5
Maternal diseases (especially eating disorders, renal disease and severe anaemia)	5
Fetal causes	**10**
Malformations, transplacental infections	
Multiple pregnancy	
Unknown	**20**

HIGH-RISK PREGNANCY

Women who have a high-risk pregnancy should be identified early if possible, and given more intensive antenatal care, particularly after the 30th week. As mentioned, in some high-risk pregnancies the fetal growth rate is normal or, in the case of pregnancy in a diabetic woman, the baby may be large (macrosomic). In other words, a large number of normal-size-for-dates babies occur in high-risk pregnancies, and their morbidity and mortality is less than if the fetus is growth restricted.

A second method of detecting fetal growth restriction is to measure the symphysiofundal height with a tape measure and refer to a chart (see Fig. 6.12, p. 46).

A third test is to use ultrasound to determine the size of the fetus, the amniotic fluid volume and Doppler umbilical blood flow velocity measurements.

TESTS FOR FETAL WELLBEING IN HIGH-RISK PREGNANCIES

Having identified that the pregnancy is high risk for the fetus, tests to determine fetal wellbeing should be started after the 30th week. In the past 10 years, biophysical tests to determine fetal wellbeing have superseded biochemical tests. These tests are:

- Fetal movement (fetal kick) counts
- Cardiotocography
- Serial ultrasound examinations
- Doppler flow velocity wave forms.

None of these has a high positive predictive value, but each has a high negative predictive value.

A note of caution should be sounded. The authors of *Effective Care in Pregnancy and Childbirth* point out that, although the tests may provide 'a minimum level of care and attention in settings where these are adequate', in other settings their use may result in 'a variety of unwarranted interventions'. It should be added that unwarranted interventions may lead to an increase in obstetric interventions and possible medicolegal problems. The doctor may be 'damned if he does and damned if he does not'. It is essential that the doctor explains to the patient what is intended and why, including the limitations of the tests.

Fetal movements

In the last half of pregnancy the fetal movements become more regular and at term the average fetus moves 40–50 times per day with a range of 10–130. The woman is asked to either report if she perceives that the fetus is moving less or to formally count the number of times the fetus kicks until she has recorded 10 kicks. Usually this number occurs in a 3-hour period, but as fetuses have different patterns of activity the woman may have to check the number of kicks during another 3-hour period that day. In one study, of those fetuses that had less than 10 movements per day, 36% of babies were subsequently stillborn, compared with none in those whose movements were more than 10 per day. If the fetus fails to kick 10 times in a day, then the woman should be instructed to contact her care giver and cardiotocographic assessment should be performed.

Cardiotocography – the non-stress test

Cardiotocography (CTG) depends on the assumption that a healthy fetus will normally be more active than an at-risk fetus, and that its heart will respond to a uterine contraction by accelerating. An external cardiotocograph is applied to the woman's abdomen as she sits in a reclining position (not on her back, as this may result in erroneous findings). The heartbeat variations in relation to the contraction are recorded. If the fetus is lethargic, it may be stimulated to move by tapping the uterus gently. CTG is usually done in hospital but can be done at home using domiciliary fetal heart monitoring and a telephone link. The term fetus sleep/wake cycle is approximately 20 minutes so if the tracing is initially non-reactive, the CTG should be continued for at least 30 minutes.

The Royal College of Obstetricians and Gynaecologists' Cardiotograph Classification is shown in Table 20.2. There are three grades:

- Normal
- Suspicious
- Pathological.

Table 20.2 RCOG cardiotocographic (CTG) classification

Normal	A CTG where all **four** features fall into the reassuring category
Suspicious	A CTG whose features fall into **one** of the non-reassuring categories and the remainder of the features are reassuring
Pathological	A CTG whose features fall into **two or more** non-reassuring categories or **one or more** abnormal categories

FETAL HEART-RATE FEATURE CLASSIFICATION	BASELINE (bpm)	VARIABILITY (bpm) ACCELERATIONS	DECELERATIONS	ACCELERATIONS
Reassuring	110–160	≥5	None	Present
Non-reassuring	100–109 161–180	<5 for ≥40 but <90 min	• early • variable • single prolonged for up to 3 minutes	Absence of accelerations with otherwise normal CTG is of uncertain significance
Abnormal	<100 >180 Sinusoidal pattern for ≥10 minutes	<5 for >90 minutes	• atypical • late • single prolonged for >3 minutes	

A normal pattern indicates that the fetus is not at risk of dying in the next 7–10 days (Fig. 20.1). Such a fetus is termed reactive. If a suboptimal pattern is found the fetus is at slightly increased risk and the test should be repeated in 3–4 days. The clinical management reaction to a suspicious or pathological CTG tracing will depend on the overall clinical picture and the gestational age of the fetus. A suspicious tracing merits closer surveillance and/or delivery if the fetus is at term, a pathological tracing intensive surveillance and, if persistent, consideration of delivery (frequently by caesarean section) if the fetus has reached viability (Fig. 20.2).

A problem with CTG is that normal patterns predict that the fetus is at very low risk, but an abnormal pattern does not give an accurate prediction of fetal danger, i.e. the false positive rate is high, the positive predictive value is low, but the false negative rate is also low.

Serial ultrasound examinations

The growth of the fetus, as a measure of its health, may be monitored by examining it using real-time ultrasound at 3-weekly intervals. The fetal abdominal circumference, head circumference, femur length and estimated fetal weight are calculated and related to the centile chart for the sex of the fetus. In addition, the longest column of amniotic fluid is measured and the amniotic fluid index (AFI) calculated (see Ch. 19, p. 150–151). In some centres customized growth or centile charts are used which make adjustment for the mother's parity, height, weight and ethnic origin. This approach has been shown to improve

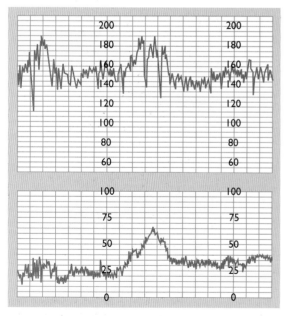

Fig. 20.1 Fetal heart acceleration during a uterine contraction (reactive).

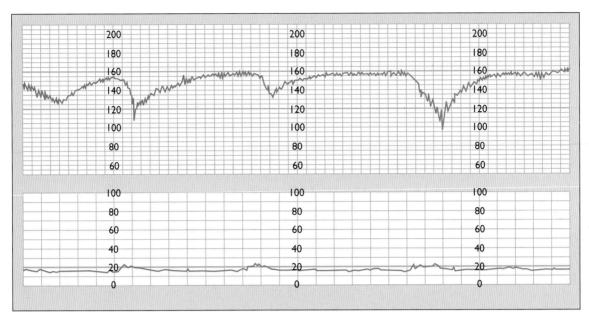

Fig. 20.2 Preterminal fetal heart rate pattern. Note marked reduction in short-term variability and repeated deceleration with Braxton Hicks contractions.

the accuracy of identification of growth-restricted fetuses and helps differentiate those fetuses from ones that are genetically small but developing normally.

Fetal blood flow velocity

Uteroplacental and fetoplacental circulations are low-resistance systems in which the flow of blood towards the placenta continues throughout the cardiac cycle, causing waveforms of different types. If fetoplacental vascular resistance increases because of acute uteroplacental atherosclerosis, fetal disease or unknown causes, the waveforms are altered. In the umbilical artery the difference between the peak systolic flow (S) and end-diastolic flow (D) can be measured (Fig. 20.3). The greater the S:D ratio the more likely it is that the fetus will be compromised, particularly if absent or reversed end-diastolic flow velocity (AEDFV) or extreme S:D ratio is found.

Fetal blood flow velocity is a useful method of determining whether the placental function is insufficient, and hence whether the wellbeing of the fetus is affected.

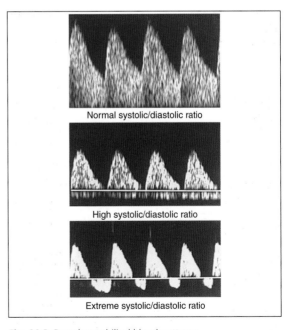

Normal systolic/diastolic ratio

High systolic/diastolic ratio

Extreme systolic/diastolic ratio

Fig. 20.3 Doppler umbilical blood patterns.

Biophysical profile

Some obstetric units, especially in North America, believe that the at-risk status of a fetus can be detected with greater accuracy if a biophysical profile is obtained. This consists of monitoring fetal movements, breathing, tone and reactivity and amniotic fluid volume by real-time ultrasound. The procedure is costly and time-consuming, and at present there is no evidence that it is superior to non-stress testing.

MANAGEMENT OF A HIGH-RISK PREGNANCY

Although fetal growth may be restricted at all stages of pregnancy (commonly in malformed fetuses), it is unusual for problems to arise before the 30th week. The effects of placental dysfunction are observable between the 30th and 35th weeks, and become more marked after that time. In three-quarters of cases the expectant mother has a clinical disorder.

A multicentre trial has demonstrated that a daily low dose of aspirin (75 mg) will reduce the risk of the develop-ment of severe pre-eclampsia and of fetal growth restriction in women who have previously had a compromised pregnancy.

All that can be done is to monitor the maternal disease if it is present, to detect deterioration and to check fetal wellbeing (Fig. 20.4). If the maternal condition worsens, for example pre-eclampsia deteriorates or if the fetal monitoring becomes grossly abnormal, e.g. ominous CTG, persistent reverse end-diastolic blood flow, the pregnancy should be terminated either by inducing labour or by caesarean section. If the gestation is less than 34 weeks then if feasible the mother should be given corticosteroids before delivery to enhance fetal lung maturity.

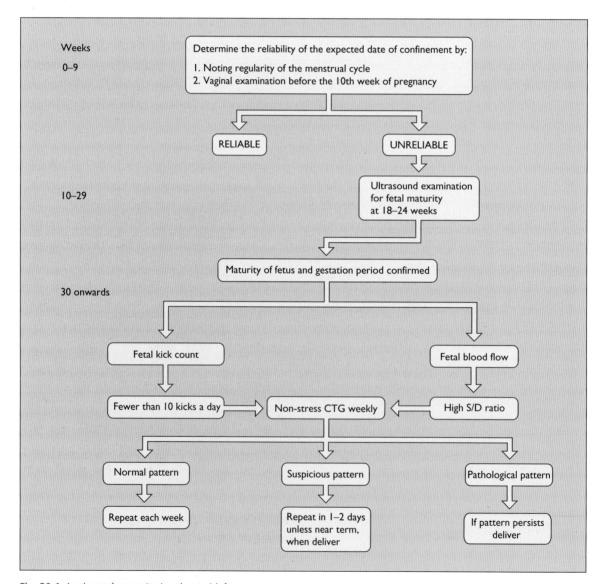

Fig. 20.4 A scheme for monitoring the at-risk fetus.

MONITORING THE AT-RISK FETUS IN LABOUR

When caesarean section is not chosen to perform an immediate delivery, the health of the mother and fetus should be monitored during the labour. The care of the woman in labour is described in Chapter 8. In this section the care of the fetus will be described.

An at-risk fetus, particularly if growth restricted, has fewer reserves on which it can draw for energy should placental gas and glucose transfer be reduced further during labour. Normally, the fetus converts glucose (released from glycogen stores) by anaerobic pathways into ketopyruvic acid, and then, in the presence of oxygen, into carbon dioxide and water via the Krebs' cycle. The process releases '30 high-energy bonds' per molecule of glucose. When the supply of oxygen is limited, the conversion cycle stops before the Krebs' cycle is initiated and only the anaerobic cycle operates. Anaerobic glycolysis releases far less energy and leads to the accumulation of lactic acid in the fetal blood, causing acidaemia. In addition, if the fetus is growth restricted and has limited glycogen and fat stored, it is at great risk of developing acidaemia and may die.

Fetuses which are at particular risk of developing hypoxia and acidaemia are those whose mother has had a pregnancy complication, or those who have been compromised either before labour or during the birth process (Box 20.1).

During labour the wellbeing of the fetus may be monitored by either external Doppler cardiotocography or by direct electronic monitoring by placement of a fetal scalp electrode once the cervix is sufficiently dilated, i.e. 2–3 cm or more.

The physiological basis of fetal heart monitoring is that when fetal hypoxia occurs the altered composition of the blood causes a rise in sympathetic and vagal tone, which differ in character and effect. In mild hypoxia the sympathetic response predominates, with resulting tachycardia; the onset of the tachycardia is delayed and it persists for 10–30 minutes after the cause of the hypoxia has ceased. In moderate or severe hypoxia the vagal response predominates. Bradycardia is rapid in onset and lasts as long as the hypoxic episode, and then disappears rapidly.

The fetal heart monitor records these changes in the fetal heart rate in relation to uterine contractions. The abnormal patterns are shown in Figure 20.5:

- **Persistent tachycardia (>160 bpm).** This may be caused by maternal or fetal pyrexia and indicates that the fetus has mild hypoxia that requires more careful fetal monitoring.
- **Early decelerations (type 1 dips).** The dip occurs in the early part of a uterine contraction and has a V shape. Early decelerations are probably due to pressure on the fetal head during a contraction and have no prognostic significance.
- **Variable decelerations.** The decelerations are variable in time of onset and severity. The deceleration pattern is U-shaped. Variable decelerations are probably caused by compression of the umbilical cord and are only prognostically significant if the dip is severe and prolonged.
- **Late decelerations (type 2 dips).** The deceleration of the fetal heart rate starts late during the contraction and persists after the contraction has ceased. The deceleration is V-shaped. Late decelerations, particularly if severe (<100 bpm) indicate impairment of the uteroplacental blood flow, a reduction in fetal oxygenation and consequent fetal hypoxia.

A further piece of information can be obtained from the heart monitor tracing, i.e. beat-to-beat variation (baseline variability). Normally the beat-to-beat heart rate shows variations of more than 5 bpm, leading to a wavy line on the trace. The diminution, or absence, of beat-to-beat variation indicates some degree of fetal hazard.

If, in addition to abnormal fetal heart tracings, the fetus passes thick, green meconium, the probability of severe fetal hypoxia is increased.

Benefits and problems of fetal heart monitoring

Fetal heart monitors are available in most obstetric units. Routine CTG monitoring has not been demonstrated to be beneficial in low-risk pregnancy. In high-risk pregnancies,

---

Box 20.1 **Fetuses at high risk of developing intrapartum hypoxia and acidaemia**

Maternal factors

Hypertensive diseases in pregnancy
Diabetes
Multiple pregnancy
Severe anaemia
Severe malnutrition

Placental factors

Abruptio placentae

Fetal factors

Growth restriction (small for dates)
Malpresentations
Cord complications
Clinical 'fetal distress'*

*Clinical fetal distress is diagnosed if the fetal heart rate is >160 but <110 beats per minute sustained for 5 minutes or meconium-stained liquor is seen.

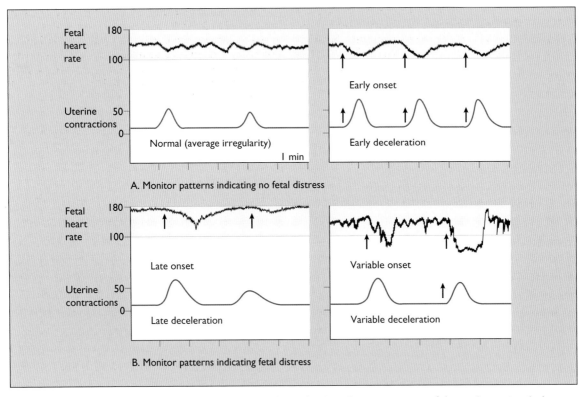

Fig. 20.5 Abnormal fetal heart patterns in labour (arrows indicate the time of commencement of the uterine contraction).

because of the low positive predictive value, abnormal tracings should be followed where possible with fetal blood sampling, unless the tracing is grossly abnormal and scalp sampling is not feasible.

Fetal scalp blood sampling

If fetal hypoxia persists, after a time acidaemia develops. The more severe the acidaemia, the higher the risk of fetal death. The degree of acidaemia can be detected by sampling the fetal scalp blood to measure either scalp pH or scalp lactate. A tubular speculum is introduced through the cervix and pressed on the fetal scalp. (If the membranes have not already ruptured, they are deliberately broken.) A small incision is made into the scalp. The blood obtained is drawn by capillary action into a specially prepared tube and its pH or lactate is measured. A pH of <7.20 or scalp lactate of >4.2 mmol/L indicates significant fetal acidosis and the need to deliver the baby expeditiously. A pH reading of more than 7.20–7.25, or a lactate of ~3.5–4.1, suggests that if there is no other indication to deliver the fetus quickly the labour may continue while close surveillance is maintained and the scalp pH repeated if indicated, and vaginal delivery may be expected.

Direct fetal pulse oximetry

Direct measurement of fetal oxygen levels is now possible by placing a pulse oximeter against the fetal cheek during labour. The membranes must be ruptured and the cervix at least 3 cm dilated. Results from a large multicentre trial showed that the number of caesarean sections performed for non-reassuring status was reduced, but this was balanced by the increased number done for failure to progress or dystocia, so its clinical effectiveness is debatable.

MANAGEMENT OF CTG ABNORMALITIES – NON-REASSURING FETAL STATUS

If the patient is in the second stage of labour and the baby is in an occipitoanterior position, then an instrumental vaginal delivery should be contemplated. If the fetal head is in a transverse or posterior position then in most circumstances the baby is best delivered by caesarean section. If the woman is in the first stage of labour she should be repositioned, preferably on her side or well propped up to reduce any pressure by the uterus on the major blood vessels; she may be given oxygen via a face mask, although the benefit of this has not been proven. If an oxytocin infusion causes very strong uterine contractions, the drip should be slowed or stopped.

After these actions have been taken, the monitor tracing is observed to see if the fetal heart pattern reverts to normal. If it does not and/or the scalp sample results indicate increasing fetal acidosis, then the baby must be delivered by urgent caesarean section. Many units use a 'code green' to signal to the operating theatre and maternity teams the urgency of the section.

Chapter | **21** |

Abnormal fetal presentations

Abnormal presentations include, in order of frequency, occipitoposterior presentations, breech presentations, face presentations, transverse presentations and brow presentations.

OCCIPITOPOSTERIOR PRESENTATIONS

In about 10% of pregnancies the fetal head enters the maternal pelvis with its occiput in one of the posterior segments of the pelvis (see Fig. 8.4, p. 70).

The diagnosis may be made on abdominal palpation when the fetal back is felt in one of the mother's flanks, the fetal heart being loudest here (Fig. 21.1). In labour, vaginal examination provides more information, the occiput and the anterior fontanelle being identified (Fig. 21.2).

During labour the fetal head is forced deeper into the pelvis, and usually flexes on the fetal neck. Once full dilatation of the cervix has occurred its progress may be in one of three ways (Fig. 21.2):

- In 65% of cases the head rotates through 135° so that the occiput lies behind the symphysis pubis.
- In 20% of cases rotation of the fetal head ceases and it becomes arrested in a transverse diameter of the pelvis.
- In 15% of cases the fetal head rotates posteriorly.

Thus, in most cases the fetal head undergoes a long or a short rotation (Fig. 21.3).

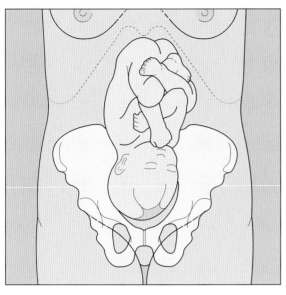

Fig. 21.1 Occipitoposterior position – abdominal findings.

Management of occipitoposterior presentations

There is no proven management that encourages rotation to an occipitoanterior position before labour starts. Once begun, the duration of labour tends to be longer in occipitoposterior positions and the mother requires more support, analgesia and hydration. Progress is monitored using a partogram. The descent of the head, and its position, are checked regularly. Any marked delay in the first stage of labour leads to prolonged labour (see p. 178–179) and a decision has to be made whether to continue or to perform a caesarean section. Delay in the second stage of labour of more than 1.5–2 hours' duration indicates the need for help to deliver the baby. If the fetal head undergoes the long rotation a spontaneous vaginal delivery may be expected. This occurs in 65% of cases. If the fetal head undergoes the short rotation and descends to the pelvic floor in the posterior position, the infant may be born spontaneously (8% of all cases) or may need help by forceps or vacuum (7%). On the other hand, the fetus may not descend much beyond the ischial spines and a manual

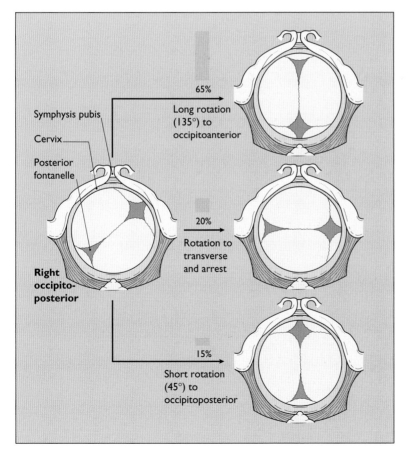

Fig. 21.2 Possible modes of rotation of the head.

Symphysis pubis

Cervix

Posterior fontanelle

Right occipitoposterior

65%
Long rotation (135°) to occipitoanterior

20%
Rotation to transverse and arrest

15%
Short rotation (45°) to occipitoposterior

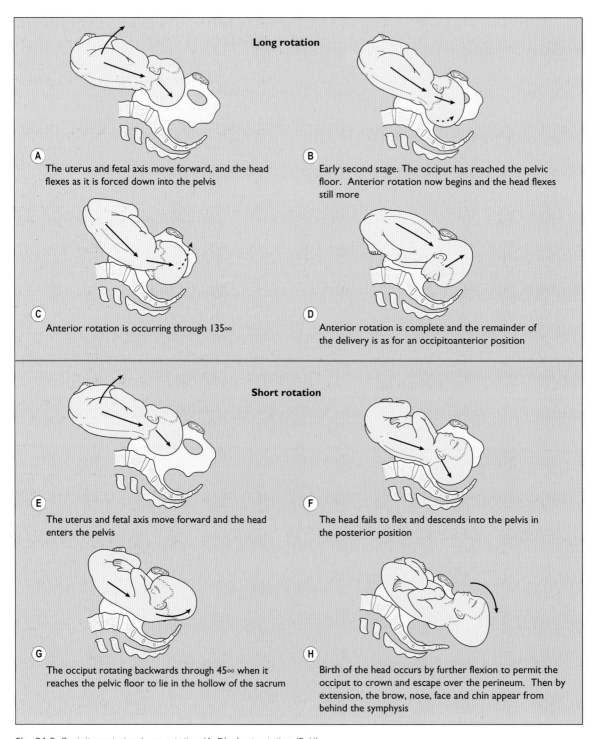

Long rotation

A
The uterus and fetal axis move forward, and the head flexes as it is forced down into the pelvis

B
Early second stage. The occiput has reached the pelvic floor. Anterior rotation now begins and the head flexes still more

C
Anterior rotation is occurring through 135∞

D
Anterior rotation is complete and the remainder of the delivery is as for an occipitoanterior position

Short rotation

E
The uterus and fetal axis move forward and the head enters the pelvis

F
The head fails to flex and descends into the pelvis in the posterior position

G
The occiput rotating backwards through 45∞ when it reaches the pelvic floor to lie in the hollow of the sacrum

H
Birth of the head occurs by further flexion to permit the occiput to crown and escape over the perineum. Then by extension, the brow, nose, face and chin appear from behind the symphysis

Fig. 21.3 Occipitoposterior. Long rotation (A–D); short rotation (E–H).

rotation and forceps delivery, Kjelland's forceps delivery or vacuum extraction may be necessary (see Ch. 22). These procedures are also required if the fetal head arrests in a transverse diameter of the pelvis. Between 5 and 10% of babies who are occipitoposterior are delivered by caesarean section.

BREECH PRESENTATIONS

The frequency of breech presentation falls as pregnancy advances. At the 30th week of pregnancy 15% of fetuses present as a breech; by the 35th week the proportion has fallen to 6%, and by term only 3% present as a breech. Most of these babies spontaneously turn to become cephalic. If the presentation is still a breech at the 37th week many obstetricians attempt a cephalic version, which is described on pages 197–199. Version is easier if the fetus has flexed legs, one of the three types of breech presentation (Fig. 21.4).

The presentation of the fetus is of no clinical importance before the 32nd–35th weeks. At this stage of pregnancy the diagnosis of a breech presentation is made by finding, on palpation, that the lower pole of the uterus is occupied by a soft, irregular mass and that in the fundal area a firm, smooth, rounded mass is present which bounces between the fingers if gently pushed. On auscultation the fetal heartbeat is loudest above the umbilicus. If any doubt remains after palpation and a vaginal examination, an ultrasound image will clarify the diagnosis and will exclude fetal malformations.

The fetus may be left as a breech or an external cephalic version may be attempted at 36–37 weeks of gestation, depending on local custom.

Problems with breech presentations

Few problems occur during pregnancy, although some expectant mothers complain of pressure beneath the diaphragm. Because breech births frequently require operative delivery there is an increased risk to the fetus, which is minimized by skilled attention and decision-making. In the absence of any other complications of pregnancy, preterm breech births (weight < 2500 g) carry a mortality of 12%, as do large postmature babies (weight > 3500 g). Mature fetuses whose weight is in the normal range have a mortality of 1%.

The main causes of morbidity are intracranial haemorrhage, asphyxia and fracture of the humerus, femur or clavicle.

Management of breech births

Elective caesarean section at term

The Term Breech Trial reported that in developed countries delivery by caesarean section was the safest option for

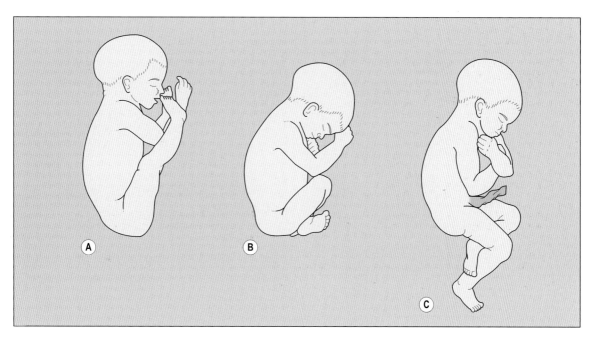

Fig. 21.4 Types of breech presentation. (A) Breech with extended legs (frank); (B) breech with flexed legs (complete); (C) footling.

the baby with a reduction in the perinatal mortality from 1.15 to 0.6%, and consequently few fetuses presenting as a breech are now electively delivered vaginally. It is noteworthy that at 2 years of age there was no difference in the development between those delivered vaginally or by caesarean section

Vaginal breech birth

It is still important to understand the management and the mechanism of a breech birth, as an unexpected breech presentation may occur at full cervical dilatation with insufficient time to organize a caesarean section. This is shown in Figures 21.5–21.14 and is described in the captions.

An algorithm for the management of breech presentations

Figure 21.15 presents an algorithm for the management of breech presentations. Not included is breech extraction, as in such cases the baby is delivered by the doctor. The main use of breech extraction is for the birth of a second twin, or if the breech is impacted in the midpelvic cavity. Unless the obstetrician is very skilled, caesarean section is safer.

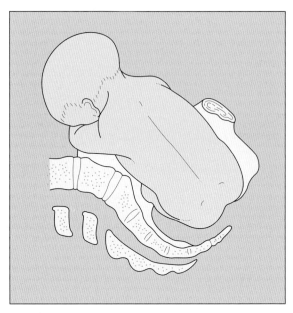

Fig. 21.6 When the buttocks reach the pelvic floor, the pelvic 'gutter' causes the buttocks to rotate internally so that the bitrochanteric diameter lies in the anteroposterior diameter of the pelvic outlet.

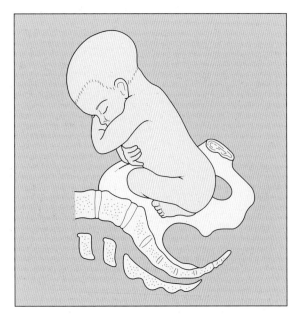

Fig. 21.5 The breech is presenting as a right sacroanterior. The bitrochanteric diameter of the buttocks has entered the pelvis in the transverse diameter of the pelvic brim. With full dilatation of the cervix, the buttocks descend deeply into the pelvis.

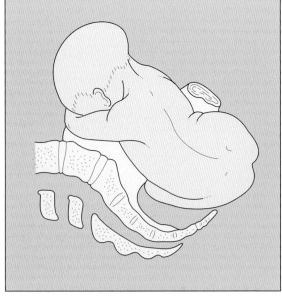

Fig. 21.7 The anterior buttock appears at the vulva. With further uterine contractions the buttocks distend the vaginal outlet. Lateral flexion of the fetal trunk takes place and the shoulders rotate so that they may enter the pelvis. At this stage the attending doctor or nurse–midwife has donned gown and gloves and is prepared to aid the delivery.

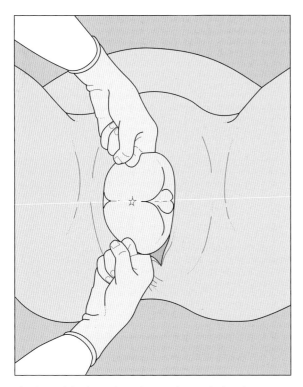

Fig. 21.8 If the buttocks make no advance during the next several contractions, an episiotomy is made and the buttocks are born by groin traction.

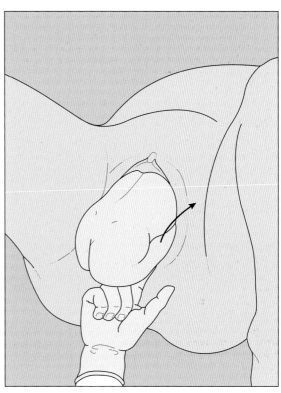

Fig. 21.10 If the fetus has extended legs, the attendant may have to slip a hand along the anterior leg of the fetus and deliver it by flexion and abduction, so that the rest of the birth may proceed.

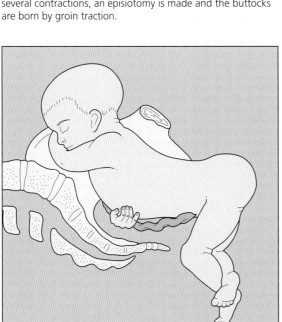

Fig. 21.9 The buttocks have been born and the shoulders have entered the pelvis in its transverse diameter. This causes the external rotation of the buttocks so that the fetal back becomes uppermost.

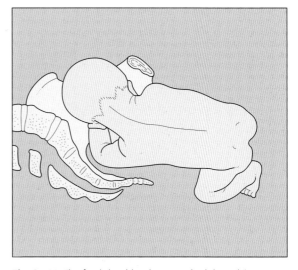

Fig. 21.11 The fetal shoulders have reached the pelvic 'gutter' and have rotated internally so that the bisacromial diameter lies in the anteroposterior diameter of the outlet. Simultaneously, the buttocks have rotated anteriorly through 90°. The fetal head is entering the pelvic brim, its sagittal suture lying in the brim's transverse diameter. Descent into the pelvis occurs with flexion of the fetal head.

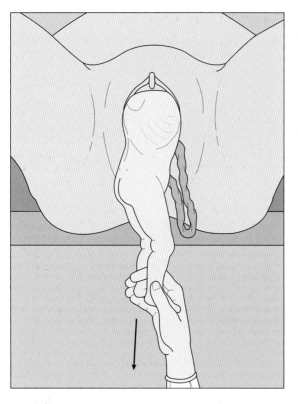

Fig. 21.12 The baby has been born to beyond its umbilicus. A loop of umbilical cord is pulled down to make sure that it is not holding back the birth. Gentle traction downwards and backwards is made by the attendant, so that the anterior shoulder and arm are born. The baby is now lifted upwards in a circle so that the posterior shoulder and arm may be born. Sometimes one arm is extended and has to be dislodged downwards. The procedure requires skill, otherwise a fractured clavicle or humerus may result. Once the anterior arm has been born, the baby's body and the posterior arm are freed in a similar manner.

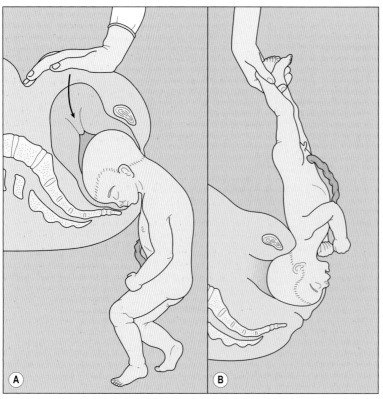

Fig. 21.13 (A) The baby hangs unsupported from the mother's vulva. The doctor applies slight suprapubic pressure to encourage further flexion of the head. When the nape of the baby's neck has appeared, the attendant holds the baby by the feet and swings it upwards through an arc. (B) This manoeuvre, by using the lower border of the sacrum, pulls the head down and rotates it through the pelvic outlet so that the chin, nose and forehead appear.

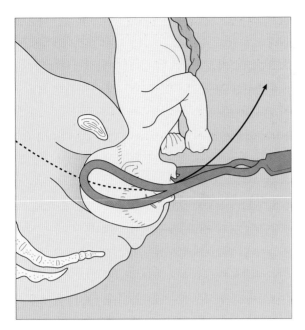

Fig. 21.14 An alternative is to deliver the fetal head by forceps.

TRANSVERSE LIES, OBLIQUE LIES AND SHOULDER PRESENTATIONS

Shoulder presentations, unstable lie, transverse lie and oblique lie may be detected in late pregnancy. These conditions occur in 1 in 200 births, usually in multiparous women. The aetiology is varied. They may occur in a lax multiparous uterus with no other complication of pregnancy, but may be associated with polyhydramnios, placenta praevia or a uterine malformation (see Fig. 36.4, p. 280). An ultrasound examination is helpful in excluding placenta praevia.

The diagnosis is made by finding a broad asymmetrical uterus with a firm, ballottable round head in one iliac fossa and a softer mass in the other (Fig. 21.16).

Management in pregnancy

When placenta praevia has been excluded a gentle cephalic version may be attempted, but in many cases the fetus returns after some time to its previous presentation. If the lie remains unstable, the expectant mother should be advised to report to hospital immediately labour starts or, if the social conditions are unfavourable, may be admitted to hospital to await labour. In some cases the presentation is corrected to cephalic and the head is held over the brim. The membranes are then ruptured and the head pressed into the pelvis as the liquor amnii is released.

Another choice is to perform an elective caesarean section.

Management in labour

If the shoulder presentation is not detected until labour has been established, caesarean section is the preferred option.

FACE PRESENTATIONS

Face presentation occurs in 1 in 500 births, usually by chance, but in 15% of cases the baby is anencephalic, or has a tumour of the neck or shortening of the neck muscles.

Face presentation is rarely diagnosed before labour, and even then may be missed until a face with swollen, distorted lips appears at the vulva. Abdominal palpation may reveal a peculiar S-shaped fetus with feet on the opposite side to the prominent occiput. The fetal head has not usually entered the pelvis (Fig. 21.17).

Vaginal examination during labour may clarify the presentation (Fig. 21.18), but in late labour, when much facial oedema has occurred, a breech may be misdiagnosed.

Mechanism and management of labour

In most cases the face enters the transverse diameter of the pelvis with the fetal chin in a mentotransverse position. Descent into the pelvis is delayed until late in the first stage or the second stage of labour (Fig. 21.19). Rotation usually occurs anteriorly so that the chin lies behind the pubis, and delivery occurs spontaneously by flexion of the head or may be aided by forceps. In a few cases the fetal chin rotates posteriorly, impacting the fetal head and preventing vaginal delivery. The impacted fetal head may be rotated using Kjelland's forceps or, preferably, the fetus may be delivered by caesarean section.

BROW PRESENTATIONS

Brow presentation is the most unfavourable and the least common (1 in 1500 births) of all malpositions and malpresentations. It may occur during late pregnancy (when it usually converts into a cephalic presentation). An ultrasound examination should be made to exclude fetal malformations, particularly hydrocephaly.

The patient should be seen each week to check the presentation, and told to come into hospital as soon as contractions start or the membranes rupture.

In labour, brow presentation is diagnosed when the fetal head is high and a sulcus can be identified between the head and the back.

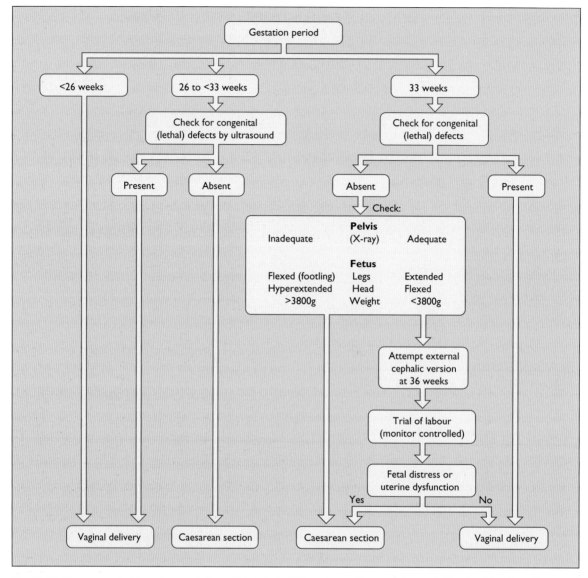

Fig. 21.15 Management of breech presentations. If detected at 36 weeks confirm gestation period by checking date of last menstrual period, visits during pregnancy and ultrasound examination. Attempt external cephalic version (ECV) without anaesthesia, using tocolytics and real-time ultrasound. If ECV fails, wait for labour.

Treatment consists of caesarean section, unless the baby is grossly abnormal or dead, when a destructive operation may be chosen (see p. 199).

MULTIPLE PREGNANCY

Multiple pregnancy occurs when two or more ova are released and fertilized (dizygotic, DZ) or when a single fertilized ovum divides early to form two identical embryos at the inner cell mass stage or earlier (monozygotic, MZ).

The incidence of twins is 1 in 90 pregnancies and that of triplets is 1 in 90 × 90 (8100) pregnancies. DZ twins are more common in older mothers, with increasing parity and where there is a maternal family history of twins. They are more common in women of African origin and less common in Asian races. Since the introduction of assisted reproductive technology, the incidence of multiple pregnancies has increased and in developed countries accounts for 50% or more of multiple pregnancies. Ultrasound examination in early pregnancy has also identified more twins, but in half of those identified one fetus dies and disappears before the second half of pregnancy – the so-called vanishing twin.

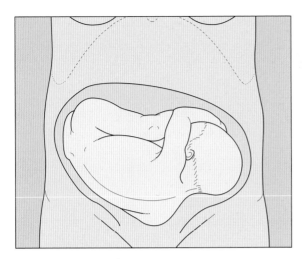

Fig. 21.16 Transverse lie.

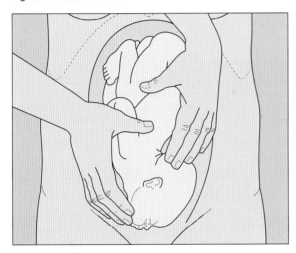

Fig. 21.17 Abdominal palpation in face presentation.

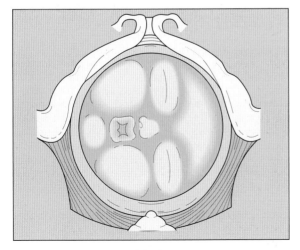

Fig. 21.18 Touch picture of the face.

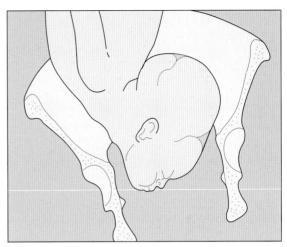

Fig. 21.19 Diagram of engagement. In the face presentation engagement occurs late, as the parietal prominences do not enter the brim until the face has reached the pelvic floor.

This occurs in 20–50% of twins, 50% of triplets and 65% of quadruplets.

In DZ multiple pregnancy each fetus is a separate individual with its own placenta, amnion and chorion. In MZ multiple pregnancy the two fetuses have a single placenta and chorion; 98% of MZ twins have their own amniotic sac (MZ diamniotic), but for the 2% who are monoamniotic this carries a high risk of cord entanglement. As there is vascular communication between the two parts of the placenta in over 75% of MZ twins it is not unusual for one twin to obtain a reduced supply of nutrients and grow more slowly than the other. In up to 35% this can cause twin-to-twin transfusion, which may result in acute polyhydramnios, anaemia, oligohydramnios and severe growth restriction in the donor, and polycythaemia, hypervolaemia, cardiac failure and polyhydramnios in the recipient twin. Occasionally one fetus dies early in pregnancy and becomes mummified (fetus papyraceous).

Because of the greater demands for nutrients, a fetus in a multiple pregnancy tends to be smaller than a singleton fetus, as its growth in utero is slower (Fig. 21.20).

Diagnosis of multiple pregnancy

Few multiple pregnancies are diagnosed in the first half of pregnancy except by ultrasound scanning. Because virtually every woman has a scan at least by 18–20 weeks' gestation it is now rare for a multiple pregnancy not to be diagnosed before it becomes clinically evident. In those rare situations when a scan has not been performed by the second half of pregnancy, a multiple pregnancy can be suspected if:

- The abdominal girth and uterine size are greater than expected from the period of amenorrhoea.
- Palpation shows an excess of fetal parts, and two fetal heads can be detected.

169

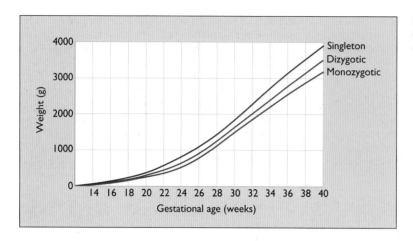

Fig. 21.20 The intra-uterine growth of multiple and single pregnancies as assessed by ultrasound fetometry.

Management of multiple pregnancy

Compared with a singleton pregnancy, a multiple pregnancy is likely to be associated with more complications (Table 21.1). For this reason the expectant mother requires additional antenatal care. She should be seen at 2-weekly intervals from the time of diagnosis. Maternal anaemia should be sought and treated, and there is a strong argument for insisting that the patient takes folic acid 4 mg and an iron salt each day. When a woman carrying twins goes into preterm labour, the decision whether to deliver the twins by caesarean section or to attempt a vaginal birth has to be made. A problem is that in 20% of twin pregnancies the weight of one twin is 20% less than that of the other. There is no consensus about the safest method to use.

A woman carrying a multiple pregnancy has an increased blood volume and an extra burden on her cardiovascular system. It is common practice to monitor fetal growth by ultrasound every 2–3 weeks from the 30th week. This is especially important in MZ twins so that twin-to-twin transfusion can be detected early. Laser ablation of the communicating placental vessels substantially improves the likelihood of a successful outcome. If growth ceases and/or Doppler blood flow indices are abnormal, delivery is expedited. The rising perinatal mortality and morbidity with increasing gestation (the nadir for mortality being 37 weeks) has led to the practice in a number of centres of electively delivering all twin pregnancies by 37–38 weeks.

Higher-multiple pregnancies

Since the development of assisted reproductive technology, the prevalence of multiple pregnancies has increased. A number of these will be triplets or higher. The perinatal mortality of these fetuses and neonates is high. To manage this problem, selective termination of some or all fetuses, by intracardiac injection, has been used. The associated medical and legal issues have not been resolved.

Triplets have an 80% risk of preterm delivery. The trend is to deliver triplets and quadruplets by caesarean section.

Management in labour

The position of the leading fetus should be checked on admission. In 45% of twin pregnancies both fetuses present as cephalic; in 25% as cephalic and breech; and as breech and cephalic or breech and breech in 10% each. If the first twin presents transversely, caesarean section is the preferable approach. If the first twin presents as a breech it is common practice (as yet unsupported by high-level evidence) to perform a caesarean section. In other cases a vaginal birth may be expected. The management of the labour is conducted in the way already described (Ch. 8). When the membranes rupture a vaginal examination is performed to check whether the umbilical cord has prolapsed.

The first baby is usually born without difficulty, if necessary following an episiotomy. Immediately following

Table 21.1 Complications of pregnancy in singleton and multiple pregnancies

COMPLICATION	SINGLETON (%)	TWIN (%)
Hypertensive disorders	5	15
Anaemia	3–5	15
Polyhydramnios	2	12
Intra-uterine growth restriction	10	25–33
Congenital anomalies	2–4	4–8
Preterm birth	5	40

the birth, the doctor makes an abdominal examination to determine the lie and presentation of the second twin. If it is transverse, the doctor may attempt external version to bring the fetus into a longitudinal position. A vaginal examination is then made to confirm the presentation, and if it is longitudinal the second amniotic sac is ruptured artificially. The fetal presenting part is led into the pelvis. A second twin which remains in the transverse presentation should be delivered either by caesarean section or by internal podalic version, depending on the skill of the obstetrician.

Following the birth of the first twin, uterine contractions may diminish for a few minutes. If they do not return soon, an intravenous oxytocin infusion may be set up. The birth of the second twin is usually uncomplicated, but postpartum haemorrhage may be expected and should be anticipated by managing the third stage actively.

Risk to mother and fetuses

There is no increased risk to a mother who has received appropriate antenatal care. The risk to a fetus of a multiple pregnancy is higher than to a singleton, mainly because of the increased incidence of preterm birth. The perinatal mortality of twin births is 50 per 1000, five times that of a singleton birth. The death of one of the twins during the birth, or in the neonatal period, presents the parents with unique problems, as they have to adjust to having one living baby who no longer has a same-age sibling. The incidence of cerebral palsy increases with the number of fetuses being 4–5 times greater in twins and 17 times in triplets and quadruplets compared with singletons.

Psychological effects of twins on the parents

The knowledge that she is carrying twins may have a considerable psychological effect on the mother and her partner, and the attending health professional needs to help and counsel the couple. If the multiple pregnancy was diagnosed in the early weeks by ultrasound scanning, the first matter to be discussed is the problem of the 'vanishing twin'. After the 20th week of pregnancy the woman and her partner should be made aware that there is a higher chance of developing complications that may require admission to hospital and which may lead to a premature birth. If the woman already has a child, or children, her absence from the home may require help from partner or relatives, and studies have shown that she has an increased chance of developing depression in late pregnancy. She also has a greater chance that the birth will be by caesarean section, which may cause anxiety, and the issue should be discussed.

In the postnatal period the demands of caring for two small babies adds to the problem of adjusting to parenthood (see p. 92–93), and usually means that the couple have little time to be with each other to enhance their general and their sexual relationship. In the period after childbirth, more women who have given birth to twins report anxiety and depression and often need support and help. Women report that discussion of these matters during pregnancy and the availability of support both during and after pregnancy reduce the stress of having twins. Fortunately, in the community there are self-help groups whose support and counselling are invaluable. However, the doctor or nurse attending the woman during and after pregnancy should be aware of the problems and of the need to talk with the woman and her partner.

PROLAPSE OF THE UMBILICAL CORD

Although prolapse of the umbilical cord is not itself a malpresentation, it is more likely to occur when there is a fetal malpresentation or position. For this reason it is included in this chapter. Prolapse of the umbilical cord occurs in 1 in 300 deliveries. The cord may be contained within the forewaters, when it is said to be presenting, or may have prolapsed to lie in front of the fetal presenting part after the membranes have ruptured (Fig. 21.21).

Aetiology

The umbilical cord is more likely to prolapse if anything prevents the snug application of the presenting part in the lower uterine segment or its descent into the maternal pelvis. For this reason, fetal malpresentations and positions, cephalopelvic disproportion and preterm births are more

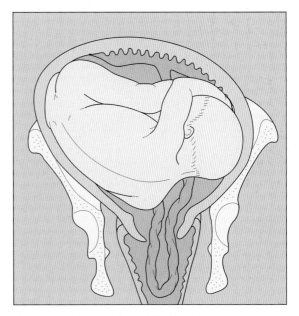

Fig. 21.21 Prolapse of the umbilical cord.

likely to be associated with cord prolapse. The cord may also prolapse at amniotomy, during version of the fetus, and in other obstetric manipulations.

Diagnosis

Presentation of the umbilical cord is rarely diagnosed. When prolapse of the cord occurs after the membranes have ruptured, it can be detected by a vaginal examination. This should be made in all cases of preterm labour, or if a fetal malpresentation or position is present. If the cord is felt on the vaginal examination, its pulsations should be sought and the fetal heart sounds checked to determine whether they are within the normal range or show tachycardia or bradycardia.

Management

The management of prolapsed cord depends on the condition of the fetus and the degree of cervical dilatation. If the fetus is dead, its birth may be awaited. If the fetus is alive and the cervix is not fully dilated, a caesarean section is safest for the baby. While arranging for the section, it may help to relieve pressure on the cord by placing the woman in the knee–chest position. The umbilical cord should be replaced in the vagina to reduce the risk of cold causing spasm of the umbilical vessels.

If the cervix is fully dilated and the fetal head or breech is deep in the pelvis, an instrumental delivery or breech extraction may be performed if an experienced obstetrician is present.

Chapter 22

Abnormal labour (dystocia) and prolonged labour

If the duration of labour exceeds the accepted norm, or if intervention is necessary either before or during labour, the condition is defined as dystocia. Dystocia may result from:

- 'Faults' in the fetus
- An abnormal size or shape of the pelvis
- Inefficient uterine contractions.

These matters are discussed in this chapter.

'FAULTS' IN THE FETUS (THE PASSENGER)

The presentation of the fetus may cause prolongation of labour (for example an occipitoposterior position), as may the size of the fetus. A large fetus (weight >4000 g) may not easily be able to be born vaginally even if the pelvis is normal in size. Some genetically programmed mothers habitually produce large babies, as do some diabetic mothers. Some babies have congenital defects that may make vaginal births difficult or impossible, for example a fetus who has hydrocephaly, or a tumour of the neck or abdomen. A fault in the fetus may be anticipated if an abdominal examination in late pregnancy reveals a large fetus whose head has not entered the maternal pelvis. The diagnosis can be established by an ultrasound examination.

ABNORMAL SHAPE OR SIZE OF THE PELVIS (THE PASSAGES)

The ideal obstetric pelvis is described on page 55. If any of the two main diameters, particularly of the pelvic brim, is reduced by 2 cm or more the pelvis is considered to be contracted. The shape of the pelvis may also be affected, for example the sacral curve may be replaced by a straight sacrum, or the pelvis may have been damaged by a serious accident.

Major pelvic abnormalities are uncommon in developed countries. The final arbiter of a successful vaginal delivery is the quality of the uterine contractions, the degree of relaxation of the pelvic ligaments and the moulding of the fetal head. Pelvimetry has little place in modern obstetric practice.

In the developing nations pelvimetry, preferably by CT scan (if available), still has a place to enable the obstetrician to make a decision about a vaginal delivery, but this prognosis is not particularly accurate, as different observers attach different prognostic values to the measurements and the shape of the pelvis. For example, if the anteroposterior diameter of the pelvic brim is less than 9 cm nearly all obstetricians will perform a caesarean section, whereas if the anteroposterior diameter is between 9 cm and 10.5 cm an obstetrician may attempt a trial of labour, provided the woman agrees, unless the sacrum is straight, when a caesarean section will be performed. If the anteroposterior diameter is more than 10.5 cm a vaginal delivery will be anticipated, unless the fetal head is very large.

CEPHALOPELVIC DISPROPORTION

Apart from the quality of the uterine contractions, the main issue with regard to vaginal birth is the size of the fetus relative to the size of the maternal pelvis; thus the concept of cephalopelvic disproportion (CPD) has arisen. The term cephalopelvic is used rather than fetopelvic, as any presentation other than cephalic would be managed by caesarean section.

In cases of CPD, if the fetal head has not entered the pelvic brim by term a caesarean section is likely to be performed because of risks to the fetus should labour proceed. On the other hand, if the fetal head has entered the pelvic brim the choice is between an elective caesarean section and a trial of labour. The decision depends on the woman's preference and the doctor's experience. For example, a woman over the age of 35, or one who has had a long history of infertility, will generally be delivered by caesarean section, as will women with medical complications.

If a trial of labour is attempted, the patient should be told that she has about a 30% chance that she will require an instrumental vaginal delivery and a 30% chance that the trial will be abandoned and a caesarean section will be performed.

In a trial of labour the aim is to determine what the woman can accomplish, not how much she can endure. As operative delivery is likely, an intravenous infusion should be established and only fluids permitted by mouth. The progress of the labour is monitored using the partogram, particular attention being paid to the speed of the descent of the fetal head and the dilatation of the cervix. A vaginal examination is made when the membranes rupture, to exclude cord prolapse. Special attention is paid

to the woman's response to the trial. The trial should be abandoned if:

- There is no increase in cervical dilatation over a period of 4 hours (or 2 hours after rupture of the membranes) in spite of strong uterine contractions.
- Non-reassuring fetal heart rate patterns develop.
- Full dilatation of the cervix is not achieved within 12 hours of labour.

ABNORMALITIES OF UTERINE ACTION

Labour will only progress normally if the contractile wave is propagated over the entire uterus in a triple descending gradient of activity (see p. 61).

If the normal pattern of uterine activity fails to occur the progress of labour will be abnormal – usually prolonged. Until the 1940s, prolonged labour was considered to be caused by 'uterine inertia'. Research since then has shown that several patterns of uterine activity may lead to delay in the birth of the child. The patterns are designated inefficient uterine activity and are divided into subgroups of abnormal uterine activity (Box 22.1). In some cases of labour the reverse occurs and the uterus is overactive, leading to a precipitate birth.

Changes in the management of labour in recent years, with the increasing use of epidural anaesthesia and of caesarean section, have rendered the description of the patterns of uterine activity less useful. They are worth recording, however, as they form the physiological basis of the modern classification.

Inefficient uterine activity

The two main types of inefficient uterine activity are:

- Hypoactive uterine activity
- Hyperactive incoordinate activity, which includes incoordinate uterine activity, 'colicky' uterus and constriction ring dystocia.

Box 22.1 Classification of abnormal uterine activity

Inefficient uterine activity

Hypoactive states
Hyperactive, incoordinate states
　Hyperactive lower uterine segment
　Colicky uterus
　Constriction ring dystocia
Cervical dystocia

Overefficient uterine activity

Precipitate labour
Tetanic uterine activity

It is difficult to determine exactly how often labour is complicated by inefficient uterine activity, but the most reliable estimates suggest that the condition is found predominantly in nulliparous women, affecting 4–6% of such labours and about 1% of all labours.

Aetiology

The aetiology of inefficient uterine action is not clear. In some cases cephalopelvic disproportion is present; in others psychological factors are postulated, as uterine dysfunction is predominantly a disorder of nulliparous labour which is not repeated in a subsequent labour.

Types of abnormal uterine action

Hypoactive states (uterine inertia)

The uterine resting tone is low and the intensity of the contraction is reduced, with the result that only a feeble contractile wave is propagated (Fig. 22.1). The contractions occur at longer intervals than usual and do not cause the patient much distress.

Hyperactive incoordinate states (incoordinate uterine action)

In normal labour the perception of pain is usually only reached when the uterine tone exceeds 25 mmHg. In hyperactive, incoordinate uterine activity the resting uterine tone is increased; in consequence, the pain threshold is reached earlier during the contraction and the pain persists for longer (Fig. 22.2). In spite of the strong contractions, cervical dilatation is slow because the triple gradient is reversed (Fig. 22.3).

If the woman has not been given an epidural anaesthetic she may complain of severe backache, which increases during each contraction when the pain radiates into her lower abdomen.

Two variations of hyperactive uterine activity may occur. Both are uncommon today and are the result of action not being taken to relieve the problem. They are colicky uterus and constriction ring dystocia. In colicky uterus, various parts of the uterus contract independently and the pain of the contraction is generalized and severe. Constriction ring dystocia occurs when an annular spasm arises at the junction between the upper and the lower uterine segments,

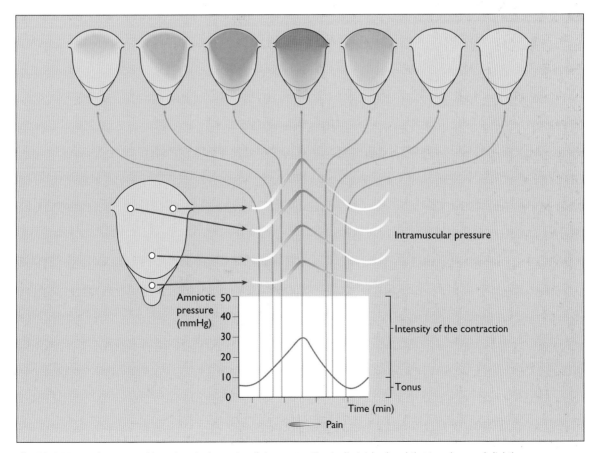

Fig. 22.1 Hypoactive uterus. Note that the intensity of the contraction is diminished and the tone lowered slightly.

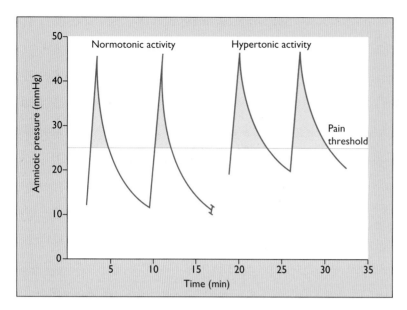

Fig. 22.2 Pain in incoordinate uterine action. Because the resting tone is raised, the pain threshold is reached earlier in the contraction and remains above the threshold for longer.

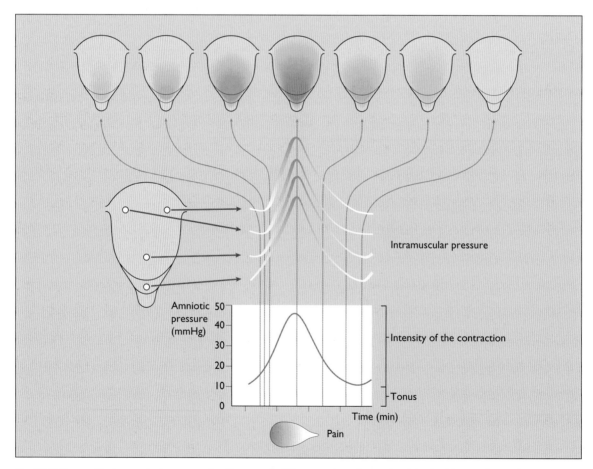

Fig. 22.3 Hyperactive lower uterine segment, with reversal of the normal gradients of activity. In this case the uterine tone is still normal but the cervix fails to dilate.

usually late in the first stage of labour or early in the second stage. It may follow the injudicious use of oxytocin or intra-uterine manipulations.

The modern classification of inefficient uterine activity

As the clinical diagnosis of the two main types of inefficient uterine activity depends on the patient's perception of the severity of the pain, its distribution and the findings on uterine palpation, the increasing use of epidural anaesthesia has limited the value of the classification.

With the introduction of the partogram, a different classification has been developed (Fig. 22.4).

- **Prolonged latent (quiet) phase.** The duration of the latent phase of labour is increased. In most cases the pattern of uterine activity shows hypoactivity.
- **Prolonged active phase.** This can be equated to the hyperactive incoordinate state of uterine activity, usually involving a hyperactive uterine lower segment (i.e. a reverse gradient of uterine activity).
- **Secondary arrest of cervical dilatation.** This pattern can be equated to incoordinate uterine activity or to the end result of obstruction to the birth in a nulliparous woman.

Management of inefficient uterine activity

Before any specific treatment is considered the course of the labour so far must be reviewed by scrutinizing the partogram, to identify, if possible, the abnormality of uterine action. The physical and psychological condition of the patient must be assessed. Dehydration and ketoacidosis should be sought and, if present, corrected by infusing 500 mL of Hartmann's solution rapidly. After this, Hartmann's solution is alternated with 5% glucose, infused at a rate of 50–100 mL/h. Fluids by mouth are avoided.

Specific treatment

Prolonged latent phase

Having established that there is no major degree of CPD and that the woman is prepared to continue with the labour, two approaches are possible. In the first, no treatment beyond reassurance is given and the onset of the active phase is awaited. The alternative is to rupture the membranes and to set up an oxytocin infusion, which is increased incrementally (see p. 190). Abdominal palpation and a vaginal examination are made at 2-hourly intervals. There are no reliable data to show that the invasive approach shortens the duration of labour significantly.

Prolonged active phase

If CPD is excluded and the woman's condition is good, the membranes are deliberately ruptured, if they are still intact, and an oxytocin infusion is set up, the rate of which is increased incrementally. Progress of labour is monitored as in the management of the prolonged latent phase. Failure of the cervix to dilate by more than 2 cm over a 4-hour period may be an indication for caesarean section.

Secondary arrest of the active stage

In this pattern of uterine activity it is essential to exclude CPD. If the woman does not have an epidural anaesthetic this should be established and an oxytocin infusion set up. (If it is not possible to provide epidural anaesthesia, an alternative is to sedate the woman with an intravenous infusion containing pethidine 300 mg and diazepam 10 mg in normal saline. The rate of the infusion is adjusted so that the woman sleeps between uterine contractions.) Monitoring of both the progress of labour and of the fetal heart rate by CTG is essential, and preparations for caesarean section are made if the cervix has not dilated by more than 2 cm over a 4-hour period.

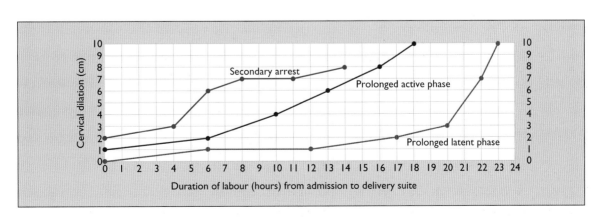

Fig. 22.4 Abnormal patterns of cervical dilatation.

Table 22.1 Classification of abnormal uterine activity and method of delivery in 684 British primigravidae

PATTERN	ALL CASES (%)	%		
		Spontaneous	Forceps	Caesarean
Normal pattern	65–70	80	18	2
Prolonged latent phase	2–5	75	10	15
Prolonged active phase	20–30	55	30	15
Secondary arrest	5–10	40	35	25

Outcome of labour

The outcome of labour treated in the above way has been reported in several studies, of which a representative is shown in Table 22.1. Since the date of that study the proportion of women delivered by caesarean section has increased but this has not led to a reduction in the perinatal mortality or morbidity, which is low.

UTERINE OVEREFFICIENCY

Precipitate labour

The birth occurs within 2 hours of the contractions starting. The contractions are intense and frequent. The problems are that the baby may be born in an inappropriate place without adequate care; may be hypoxic in utero because of the frequent, intense contractions; may suffer intracranial haemorrhage during its rapid descent through the birth canal; or may be injured by falling on the floor.

Management

If the baby has been born before the arrival of a medical attendant, mother and baby should be examined for any injury.

Because precipitate birth tends to recur, in her next pregnancy consideration should be given to admitting the mother to hospital just before the estimated date of birth and inducing labour by artificial rupture of the membranes when the cervix is favourable.

Tetanic uterine activity

This follows the uncontrolled use of oxytocin. Treatment consists of stopping the oxytocin infusion and if the uterus remains contracted and/or the fetal heart rate is bradycardic intravenous administration of a uterine relaxant such as salbutamol or terbutaline. This complication should not occur in today's obstetric practice.

SHOULDER GIRDLE DYSTOCIA

Shoulder dystocia is frequently unanticipated as it can occur in the absence of known risk factors which include maternal diabetes, macrosomia, maternal obesity, prolonged second stage, a rotational operative vaginal delivery, or previous shoulder dystocia. The fetal head may be born but the head burrows back into the perineum (turtle sign) as the bisacromial diameter of the fetal shoulders fails to rotate to enter the transverse diameter of the pelvic brim. The baby must be delivered quickly or it will die (Fig. 22.5A–D). Shoulder girdle dystocia occurs in 1% of births and the delivery requires considerable experience: damage to the lower genital tract is a usual occurrence, and damage to the baby not uncommon. Most often the damage is to the brachial plexus, or the clavicle or humerus can be fractured. The latter two will heal without sequelae, but a brachial plexus palsy can be permanent. Only 50% of brachial plexus palsies actually follow shoulder dystocia and some 5% occur in association with a caesarean delivery which implies that at least some have an antepartum aetiology.

PROLONGED LABOUR

By convention, a labour which has lasted more than 12 hours after the woman has been admitted to hospital in labour is considered to be prolonged. Between 5 and 8% of labours are classified as prolonged, and the incidence is twice as common among nulliparous women than among multipara. Cephalopelvic disproportion and inefficient uterine action are the usual causes of prolonged labour, but in a few cases no cause can be identified.

Fifty years ago, labour was defined as being prolonged if it had lasted for more than 48 hours. Labours of this length were associated with increased maternal morbidity. During these labours dehydration often occurred, infection was not uncommon, and the risk of postpartum

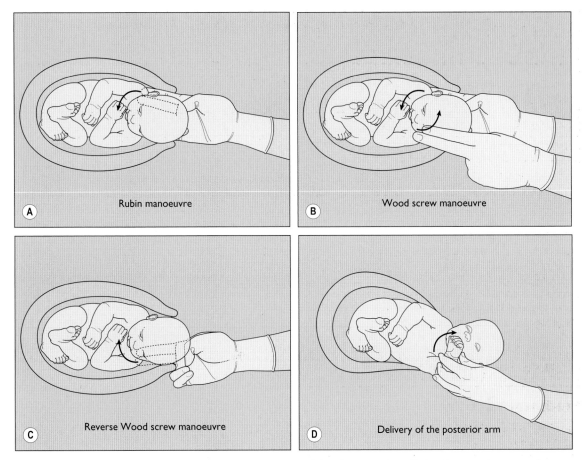

Fig. 22.5 (A) The accoucheur's hand is inserted into the vagina and digital pressure is applied to the posterior aspect of the anterior shoulder pushing it towards the fetal chest. This rotates the shoulders forward into the more favourable oblique diameter. Attempt delivery. (B) While maintaining pressure as for Rubin manoeuvre, the accoucheur introduces their second hand and locates the anterior aspect of the posterior shoulder. Pressure is applied to rotate the posterior shoulder. Attempt delivery once the shoulders move into the oblique diameter. If this movement is unsuccessful, continue rotation through 180° and attempt delivery. (C) Apply pressure to the posterior aspect of the posterior shoulder and attempt to rotate it through 180° in the opposite direction to that described in the Wood screw manoeuvre. (D) The accoucheur passes their hand into the vagina over the chest of the fetus to identify the posterior arm and elbow. Apply pressure to the antecubital fossa to flex the elbow in front of the body, and/or grasp the posterior hand to sweep the arm across the chest and deliver the arm. This is followed by rotation of the fetus into the oblique diameter of the pelvis, or through 180°, bringing the anterior shoulder under the symphysis pubis.

haemorrhage was increased. These problems should not arise in the developed countries today, but they still occur in some developing countries. Perinatal morbidity and mortality also increase in prolonged labour. The main causes are pneumonia following intra-uterine infection, increased fetal acidaemia, and trauma from an operative delivery.

Earlier intervention has reduced or eliminated these problems, but care must be taken to monitor women in labour to ensure they do not become dehydrated, ketoacidotic or infected. If the woman is anxious and distressed this should be attended to by reassurance and explanation of the progress of the labour.

PSYCHOLOGICAL EFFECTS OF DYSTOCIA AND PROLONGED LABOUR

The memory of a difficult labour, attended by unsympathetic, uncommunicative medical personnel and terminated by an operative delivery, may leave a scar on the woman's mind deeper than the scar on her abdomen or perineum.

The woman and her partner need explanation and reassurance. Most couples are anxious to know whether the next childbirth will be as difficult and painful as the last one. As inefficient uterine action is the only identified cause in many cases of prolonged labour, and as this is less likely to occur in a subsequent labour, the woman can be given some reassurance. When she becomes pregnant again, the doctor or midwife responsible for her antenatal care needs to listen to her concerns, to reduce her anxieties and to communicate with her, so that she reaches labour in a positive frame of mind. The use of adequate anaesthesia should be discussed and the patient given the choice of having an epidural anaesthetic if she so wishes.

OBSTRUCTED LABOUR

Obstructed labour is the end result of a poorly managed or neglected labour, in which CPD or a shoulder presentation has not been detected early and timely intervention effected.

During an obstructed labour, uterine contractions attempt to overcome the obstruction. In a first labour the uterus contracts strongly for a while and then, failing to overcome the obstruction, becomes hypoactive, developing secondary arrest. In contrast, if the obstruction occurs in a subsequent labour, the uterus continues to contract strongly in an attempt to push the fetus through the maternal pelvis. With each contraction there is some myometrial shortening (retraction), the upper uterine segment becoming progressively thicker and shorter, and the lower segment becoming progressively stretched and thinner. The junction between the two segments becomes obvious, forming a pathological retraction ring – Bandl's ring (Fig. 22.6). The pathological retraction ring may be confused with a distended urinary bladder, but the oblique line is diagnostic. The patient becomes dehydrated, with a coated tongue and

dry lips. She has tachycardia and concentrated urine, and faces the risk of a ruptured uterus at any time.

Treatment is urgent. The dehydration should be corrected rapidly and a caesarean section performed under antibiotic cover as soon as possible, even if the fetus is dead.

RUPTURE OF THE UTERUS

The end result of obstructed labour, unless intervention is made, is rupture of the uterus. Rupture may also occur in late pregnancy, when it may follow trauma to the uterus, or derive from a caesarean scar. In labour, as well as following an obstructed labour (Fig. 22.7), rupture of the uterus may be caused by the inappropriate use of oxytocics and the dehiscence of a caesarean section scar.

In modern obstetric practice the most common cause of uterine rupture is dehiscence and extension of a previous caesarean scar. Three per cent of classic scars rupture, most of them during labour, which is the reason for performing an elective caesarean section on a woman who has a classic caesarean scar. Rupture of a lower segment caesarean scar is less common, 0.5% rupturing, mostly during labour.

In cases of uterine rupture following trauma or obstructed labour, the rupture usually involves one or other lateral wall and extends into the upper uterine segment (Fig. 22.8).

Rupture of a lower segment caesarean scar is usually quiet. The first sign is most commonly changes in the fetal heart pattern and for this reason all such labours should be monitored by cardiotocography (CTG). Slight vaginal bleeding may occur and the patient complains of pain,

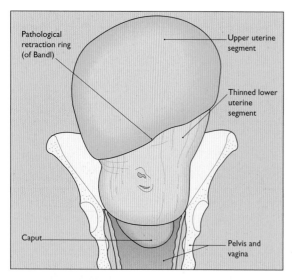

Fig. 22.6 Threatened rupture of the uterus in a case of cephalopelvic disproportion and obstructed labour.

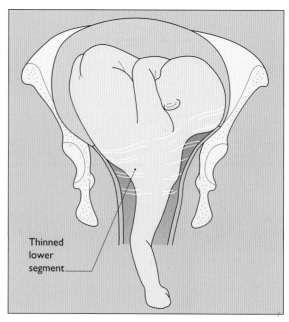

Fig. 22.7 Threatened rupture of the uterus in a neglected shoulder presentation.

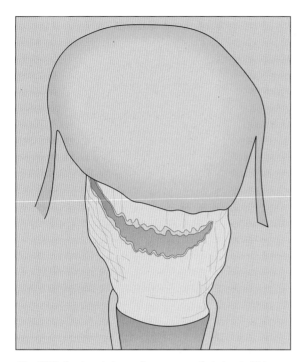

Fig. 22.8 Ruptured uterus, from a case of obstructed labour.

which becomes constant. The patient's pulse begins to rise, and in some cases shock supervenes. In some patients no symptoms or signs occur and the ruptured uterus is only detected by intra-uterine palpation following the birth.

Treatment

Rupture following obstructed labour or trauma frequently requires hysterectomy, although in a few cases the uterine tear can be sutured. Rupture of a caesarean scar generally can be sutured.

CLASSIFICATION OF PELVIC ABNORMALITIES

In the developed nations of the world, contracted pelvis has diminished as a cause of dystocia. However, among the less privileged groups in the rich nations and among the urban poor in the developing nations, contracted pelvis still occurs and may lead to a difficult labour.

Major defects of nutrition or environment

Rickets

In the past 50 years, in most developed countries rickets has largely disappeared as increasing attention has been

given to social and preventive medicine. Because in many of the developing countries they have an abundance of sunshine (which converts ergosterol in the skin into vitamin D), and most of the drinking water is rich in calcium, rickets is not common among children.

In a young child suffering from rickets the weight of the upper body presses down through the spine on to the softened pelvic bones. The sacral promontory is pushed forwards and downwards, and the sacrum itself pivots backwards. At the same time, the ligaments of the back draw the spinous process medially and the ilia flare outwards, as do the ischial tuberosities. In extreme cases the softened acetabula may be forced inwards. The main alteration in pelvic shape is a marked reduction of the anteroposterior measurement of the brim, with some irregular widening of the cavity (Fig. 22.9).

Osteomalacia

This is due to an acquired deficiency of calcium and, encountered in adult life, causes the same deformities as rickets, but is rare, except in certain inland parts of northern India and China (Fig. 22.10).

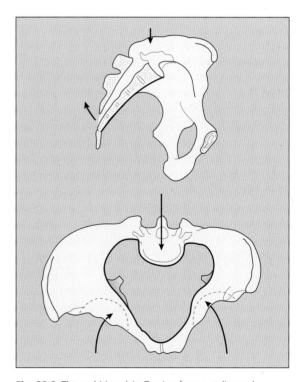

Fig. 22.9 The rachitic pelvis. Tracing from a radiograph showing the anteroposterior diameter of 8 cm, the widest transverse diameter of 11.7 cm and a brim index of 69. The arrows show how pressure on the softened bones alters the shape of the pelvis.

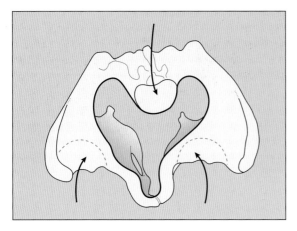

Fig. 22.10 Osteomalacic pelvis. The arrows show how pressure deforms the softened bones.

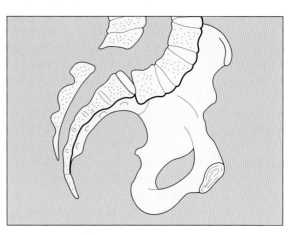

Fig. 22.12 Spondylolisthesis. Tracing from the radiograph showing the subluxation of the fifth lumbar vertebra upon the sacrum. The diagnosis can only be made by radiography.

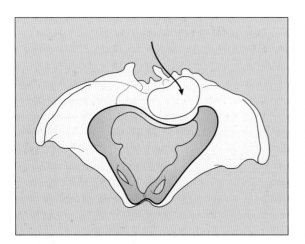

Fig. 22.11 Scoliosis and kyphosis.

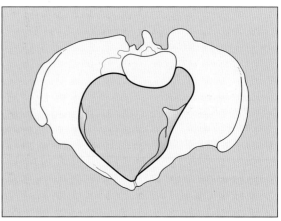

Fig. 22.13 Naegele's pelvis. Note the absence of the sacral alae.

Disease or injury

Spinal

Kyphosis of the lower dorsal or lumbar region that started in childhood may alter the shape of the brim of the pelvis, as the weight of the body pushes the upper part of the sacrum backwards and the lower part forwards. The side walls of the pelvis converge, forming a funnel. In scoliosis the altered pressure distribution on the soft bones may cause bays on each side of the sacral promontory, rendering the shape of the brim asymmetrical (Fig. 22.11). Spondylolisthesis, which means the slipping forward of the fifth lumbar vertebra to project beyond the sacral promontory, is rare (Fig. 22.12).

Pelvic

Osteomata may develop, or an injury may lead to excessive bone formation over the site of the fracture.

Limbs

Poliomyelitis in childhood, or congenital dislocation of the hip, may cause pelvic deformity. The child puts most of its weight on the stronger leg, and on this side the pelvis is pressed in, with flattening of the brim on the same side.

Congenital malformations

These include Naegele's pelvis and Robert's pelvis, and are due to the defective development of one or both sacral lateral masses, causing the sacrum to fuse with the ilium on one or both sides (Fig. 22.13). The high assimilation pelvis occurs when the fifth lumbar vertebra is fused to the sacrum, thus increasing the inclination of the pelvic brim. This hinders engagement of the fetal head.

Chapter | 23 |

Disorders in the puerperium

POSTPARTUM HAEMORRHAGE

Primary postpartum haemorrhage is a blood loss per vaginam of more than 500 mL in the first 24 hours after birth. Secondary postpartum haemorrhage is defined as abnormal bleeding from 24 hours after birth until 6 weeks postpartum.

Primary postpartum haemorrhage (PPH)

Recently many centres are reporting an increase in the rates of postpartum haemorrhage. The reasons for this are not resolved but factors such as increased operative deliveries, multiple pregnancies, obesity and changes in obstetric practice including longer duration of labour and delays in administering prophylactic oxytocics have been postulated as possible contributors.

Aetiology

In normal labour, following the birth of the baby a blood loss of 200–600 mL occurs before myometrial retraction, supplemented by strong uterine contractions. This causes shortening and kinking of the uterine blood vessels and a retraction of the placental bed. These changes prevent further blood loss (Fig. 23.1). Some discussion arises as to whether this traditional quantity of blood loss is an underestimate, when blood loss is measured accurately. Provided the blood loss is less than 800 mL, the woman should have no problems.

If the uterus does not contract effectively (atonic uterus) or if placental remnants prevent good placental site retraction, haemorrhage may occur ('an empty contracted uterus does not bleed!'). These two causes account for 80% of cases of PPH.

In 20% of cases the cause of bleeding is a laceration of the genital tract, usually of the vagina or cervix, but rarely following uterine rupture (see p. 180). In a few instances PPH follows a blood coagulation defect, such as may occur following abruptio placentae.

PPH is more likely to occur following a prolonged labour; overdistension of the uterus (multiple pregnancy or polyhydramnios); antepartum haemorrhage;

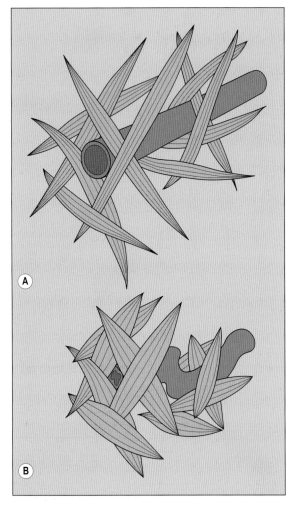

Fig. 23.1 'Living tourniquet' of contracted uterine muscle. (A) Uterine muscle fibres relaxed. (B) Contraction of muscle fibres restricts blood flow through the uterine vessels.

with operative deliveries, and deep general anaesthesia. In these cases action is taken to prevent PPH: either prophylactic oxytocics are given following the birth or, if the third stage is managed traditionally, 'fundal fiddling' is avoided. If an oxytocic is not routinely administered, the PPH rate is quadrupled to 16%.

Diagnosis

The diagnosis is usually obvious, excessive blood loss occurring before the placenta has been delivered (third-stage bleeding) or following its expulsion. After delivery of the placenta, blood may clot inside the uterus and not be expelled, causing the fundus to rise in the abdomen; if a contraction is rubbed up, the uterus contracts and the clots are expelled. The bleeding tends to be intermittent, as the uterus contracts periodically.

Management

PPH must be dealt with expeditiously, as it is a cause of maternal death. The management differs depending on whether the placenta is still in the uterus or if it has been expelled.

Third-stage bleeding (placenta in the uterus)

Two stages are involved:

- A contraction is rubbed up and fundal pressure combined with controlled cord traction is generated with the aim of delivering the placenta. If bleeding continues in spite of a contracted uterus, the lower vaginal tract should be inspected to see if there is any damage.
- If the placenta cannot be delivered or if, when it is delivered, inspection shows that it is incomplete, the uterine cavity must be explored. Unless the patient already has an epidural anaesthetic, a general anaesthetic is given and manual removal of the placenta is effected by inserting a gloved hand into the uterine cavity and controlling its actions with the other hand placed on the fundus (Fig. 23.2). The umbilical cord is followed to its insertion and the lower placental edge is identified. With the palm of the intra-uterine hand facing the uterine cavity, the obstetrician separates the placenta from its attachments with a sawing motion. When the placenta has been completely detached, the remainder of the uterine cavity is explored

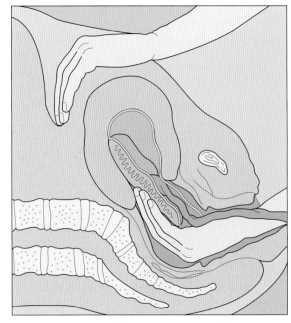

Fig. 23.2 Manual removal of the placenta.

for further placental remnants and damage. This completed, the placenta is grasped by the hand in the uterus and the membranes are pulled out of the birth canal while the external hand massages the fundus. The placenta is inspected carefully to ensure that it is complete. Ergometrine 0.5 mg is then injected intravenously and 0.5 mg is given intramuscularly.

True postpartum haemorrhage (placenta expelled)

Several stages are involved:

- Check the placenta to determine if it is complete.
- Massage the uterus with a slow, rotary movement.
- Set up an infusion of Hartmann's solution and give 0.25 mg of ergometrine intravenously or Syntocinon by continuous infusion (10 IU in 500 mL Hartmann's solution). Alternatives are Syntometrine or misoprostol 800 μg given rectally. As Syntometrine is contraindicated if the mother has hypertension, misoprostol may be preferred. In cases of severe PPH (a loss estimated at over 1000 mL) due to a hypotonic uterus, carboprost (15-methyl-$PGF_{2\alpha}$) 5 mg diluted in 20 mL saline, i.e. 1 mg/4 mL, is given; 1 mL is injected directly into the myometrium and repeated every 15 minutes if there is no response. Gemeprost pessaries can be placed directly into the uterine cavity and are another effective uterotonic agent.
- If the blood loss is more than 1000 mL, a blood transfusion may be needed.
- Check blood samples for coagulation defects and, if present, treat.
- If bleeding continues in spite of firm uterine contractions induced by the oxytocics mentioned, inspect the genital tract for lacerations.
- If bleeding persists, try bimanual compression of the uterus (Fig. 23.3). This is painful to the patient and tiring to the obstetrician.
- If bleeding persists, insertion of an intrauterine balloon catheter can provide effective compression on the placental bed
- If bleeding persists then operative intervention including the placement of a B-Lynch suture to compress the uterine fundus, internal iliac artery ligation or hysterectomy may have to be performed.
- In situations where the bleeding is persistent or when major haemorrhage is anticipated such as with placental percreta, cannulation of the uterine arteries followed by embolization can be life saving and also enable retention of the uterus.

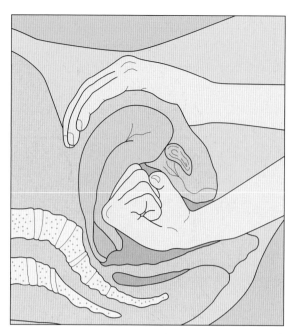

Fig. 23.3 Bimanual compression of the uterus.

Secondary postpartum haemorrhage

The most common causes of secondary postpartum haemorrhage are:

- Poor epithelialization of the placental site (80% of cases)
- A retained placental fragment and/or blood clots.

An ultrasound scan of the uterus will identify placental tissue or clots. The uterus may be bulky and tender and the cervix open. The initial treatment is to give ergometrine 0.5 mg intramuscularly, repeated if needed; and antibiotics are given to control any infection present. Curettage is only needed if placental tissue or clots are found in the uterus by ultrasound scanning, or if bleeding persists in spite of the oxytocics.

PUERPERAL INFECTION

Puerperal infection (puerperal pyrexia) is defined as a rise in temperature to 38 °C or more, maintained for 24 hours or recurring during the period from the end of the first to the end of the 10th day after childbirth or abortion. In recent years, because of better obstetric care, better hygiene and better control of infection in hospitals, the incidence of puerperal pyrexia has fallen to 1–3% of all births or abortions.

The infection may be genital or non-genital. The main causes and the probable infecting agent are shown in Table 23.1.

Table 23.1 The main bacterial causes of infection in the puerperium

Genital infection	%
Potential pathogens which normally inhabit the vagina:	
Anaerobic streptococci	65–85
Anaerobic Gram-negative bacilli	5
Haemolytic streptococci (other than group A)	1
Bacteria introduced from adjacent viscera:	
E. coli	5–15
Cl. welchii	Rare
Bacteria introduced from distant organs or from outside:	
Staphylococci	5–15
Streptococcus haemolyticus (group A)	3
Mycoplasma hominis	Rare
Non-genital infection	
Urinary tract infection:	
E. coli	
Breast infection:	
Staphylococci (mainly from the baby)	

Site and spread of the infection

Most cases of puerperal infection arising in the genital tract are ascending infections from the vagina or cervix that infect the placental bed. Spread from here is either into the parametrium or, via the uterine cavity, to the Fallopian tubes and, in some cases, onwards to cause pelvic peritonitis.

The severity of the infection depends on the virulence of the infective agent and the patient's immune response.

Diagnosis

Any woman who develops puerperal pyrexia should be investigated and may require to be isolated. The breasts are examined for signs of mastitis and a midstream urine specimen is examined to exclude urinary tract infection. An abdominal examination may reveal a tender, bulky uterus. The lower genital tract is inspected for infected lacerations, tears or episiotomy wound. A high vaginal swab is made for bacteriological examination, and the lochia smelt for an offensive odour.

Treatment

Treatment consists of giving broad-spectrum antibiotics appropriate for the infecting agents. The combination of intravenous once-daily gentamicin (5 mg/kg) and clindamycin (2700 mg) or three times daily gentamicin 1.5 mg/kg and clindamycin 900 mg until the woman has been afebrile for 24–48 hours are both effective in most cases. If there is not a rapid response then the hospital infection disease control officer should be consulted, whether the woman is in hospital or is being treated by her general practitioner at home.

THROMBOEMBOLISM

Thrombosis of a vein may occur in pregnancy (see p. 125) or, more commonly, in the puerperium, usually between days 5 and 15 of the puerperium. With better obstetric care and early ambulation, fewer women nowadays develop thromboembolic disorders in the puerperium. The incidence is fewer than 1 per 1000 births. The condition is more likely to occur in women who are overweight, over the age of 35, or who have had a caesarean section. Other risk factors include cardiac disease, diabetes and smoking. In 50 % an inherited or acquired thrombophilia can be identified.

The thrombotic process usually starts in the deep veins of the lower leg, but may extend into the femoral or pelvic veins before being detected, or may arise de novo in the pelvic veins. If these veins are involved, pulmonary embolism may occur. Pulmonary embolism affects 1 puerperal woman in 6000 in most developed western nations, and 1 affected woman in 5 dies.

Diagnosis of deep vein thrombosis (DVT)

The clinical signs are the presence of low-grade pyrexia, a raised pulse rate and a feeling of uneasiness. The clinical signs are a poor guide to the diagnosis of DVT and do not give any indication whether the thrombus is stationary, lysing or progressing. If the calf muscles are examined and are found to be tender and painful on firm palpation, DVT may be suspected. The diagnosis should be confirmed by compression ultrasound scanning, preferably using colour-enhanced Doppler imaging, in which the tibial and femoral veins are imaged in longitudinal and lateral planes and the lumen of each vein is inspected.

Diagnosis of pulmonary embolism

The woman complains of dyspnoea and, later, pleural pain. Cyanosis may develop. Examination of the chest may reveal a friction rub. A lung scan will confirm the clinical diagnosis. It should be made urgently, as two-thirds of women dying from pulmonary embolus do so within 2–4 hours.

Treatment

DVT

Heparin is given by an intravenous infusion pump (25 000 U in 500 mL normal saline) A loading dose of 5000 U is followed by infusion at a rate of 30 U/h. The rate is adjusted after 4 hours to maintain the active partial thromboplastin time (APTT) at 2.5 times the baseline APTT. Heparin is continued for 5 days. Warfarin is started at the same time as the heparin, which is continued until warfarin has prolonged the prothrombin time (international normalized ratio) to 2.5–3.5. Warfarin is continued for 6–12 weeks in cases of proven DVT, and for 12–24 weeks in cases of pulmonary embolism.

The patient remains in bed with her leg elevated until fully heparinized and until the limb ceases to be tender. She may then walk about, but should wear a properly fitted elastic stocking.

Pulmonary embolism

The same regimen of heparin is used as in the treatment of DVT. The idea of the heparin bolus is to reverse the bronchoconstriction and vasoconstriction that follow the release of serotonin from platelets. An alternative is to give streptokinase. Pulmonary embolism is so serious that expert help should be obtained.

Long-term consequences of DVT

The long-term follow-up of women who have DVT in pregnancy or the puerperium, which is adequately treated, shows that, after a median of 10 years, only 25% are without symptoms of deep vein insufficiency. Half of the women have a swollen leg, 40% have leg cramps, 25% leg discoloration and 4% leg ulceration.

POSTPARTUM PSYCHIATRIC PROBLEMS

Three psychiatric conditions affect women after childbirth: third-day blues, postpartum depression and postpartum psychosis. Post-traumatic stress disorder can also occur secondary to traumatic birth experiences, particularly if the woman does not understand what is happening.

Third-day blues

Between 50 and 70% of mothers experience a transient state of heightened emotional reactivity and feel either irritable, miserable or elated. Episodes of crying are common. The cause is not known. The symptoms start between the third and fifth days after the birth of the baby. The emotional lability usually lasts for less than a week, but may persist for a month. This is discussed on page 92.

Postnatal non-psychotic depression

Between 8 and 20% of women develop clinically diagnosed depression in the year following the birth. Usually this occurs in the first 6 months after childbirth. Women at increased risk are those who:

- Are under the age of 16 when giving birth
- Have unrealistic ideas of motherhood
- Suffered from depression during the pregnancy
- Have a history of depression or other psychological (Ch. 29) or psychiatric illness
- Have a family history of depression or other psychiatric illness
- Had an unstable, absent or abusive family (no adequate role models)
- Lacked positive support from husband or partner during and after pregnancy
- Lack support from a relative or friend who could care for the baby from time to time
- Had poor or inadequate antenatal care, which lacked accurate information and good communication with health professionals
- Experienced a complicated pregnancy (for example pre-eclampsia, placenta praevia, preterm birth, multiple birth).

In other words, women are more likely to develop postnatal depression if they are socially and emotionally isolated, or have had recent stressful life events and a genetic vulnerability.

There is no persuasive information, however, that postnatal depression is related to any hormonal or biochemical change or to any nutritional deficiency.

It is likely that women who develop postnatal depression may develop problems in maternal–infant relationships, and adverse effects on infant cognitive development may occur. Because of potential problems to the mother and infant, signs of postnatal depression should be sought early and help provided.

Women developing postnatal depression show the symptoms of ordinary depressive illness, although fatigue, irritability and anxiety are more common than in most clinically depressed women. Some psychiatrists recommend that all women presenting at a postnatal clinic 6–8 weeks after the birth should be screened using the Edinburgh Postnatal Depression Scale.

Management

The woman needs support and encouragement initially, not drugs. The doctor should listen to what she is saying, help her resolve her anxieties and conflicts about her ability to be a parent, and arrange for assistance in caring for the baby so that she may have 'time out'. Her decision to continue or cease breastfeeding should be supported. Cognitive behavioural therapy, supportive psychotherapy and couple therapy have been shown to help. In some cases, admission to hospital for a few days for support and group therapy may help; in others antidepressants should be prescribed. Parents should be reassured that if the mother is breastfeeding and takes an antidepressant drug (SSRI, selective serotonin reuptake inhibitor) the medication will have no effect on the neurological development or intelligence of her child. In more severe depression a psychiatric consultation should be obtained.

If hospital treatment is needed, admission should be to a 'mother and baby' unit if one is available, rather than to a psychiatric ward. It is important that the treatment is given early, as women whose postnatal depression lasts for more than 4 months are more likely to have depressive episodes in a subsequent pregnancy and at other times.

Postnatal psychotic depression

Between 1 and 3 per 1000 women develop a postnatal psychosis. This is manifested by delusions or hallucinations or both, which occur for the first time or as part of a recurrent illness, usually a mood disorder, such as depression or bipolar disorder (manic and depressive features), and sometimes schizophrenia. The illness starts abruptly within 3 weeks of the birth. In the beginning the woman is confused, anxious, perplexed, restless and sad. Delusions (that the baby has died or is deformed) or hallucinations develop rapidly. Just before the psychosis the woman with psychotic depression can appear well, and health professionals may inadvertently believe she has recovered.

Management

Admission to hospital is essential, preferably with the baby so that the woman's delusions may decrease. This throws a considerable strain on the staff, who have to make sure that the baby will not be harmed. Psychotropic drugs are given, haloperidol being currently preferred. Most women respond well and relatively quickly. About 15% develop the illness in a subsequent pregnancy, and one woman in three develops a non-puerperal psychosis.

Chapter | 24 |

Obstetric operations

INDUCTION OF LABOUR

Induction of labour may be required to 'rescue' the fetus from a potentially hazardous intra-uterine environment in late pregnancy for a variety of reasons, or because continuation of the pregnancy is dangerous to the expectant mother. Indications for induction of labour are listed in Table 24.1.

The method adopted depends on:

- The duration of the pregnancy
- The condition of the cervix (i.e. favourable or unfavourable) (Fig. 24.1)
- The position of the fetal head in relation to the pelvis.

The highest rate of success, (i.e. that the induction is followed by a vaginal birth within 24 hours) occurs in a woman whose cervix is favourable and whose Bishop score is 5 or more (Table 24.2).

If the chances of success are evaluated as low, the doctor may recommend caesarean section.

Techniques of inducing labour

Labour may be induced by drugs, by the surgical technique of amniotomy, which is also known as artificial rupture of the membranes (ARM), or by mechanical stimulation of the cervix.

Induction of labour using drugs

Two agents are available: prostaglandins and oxytocin.

Prostaglandins

Three prostaglandins with different properties are used.

- PGE_1 gemeprost is available in pessary form or as an intracervical injection system. It is used in the second trimester of pregnancy for the termination of pregnancy and for the induction of labour in cases of fetal death in utero. It should be avoided in the third trimester because of the risk of uterine hypertonicity. Misoprostol is a synthetic PGE_1 analogue which compares favourably with PGE_1 and PGE_2 in its efficacy in inducing labour. It can be administered by placing a tablet ($25\,\mu g$) in the posterior vaginal fornix every 4 hours. Oral administration appears to be less effective and has been reported to be associated with higher rates of uterine hyperstimulation.
- PGE_2 is available as a gel or in pessary form and may be introduced intravaginally or intracervically. The gel appears to be more effective and is associated

Table 24.1 Indications for induction of labour: Australia

INDICATION	PROPORTION OF INDUCTIONS
Prolonged pregnancy (41 or more weeks)	26%
Hypertensive disorders	12%
Prelabour/prolonged rupture of membranes	10%
Diabetes – pregestational and gestational	7%
Intra-uterine growth restriction	5%
Non-reassuring fetal status	2%
Fetal death in utero (FDIU)	1%
Blood group isoimmunization	0.2%
Chorioamnionitis	0.1%
Social induction	16%
Others	21%

with a lower risk of producing uterine hypertonicity. PGE$_2$ softens the cervical connective tissue and relaxes cervical muscle fibres, 'ripening' the cervix. PGE$_2$ may stimulate the production of PGF$_2\alpha$, which will induce uterine contractions. PGE$_2$ produces cervical ripening when the cervical (Bishop) score is less than 5, and therefore amniotomy is contraindicated. It is available in a prefilled syringe in a dose of 1–2 mg, which is introduced into the posterior vaginal fornix. The patient's pulse rate, fetal heart rate and uterine activity are monitored for 30 minutes, after which time she may walk about if she wishes, provided the pregnancy is not at high risk. If labour is not established within 6 hours the woman is reassessed. If the cervix is now favourable ARM is performed, otherwise a further dose of PGE$_2$ is given.

- A slow-release pessary (Cervidil). It releases a mean of 4 mg over 12 hours and can easily be removed by its tape if necessary.

Oxytocin (Syntocinon)

Oxytocin should always be administered by intravenous infusion, preferably using an infusion pump. If it is used alone, 50% of women will be in labour within 12 hours. Induction is more effective if preceded by PGE$_2$ vaginal pessaries or following amniotomy.

The infusion rate is increased by 5 mU/min every 30 minutes until contractions lasting longer than 60 seconds recur at 3–5-minute intervals. The maximum rate used is 60 mU/min. Because of the risk of water intoxication, the quantity of fluid infused should not exceed 1500 mL in 10 hours.

Surgical induction of labour (amniotomy)

Surgical induction of labour (amniotomy) is more effective if the cervix is favourable (Bishop score 5+). The patient is placed in the dorsal or lithotomy position and the vagina swabbed with antiseptic. Two of the doctor's fingers are inserted to reach the cervix and, if practicable, one is inserted through the cervix to 'sweep' the membranes. An amnihook, or a Kocher forceps, is introduced along the intravaginal fingers and the membranes below the fetal head (the forewaters) are broken with the instrument.

The problems following amniotomy are:

- Prolapse of the umbilical cord (0.5% of cases)
- Infection, if the induction–delivery interval is >24 hours.

A suggested schema (flow chart) for the induction of labour is shown in Figure 24.2.

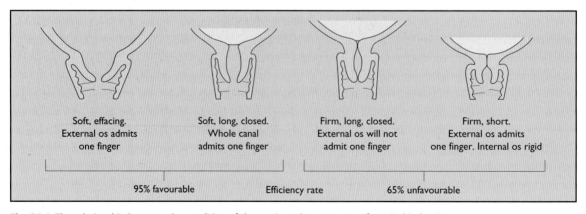

| Soft, effacing. External os admits one finger | Soft, long, closed. Whole canal admits one finger | Firm, long, closed. External os will not admit one finger | Firm, short. External os admits one finger. Internal os rigid |

95% favourable   Efficiency rate   65% unfavourable

Fig. 24.1 The relationship between the condition of the cervix and success rate of surgical induction.

Table 24.2 A method of cervical 'scoring' (Bishop score)

FACTOR	SCORING RATING			
	0	1	2	3
Cervix				
Length (cm)	>4	>2	1–2	<1
Dilatation (cm)	<1	<2	2–3	>4
Consistency	Firm	'Average'	Soft	Soft
Position	Posterior	Other (mid, anterior)	Other	Other
Fetal head				
Position relative to ischial spines (cm)	−3	−2	−1 or 0	+1 or more

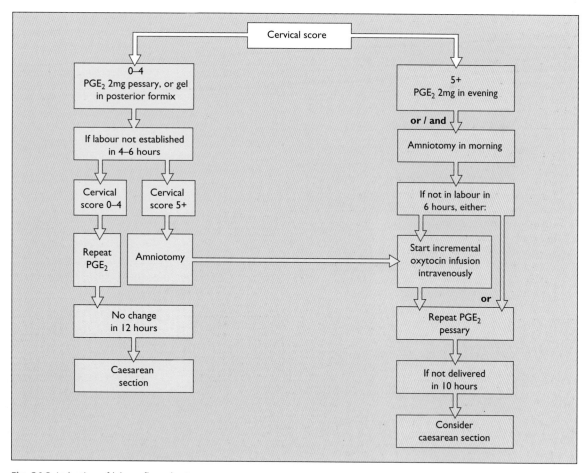

Fig. 24.2 Induction of labour flow chart.

As can be seen from the flow chart, if the cervix is 'unfavourable' (i.e. a low Bishop score), the drugs mentioned may be used to ripen the cervix so that surgical induction, if needed, will be more effective. In the flow chart PGE_2 is featured, but the other prostaglandins listed above are equally effective.

Mechanical methods

A single (e.g. Foley) or double (Atad) balloon catheter is also an effective method of inducing labour. The catheter is passed aseptically through the cervix and the balloon(s) are inflated with sterile saline. The woman is then free to ambulate and is assessed 6 or so hours later, unless she goes into labour or the membranes rupture. Other devices, such as the hydrophilic laminaria tent have been used. They swell by absorbing fluid and so slowly dilate the cervix.

The principal benefits of balloon catheters are the induction of labour in women who have previously had a caesarean section; this avoids the potential hyperstimulation that may occur with prostaglandins, or the theoretical softening of the collagen fibres in the uterine scar.

AUGMENTATION OF LABOUR

In cases where the quality of the uterine contractions is poor (see p. 174), their strength may be augmented by performing ARM and, if necessary, by setting up an incremental oxytocic infusion, or both.

INSTRUMENTAL DELIVERY

In the second stage of labour situations may arise wherein it becomes necessary to deliver the baby. These are:

- Delay in the birth of the baby when the second stage of labour has exceeded 2 hours without regional anaesthesia or 3 hours with regional anaesthesia in a nulliparous woman or the fetal head has been delayed on the perineum for more than 30 minutes. The delay usually occurs because:
  - The fetal head has not rotated and is arrested in the transverse diameter of the midpelvic cavity (deep transverse arrest of the head).
  - The head has rotated into the posterior position in the midcavity or in the lower pelvic strait (posterior arrest of the head).
  - A minor degree of cephalopelvic disproportion is present.
  - The uterine contractions have become weaker.
- The fetus shows signs of distress (i.e. bradycardia or the passage of meconium).
- The mother has become distressed, either physically or mentally, in the second stage of labour.
- The mother has an existing obstetric condition, or a medical one (e.g. pre-eclampsia, chronic hypertension, cardiac disease), that may deteriorate during the expulsive stage of labour.
- To aid in the delivery of the aftercoming head in a breech presentation.

Methods and conditions of instrumental delivery

The incidence of instrumental delivery varies between 5 and 12% of all deliveries. Two methods are available. The first, delivery by obstetric forceps, was introduced 400 years ago; the second, delivery by vacuum extraction, was introduced 70 years ago.

The conditions for instrumental delivery are:

- The greatest diameter of the fetal head must have passed the pelvic brim.
- The cervix must be fully dilated.
- The membranes must have ruptured and the bladder must be empty.
- The patient must receive adequate anaesthesia or analgesia. Women requiring a vacuum extraction or a low forceps require a perineal nerve block at the very least. Women requiring a midforceps delivery should have an epidural block, a pudendal nerve block or a general anaesthetic.

Obstetric forceps

From crude beginnings the obstetric forceps has developed into a precision instrument that must be used with great skill to avoid damage to the woman or her fetus. More than four-fifths of forceps deliveries are by low or outlet forceps, which are relatively safe.

Types of forceps delivery

As shown in Figure 24.3, the station of the fetal head is used to describe the type of forceps delivery.

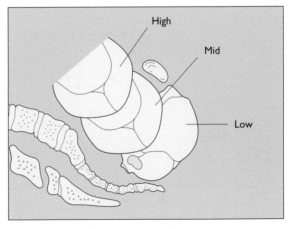

Fig. 24.3 Types of forceps delivery, showing the station of the head when the forceps is applied.

- **High forceps** deliveries are no longer performed because of the high risk of causing serious fetal and maternal damage. Delivery should be by caesarean section.
- **Midforceps.** The forceps blades are applied to the sides of the fetal head, whose biparietal diameter has entered the pelvis but has not advanced much beyond the ischial spines. Usually the occiput lies in one or other transverse diameter of the maternal pelvis.
- **Low forceps.** The forceps blades are applied to the sides of the fetal head, whose biparietal diameter has advanced to or beyond the ischial tuberosities and has rotated so that the sagittal suture lies in the anteroposterior diameter of the maternal pelvis.
- **Outlet forceps.** The fetal head distends the vaginal introitus, but the perineum is holding it back.

The short-shanked forceps is used for low or outlet forceps procedures (Fig. 24.4). The long-shanked forceps is used for midforceps delivery after manual rotation of the fetal head if it is arrested in the transverse diameter of the pelvis (Fig. 24.5). They are also suitable for low or outlet deliveries. Kjelland's forceps has a sliding lock and can be used to rotate the fetal head and deliver it (see Fig. 24.6).

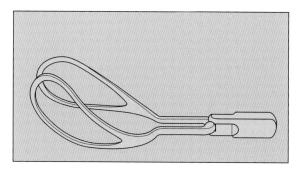

Fig. 24.4 Wrigley's forceps (scale ×2 that of Figs. 24.5 and 24.6).

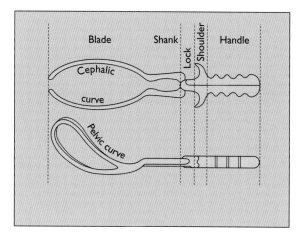

Fig. 24.5 Simpson's obstetric forceps.

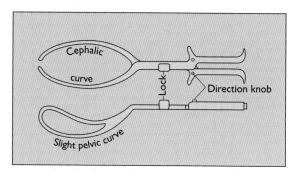

Fig. 24.6 Kjelland's forceps.

All forceps compress the fetal head to some extent and apply traction to effect the birth.

Technique of forceps delivery

The technique of forceps delivery is shown in Figures 24.7–24.15.

Low or outlet forceps

The use of these is described in Figures 24.7–24.10.

Midforceps

The technique for applying the long-shanked curved forceps is the same as that used to apply the short-shanked forceps. As the forceps blades have to be introduced further into the vagina, great care must be exercised to avoid damaging the

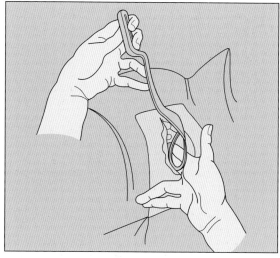

Fig. 24.7 The assembled forceps are held in front of the woman's vulva, with the pelvic curve uppermost. The left blade is introduced, without force, into the vagina between the fetal head and the vaginal wall, which is protected by the doctor's fingers; the blade is steered to lie along the left side of the baby's head.

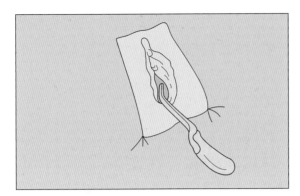

Fig. 24.8 When correctly applied the shank will press on the mother's perineum.

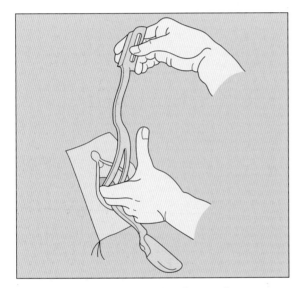

Fig. 24.9 The right blade is introduced in a similar manner and the two blades are assembled in the lock. If they do not fit easily into the lock there is a misapplication, and if they cannot be made to adjust easily, the forceps is removed and the procedure is repeated.

vaginal wall and to ensure that the forceps blades are correctly applied along the sides of the fetal head.

Because the head has to be pulled through the pelvic curve, the mother should be positioned correctly, with her legs in stirrups and her buttocks projecting over the end of the bed (see Fig. 24.11). This is because the pull required to deliver the baby has to be downwards initially and then curving upwards (see Fig. 24.12). Some obstetricians use the axis traction device, but skill is required to use it properly (see Fig. 24.13).

If the baby's head is arrested in the transverse diameter of the midpelvis manual rotation may be attempted (see Fig. 24.14), followed by midforceps delivery. Alternatively, Kjelland's forceps may be used or a caesarean section performed.

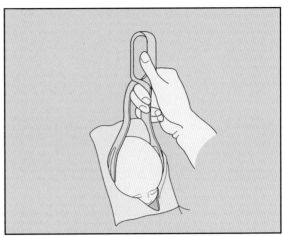

Fig. 24.10 The forceps are held as shown and the baby's head is delivered in a smooth curve, using controlled traction, preferably during a uterine contraction. An episiotomy is often needed to prevent a perineal tear.

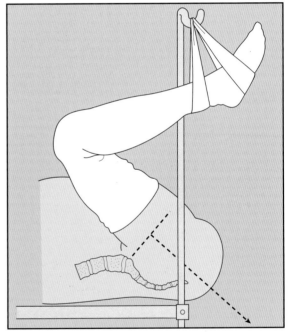

Fig. 24.11 Position of the patient for midforceps delivery.

Kjelland's forceps

This instrument is used to rotate a head arrested in the transverse diameter of the midpelvis. It requires considerable skill and the woman should ideally be delivered in an operating theatre so that, if any difficulty is experienced, a caesarean section can be done immediately.

The forceps is held in front of the woman's vulva and positioned so that the dot on the shoulders of the instrument

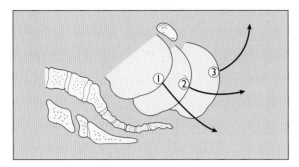

Fig. 24.12 Direction of traction in forceps delivery. In midforceps delivery (1) the initial direction of pull is downwards, in low forceps (2) horizontal, and in outlet forceps (3) slightly upwards.

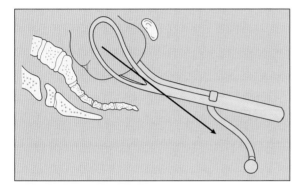

Fig. 24.13 The mechanics of forceps delivery. Midforceps: with axis traction the force is resolved and the pull is in the axis of the birth canal.

points to the side of the pelvis where the baby's occiput lies. The remainder of the application of Kjelland's forceps is shown in Figure 24.15. Usually a wide episiotomy is made, as perineal damage is almost inevitable. Alternative methods of delivery are vacuum extraction, manual rotation of the fetal head and forceps delivery, or caesarean section.

Dangers of a difficult forceps delivery

The vagina and cervix may be damaged, causing haemorrhage. Following a midforceps delivery the entire vagina should be inspected with good illumination, and lacerations looked for and sutured.

The dangers to the fetus are trauma, compression of the brain, and tentorial tearing caused by too strong compression and traction. Fracture of the fetal skull and facial paresis may occur if the forceps has been incorrectly applied and compresses the nerve where it nerve emerges in front of the mastoid process.

Vacuum extractor or ventouse

The vacuum extractor, or ventouse, consists of a cup, either metal or plastic (the 'soft cup') with a handle. The cup is attached to a tube, which connects with the suction apparatus. The cup is positioned over the flexion point of the

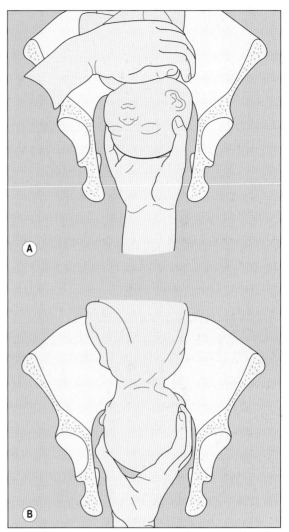

Fig. 24.14 Manual rotation of the head from a left occipitoposterior position. (A) The left hand is placed on the abdomen and pulls the right shoulder of the baby towards the mother's right side. Simultaneously, the right hand, in supination, holds the head by its biparietal diameter and rotates it through 180° to a position of pronation. (B) At the end of the manoeuvre the occiput becomes anterior.

head, which is located along the sagittal suture 3 cm from the posterior fontanelle of the fetal head, and is held firmly against the scalp while a vacuum is slowly built up. This sucks some of the scalp into the cup, forming a firm attachment. Once a vacuum of 0.8 kg/cm^2 is obtained, the perimeter of the cup is checked to ensure that no vaginal tissue is included and traction is applied by pulling the handle at right-angles to the pelvic curve, concurrently with a uterine contraction and with the mother's own expulsive efforts.

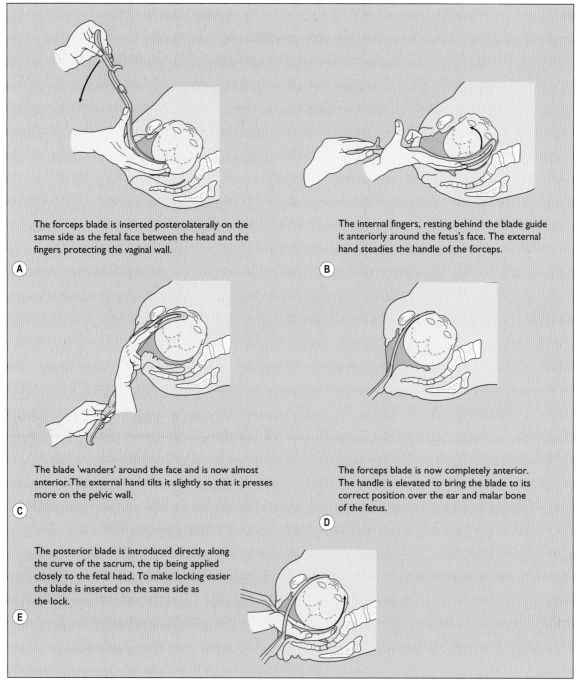

The forceps blade is inserted posterolaterally on the same side as the fetal face between the head and the fingers protecting the vaginal wall.

(A)

The internal fingers, resting behind the blade guide it anteriorly around the fetus's face. The external hand steadies the handle of the forceps.

(B)

The blade 'wanders' around the face and is now almost anterior. The external hand tilts it slightly so that it presses more on the pelvic wall.

(C)

The forceps blade is now completely anterior. The handle is elevated to bring the blade to its correct position over the ear and malar bone of the fetus.

(D)

The posterior blade is introduced directly along the curve of the sacrum, the tip being applied closely to the fetal head. To make locking easier the blade is inserted on the same side as the lock.

(E)

Fig. 24.15 Application of Kjelland's forceps in cases of deep transverse arrest.

If the head is in a transverse or posterior position a manoeuvrable cup, such as the Bird posterior cup or the Omnicup (Fig. 24.16), is used as it allows accurate placement over the flexion point.

The hard cups (e.g. Malmstrom, Bird, O'Neil and Omnicup) have a lower failure rate than the soft cups (e.g. Silc, Silastic) – 5% versus 14% – and a lower detachment rate, 13% versus 33%.

Systematic reviews comparing the vacuum extractor with forceps delivery have concluded that the vacuum extractor:

- Is less likely to deliver the baby
- Is associated with a lower caesarean section rate

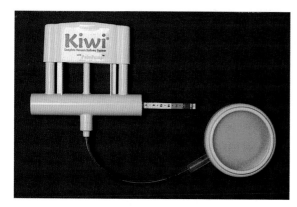

Fig. 24.16 Omnicup vacuum extractor system. Note that the vacuum tubing is attached to the side of the cup, which allows the cup to be placed over the flexion point in deflexed (occipitoposterior and lateral) positions, enabling rotation of the fetal head as it descends. The system incorporates a palm pump.

- Is less likely to cause serious maternal injury
- Requires less anaesthesia, both regional and local
- Is associated with less maternal pain at delivery and at 24 hours
- Is associated with more cephalhaematomas, subgaleal haemorrhage and retinal haemorrhages
- Is not associated with significant differences in neonatal morbidity
- Results in more maternal concerns about the appearance of the baby.

The ventouse cannot be used to aid the delivery of the aftercoming head of a breech presentation, or if the baby is preterm. Early reports suggested that it should not be used after fetal scalp blood sampling, but larger reviews have not supported this. The most serious injury associated with vacuum extraction is a subgaleal (subaponeurotic) haemorrhage. This almost always follows poor application of the cup, prolonged extraction, and multiple cup detachments and reapplications. It is important that all babies delivered by vacuum extraction or forceps are carefully examined after delivery and monitored at regular intervals if the delivery was difficult.

CAESAREAN SECTION

Caesarean section means that the baby is removed from an intact uterus by abdominal operation. In many developed countries the caesarean section rate has risen from 5% 30 years ago, to 15–35%. This increase is due to:

- Fashion
- Fear of litigation if a perfect baby is not born
- The changing pattern of conception: women are delaying the conception of their first child and are limiting the number of children they have

- The trend to deliver all breeches and a high proportion of multiple pregnancies abdominally.

Indications for caesarean section

These have broadened in recent years and are listed in Box 24.1.

Technique of caesarean section

There are two types of caesarean section. In the first, a transverse incision is made through the stretched lower uterine segment. In the second – the classic section – a vertical incision is made through the myometrium. The classic section is now rarely used, except when the lower uterine segment is excessively vascular, cannot be reached because of extensive adhesions, or if the fetus presents as a transverse lie, with an impacted shoulder. Caesarean hysterectomy may be required if intractable bleeding occurs, for placenta accreta, or if the uterus has ruptured.

The operative technique is shown in Figure 24.17. As blood loss is unpredictable, cross-matched blood should be available.

Postoperative care is no different from that for any other abdominal operation. Early ambulation is encouraged, especially as in some hospitals the neonate is kept in the nursery for 24–48 hours. Maternal morbidity varies between 3 and 12%, depending on the reason for the caesarean section.

Box 24.1 Indications for caesarean section

- Failure of labour to progress (dystocia)
    - abnormal uterine action
    - cephalopelvic disproportion
- Malpresentation or malpositions
    - breech
    - face and brow
    - transverse lie
    - occipitoposterior
    - prolapse of umbilical cord
    - multiple pregnancy
- Antepartum haemorrhage
    - abrupto placentae
    - placenta praevia
- Hypertensive disease in pregnancy
- Diabetes mellitus
- Fetal conditions
    - fetal distress
    - isoimmunization
    - very low birthweight
- Older primigravidae
- Failed induction of labour
- Repeat caesarean section

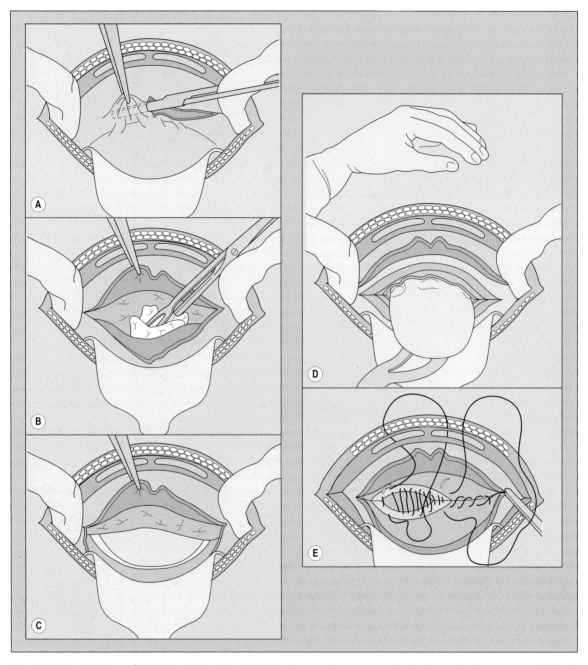

Fig. 24.17 The technique of caesarean section. (A) and (B) The loose peritoneum covering the lower uterine segment is divided and pushed down. (C) The exposed muscle of the lower segment is incised so that the membranes bulge into the wound. The incision may be extended with a knife, or the muscle fibres separated with the fingers. (D) The membranes are ruptured and the head delivered using a forceps blade as an inclined plane, counterpressure being exerted on the fundus. (E) The placenta has been expelled and the wound sutured in layers. Great care must be taken at the angles.

Endometritis accounts for two-thirds of morbidity. For this reason, prophylactic antibiotics are routinely given during the operation. Women at higher risk of developing thromboembolism are prescribed prophylactic anticoagulants.

Caesarean section is a very safe operation, the overall mortality rate being about 0.4 per 1000 sections and 0.1 per 1000 sections performed electively.

VAGINAL BIRTH AFTER PREVIOUS CAESAREAN SECTION

When a caesarean section is performed for a non-recurrent condition, the next baby may be born vaginally or by caesarean section depending on the wishes of the woman and the advice of the obstetrician. Studies from countries outside North America show that nearly half the women who had a previous caesarean section deliver their next baby vaginally. In North America less than one-third deliver vaginally. The expected rate for achieving a vaginal birth is between 60 to 80%. This is reduced by about 10% if labour is induced and for women with a BMI >30 the success rate is 55%.

If a woman chooses a vaginal birth after a caesarean section (VBAC), the birth should take place in a well-equipped hospital staffed by experienced obstetricians. The reason for this is that the trial of vaginal delivery is terminated by caesarean section in one-fifth of all cases, 0.25% of women suffering a ruptured uterus. Induction of labour using prostaglandins is associated with an increased risk of uterine rupture by comparison with ARM and Syntocinon and therefore should be used only with close supervision.

If an elective caesarean section is chosen, the maturity of the fetus must be established so that the operation is performed when the gestation period is greater than 38 weeks, to obtain the lowest neonatal respiratory morbidity.

VERSION

External cephalic version may be chosen when a fetus presenting as a breech has not turned cephalically by the 37th week of pregnancy. Before attempting the version the doctor must be sure that the pelvis has normal dimensions and that the placenta is not praevia. The mother should not have hypertension or a multiple pregnancy.

Some doctors give a tocolytic drug intravenously before the attempt. The version is performed gently. The breech is mobilized and the version attempted by lifting it with one hand and pushing the fetal head down with the other (Fig. 24.18). The fetal heart rate is either monitored continuously or every 2 minutes during, and for 30 minutes after, the version. If the fetal heart rate falls below 90 bpm

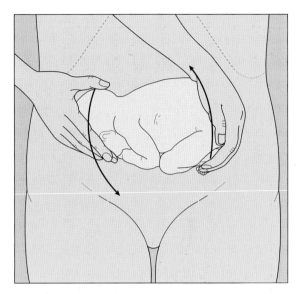

Fig. 24.18 External version. The obstetrician has lifted the buttocks out of the pelvis; his right thumb controls the baby's head and the direction in which the child is moved encourages flexion.

during the version, the attempt is abandoned. Short-term bradycardia occurs in 20% but delivery by emergency caesarean section, because of persistent bradycardia, is required in only 0.2%.

Other problems associated with version are uncommon. They include rupture of the membranes, cord entanglement around a limb of the fetus, and the onset of premature labour.

There is insufficient evidence to support moxibustion (burning of *Artemisia vulgaris* to stimulate acupuncture point lateral to the small toe), acupuncture alone or maternal postural positioning, to effect conversion of the breech to a cephalic presentation.

Internal podalic version, in which the doctor's hand is introduced into the uterus to grasp a limb and pull it through a fully dilated cervix, is rarely performed today. It may find use in cases of the delayed birth of a second twin which is lying transversely in the uterus, but in most cases caesarean section is safer.

DESTRUCTIVE OPERATIONS ON THE FETUS

There is very little place for these procedures in modern obstetric practice. An exception may be when a hydrocephalic fetus has died during labour. In this case the head is perforated with a perforator and the fluid allowed to drain, making the fetus easier to deliver.

The epidemiology of obstetrics

The quality of obstetric care in a country can be measured by the maternal and the perinatal mortality rates. The death of a woman in pregnancy or childbirth is one of the greatest tragedies that can happen to a family.

MATERNAL MORTALITY

A maternal death is defined by the International Classification of Diseases, Injuries and Causes of Death (ICD-10) as the death of a woman while pregnant or within 42 days after abortion, miscarriage or delivery that are due to direct or indirect maternal causes. These deaths are divided into direct, indirect, late and incidental (Box 25.1). The maternal mortality rate is the number of such deaths per 100 000 maternities.

In most developed countries the maternal death rate remained about the same from 1850 to 1934, when it began to fall. In the period before the mid-1930s it was about 500 per 100 000; by the mid-1980s, in many industrialized countries it had fallen to fewer than 10 per 100 000 maternities (Fig. 25.1). The initial fall was due to the control of infections by better obstetric care and the introduction of antibiotics. The second factor was that most women availed themselves of good-quality antenatal care, which enabled complications to be detected early and treatment to be offered, usually in well-equipped hospitals staffed by trained medical attendants. Blood became increasingly and quickly available from blood banks, which considerably reduced the deaths due to haemorrhage. Sociological changes have also occurred in the past 60 years: fewer women now have more than three children, and most have their pregnancies before the age of 35. Higher parity and advancing age increase the risk of maternal death. There has been a small rise in the maternal mortality rates in some developed countries in the last decade. Whether this is due to women with medical conditions that previously precluded pregnancy having children, increasing maternal age, the rise in obesity or better ascertainment of cases is not clear.

In the developing countries the maternal mortality rate is much higher. In sub-Saharan Africa it averages 600 per 100 000 live births; in south Asia, 500 per 100 000 births; in southeast Asia and Latin America 300 per 100 000 live births. The reasons for these high rates are: frequent pregnancies, with short intervals between them; the resort to unsafe abortion performed in unhygienic surroundings; a relative lack of prenatal care and a lack of the perception of its value by poorly educated and poorly informed women; a lack of access to skilled medical help; and a lack of government support to make changes to the status, education and empowerment of women. Worldwide a woman dies every minute as a result of pregnancy.

Box 25.1 Definitions of maternal deaths

International Classification of Diseases (ICD-10): Deaths of women while pregnant or within 42 days of delivery, miscarriage or termination of pregnancy irrespective of the cause of death.

World Health Organization (WHO): Death of a woman during pregnancy, childbirth or in the 42 days of the puerperium irrespective of the duration or site of the pregnancy, from any cause related to or aggravated by the pregnancy or its management. Excludes incidental deaths from causes unrelated to pregnancy such as death from injury or malignancy.

Direct: Deaths resulting from obstetric complications of the pregnant state (pregnancy, labour and puerperium), from interventions, omissions, incorrect treatment or from a chain of events resulting from any of the above.

Indirect: Deaths resulting from previous existing disease or disease developed during pregnancy and which was not due to direct obstetric causes, but was aggravated by the physiological effects of pregnancy. Includes deaths consequent on psychiatric disease, suicide and homicide.

Late: Deaths occurring between 42 days and 1 year after termination of pregnancy, miscarriage or delivery that are due to direct or indirect maternal causes.

Incidental: Deaths from unrelated causes which happen to occur in pregnancy or the puerperium, e.g. passenger in a motor vehicle accident.

Causes of maternal death

Several developed countries publish the results of confidential enquiries into maternal deaths at intervals of about 3 years. In these reports the causes of and contributing factors to the deaths are analysed and suggestions are made that might prevent such deaths occurring.

These reports have been published in the UK since 1952 and in Australia since 1965. The total direct and indirect deaths per 100 000 maternities had risen from 9.83 in the 1985–7 triennium to 12.45 in 2003–5. This may be due to underreporting in earlier years, but emphasizes that there is no room for complacency in modern maternity units in the developed world. The major contributing factors to suboptimal care are poor liaison between healthcare professionals, failure to appreciate the severity of the condition, and wrong diagnosis. Table 25.1 shows the most common causes of death, Table 25.2 the percentage associated with substandard care, and Figure 25.2 illustrates the changes with time in the major causes of maternal death in England and Wales. Maternal deaths can be reduced further, particularly those associated with anaesthesia, ectopic gestation, sepsis and pulmonary embolism.

Table 25.1 Major causes of maternal deaths per million maternities in the UK 1985–2005

CAUSE	DEATHS
Direct	
Thrombosis and thromboembolism	14–22
Pre-eclampsia and eclampsia	7–12
Haemorrhage	3–9
Amniotic fluid embolus	4–8
Early pregnancy (ectopic and miscarriage)	5–8
Sepsis	4–9
Anaesthetic	1–3
Indirect	
Cardiac	8–23
Psychiatric	4–9
Malignancies	3–5
Coincidental	12–26
Late	10–40

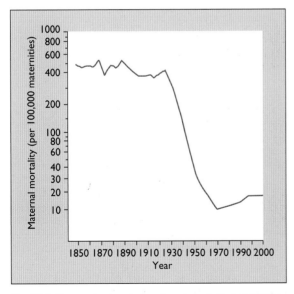

Fig. 25.1 The secular trend of maternal mortality in Australia and the United Kingdom.

Table 25.2 Direct and indirect maternal deaths United Kingdom 2003–2005 assessed as having substandard care

CAUSE OF DEATH	% WITH SUBSTANDARD CARE
Direct	
Thromboembolism	56
Pulmonary embolism	67
Cerebral embolism	13
Pre-eclampsia/eclampsia	72
Haemorrhage	59
Amniotic fluid embolism	41
Early pregnancy	79
Sepsis	78
Anaesthetic	100
All direct	64
Late direct	55
Indirect	
Cardiac	46
Psychiatric	42
Malignancy	50

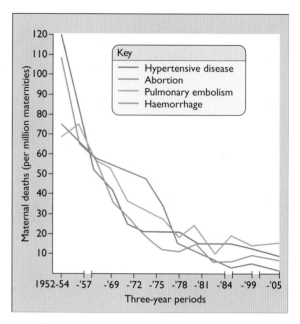

Fig. 25.2 Main causes of maternal deaths directly due to pregnancy or childbirth (England and Wales) per million maternities.

- Late fetal death is fetal death at 28 completed weeks of gestation and over. The fetus usually weighs 1000 g or more (also called stillbirth).
- Neonatal death is the death of a liveborn infant, less than 28 completed days after birth, of at least 20 weeks' gestation or if the gestation is unknown weighing at least 400 g. Neonatal deaths can be divided into two groups: early neonatal deaths and late neonatal deaths.
  - Early neonatal or postnatal death is the death of a liveborn baby in the first 7 completed days (168 hours) of life.
  - Late neonatal death is the death of a liveborn infant after 7 completed days but before 28 completed days of life.

Perinatal death is a stillbirth (or fetal death) or neonatal death

The definitions of the mortality rates and ratios is summarized in Box 25.2. For international comparison the WHO perinatal mortality rate refers to all births of at least 1000 g birthweight or when the birthweight is unknown, of at least 28 weeks' gestation and neonatal deaths occurring within 7 days of birth. In many developed nations the PMR is around 6 per 1000 births. In the few developing countries that have been able to publish reasonably reliable data the PMR is between 35 and 55 per 1000 births.

Social factors affecting the PMR

The most exact information about the effect of sociological factors on the PMR is obtained from the British Perinatal

PERINATAL MORTALITY

The death of a fetus in utero or its death in the neonatal period causes much distress to the parents and is a measure of the quality of obstetric care.

Before perinatal mortality can be discussed, some terms need to be clarified.

- Live birth is the birth of an infant, regardless of maturity or birthweight, who breathes or shows any other signs of life after being born.
- Stillbirth or fetal death is the birth of an infant of at least 20 weeks' gestation or if gestation is unknown weighing at least 400 g, which shows no signs of life after birth.
- Early fetal deaths equate to abortions, and intermediate fetal deaths are those occurring between the 22nd and 27th completed gestational weeks, the fetus weighing 500–999 g (also called stillbirth).

Box 25.2 Definitions of mortality rates and ratios

$$\text{Stillbirth rate (per 1000 total births)} = \frac{\text{Number of stillbirths} \times 1000}{\text{Total (stillbirths + livebirths)}}$$

$$\text{Neonatal mortality rate (per 1000 livebirths)} = \frac{\text{Number of neonatal deaths} \times 1000}{\text{Total livebirths}}$$

$$\begin{array}{l}\text{Perinatal mortality rate (PMR)}\\\text{(per 1000 total births)}\end{array} = \frac{(\text{Number of stillbirths + neonatal deaths}) \times 1000}{\text{Total (stillbirths + livebirths)}}$$

$$\text{Infant mortality rate (per 1000 live births)} = \frac{\text{Number of infant deaths} \times 1000}{\text{Total live births}}$$

$$\text{Maternal mortality ratio} = \frac{\text{Number of direct and indirect maternal deaths} \times 100\,000\text{ confinements}}{\text{Total number of confinements}}$$

Mortality Surveys published in 1958 and 1970. All births occurring during 1 week and all singleton fetal deaths and neonatal deaths over a 3-month period were surveyed.

The findings were that:

- The lower the social class the higher the standard PMR, which rose from 7.5 per 1000 in social class 1 to 26.8 per 1000 in social classes IV and V.
- The mother's age affected the PMR. It was highest among the infants of mothers younger than 17 years and older than 35 years.
- Women who did not avail themselves of antenatal care had 5–10 times the mean PMR.
- The management of the labour affected the PMR. One-third of the perinatal deaths were due to intrapartum anoxia alone or were associated with birth trauma. In some cases the intrapartum anoxia was a sequel to antepartum conditions, the fetus entering labour in poor health; in other cases, mismanagement of labour or the misuse of forceps damaged the baby which was either stillborn or died in the early neonatal period.

Analysis of perinatal mortality

Perinatal deaths are classified according to their aetiology and not by the immediate cause of death. The accurate determination of the specific factors leading to the neonatal death enables health professionals to identify correctable problems. The principal causes of perinatal deaths in Victoria, Australia are shown in Table 25.3.

Reduction of perinatal mortality

Many of the measures that have been effective in reducing maternal deaths are also effective in reducing perinatal deaths. In addition, the provision of well-equipped, well-staffed neonatal intensive care units (NICU) will enable a number of low-birthweight babies to survive and grow.

MANAGEMENT OF FETAL INTRA-UTERINE DEATH

Clinical aspects

The mother notices that fetal movements have ceased and Doppler or ultrasound examination fails to detect any fetal heart activity. When she realizes that her baby has died the expectant mother is distressed and concerned that the dead fetus, if it remains in her uterus, will decay and cause infection. Medical problems are unlikely, at least in the first 3 weeks after the fetal death has been diagnosed. After this time, disseminated intravascular coagulation and hypofibrinogenaemia may arise, with potentially serious consequences to the woman.

Management

The parents need support, information, and their immediate questions answered. They should be offered bereavement counselling. They should be reassured that the dead fetus, if left in the uterus, will not cause any harm in the following 3 weeks, and that usually labour will start during this time. The woman may choose to await spontaneous labour or to have labour induced. The management of the labour should be discussed with her and she should be assured that she will be given analgesics to reduce or eliminate the pain of childbirth. If she and her partner wish to view and hold the fetus after delivery they should be made aware that it may be macerated, depending on when the death occurred.

Table 25.3 Causation of perinatal mortality: Victoria, Australia 2006

CAUSE OF DEATH	FETAL DEATH	NEONATAL DEATH	TOTAL
Congenital abnormality	22.4	36.1	26.1
Infection	1.5	0.9	1.3
Hypertension	2.8	2.6	2.8
Antepartum haemorrhage	7.2	7.9	7.4
Termination for psychosocial indications	24.7	0	18.0
Twin-to-twin transfusion	2.1	7.0	3.5
Hypoxic peripartum death	1.0	6.2	2.4
Fetal growth restriction	6.4	1.8	5.2
Spontaneous preterm	10.5	29.1	15.6
Unexplained antepartum death	15.0	0	10.9

If spontaneous labour has not started 3 weeks after the diagnosis, or if the woman chooses immediate treatment, labour is induced by prostaglandin E_2 vaginal pessaries or gel, as described on page 189. Alternatives are to prescribe mifepristone 600 mg/day for 3 days, misoprostol 100–200 μg 12-hourly for four doses, or the prostaglandin analogue sulprostone, 1 μg/min IV, until the fetus is expelled. Using any of these methods, 50% of women will expel the fetus in 12 hours and 90% in 24 hours.

If the woman chooses to await the spontaneous onset of labour, frequent blood checks should be made by observing the clotting time of the blood or by estimating fibrinogen levels.

Investigations

The basic investigations to determine the cause of death that should be offered are listed in Box 25.3. An autopsy should be offered, as the reason for the death is changed by the autopsy findings in up to 25% of cases. The findings can have significant implications for counselling and for the management of another pregnancy.

Psychological effects on the parents

The loss of a fetus or of a neonate usually causes a considerable grief reaction in the mother, including postpartum depression. The father is also affected. The more mature the fetus or neonate at the time of death the greater the grief reaction. This reaction is reduced if the parents touch and hold the infant for as long as they wish; if keepsakes are available, including a lock of hair and a photograph;

and if a health professional is readily available if the parents want more information.

Box 25.3 **Investigating a perinatal death**

Baby and placenta

- Routine cord blood tests (unless macerated)
- Detailed, documented, external examination of infant
- Placenta and cord documented, macroscopic description and pathological examination and microbiological culture
- Autopsy should be discussed and offered in all cases of perinatal death and recommended especially when no explanation for cause of death is apparent

Mother

- Full blood count
- Kleihauer test (preferably prior to onset of labour)

Other tests

The following may be indicated under specific circumstances:
- Antinuclear antibody screen
- Lupus anticoagulant
- Parvovirus B_{19}
- Syphilis serology
- Cytomegalovirus
- Toxoplasmosis
- Hepatitis B and rubella if status is unknown
- HbA_{1c}
- Cardiac puncture or skin biopsy for karyotype

Chapter | 26 |

The newborn infant

TRANSITION TO EXTRA-UTERINE LIFE

Following birth the neonate undergoes several physiological changes so that it can adapt to extra-uterine life. Two main changes affect respiration and cardiovascular function.

First breaths

The several control systems that regulate breathing are already present in fetal life. Most of them operate mainly in fetal active states, such as REM (rapid eye movement) sleep. In quiet sleep, long periods without breathing occur. At birth there is a need to exchange oxygen and carbon dioxide. Breathing is augmented by an elevated carbon dioxide. Non-specific stimuli, such as pain, cold and light also lead to stimulation of breathing. In most infants the first breathing efforts occur within 30 seconds of birth and are forceful enough to overcome the high resistance of the liquid in the airways and to inflate the lungs. In immature and abnormal infants the breathing efforts may be reduced.

Changes in the pattern of blood circulation

The second change is the redirection of the blood flow following the cessation of the high blood flow through the umbilical arteries that perfused the placental villi, and a lowering of the large volume of blood returning through the umbilical vein and the vena cava. The venous pressure in the vena cava falls and the ductus venosus closes. The lungs expand with the first breath and the pulmonary vascular resistance falls abruptly. The infant's systemic blood pressure rises slightly at the same time, which results in a temporary reversal in the direction of the blood flowing through the ductus arteriosus. As the infant breathes, the oxygen tension in the blood rises and the muscular walls of the ductus contract, the passage of blood through it ceasing. At the same time, the pressure in the right atrium falls. There is a simultaneous increase in the blood flow through the lungs. This blood enters and increases the pressure in the left atrium. Because of the changes in pressure between the two atria, the foramen ovale closes.

With the closure of the ductus venosus, the foramen ovale and the ductus arteriosus, the adult pattern of circulation of the blood is established (Fig. 26.1; compare with Fig. 4.1, p. 29).

Changes in liver function

After the cardiovascular changes have taken place the infant's liver perfusion is increased. The liver can efficiently convert glucose into glycogen and vice versa, but some of its enzymatic functions are immature. The most important is its limited ability to conjugate bilirubin. In consequence, physiological jaundice may occur in the first week of life.

Most of the glycogen stored in the liver is laid down in the last 8 weeks of intrauterine life. Glucose from glycogen and the metabolism of ketone bodies contribute significantly to the energy needs of the first few days of life. Preterm and growth restricted babies have smaller liver glycogen stores and may develop hypoglycaemia. After a few days the neonate obtains energy from food and by oxidizing fats stored in adipose tissue.

Temperature control

At birth, vasoconstriction of the skin vessels preserves body heat, but temperature maintenance is made difficult because of the newborn infant's relatively large surface area. The body temperature of newborn infants may fall by up to 1.5 °C immediately after the birth, especially if wet skin is exposed allowing rapid heat loss. A mature infant

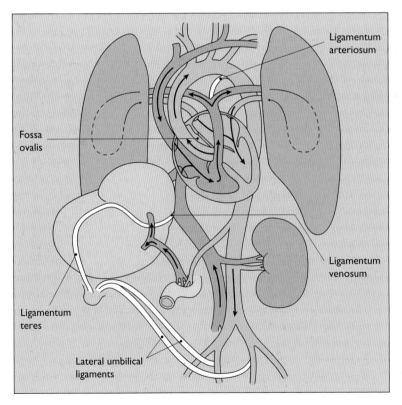

Fig. 26.1 Normal circulation in the newborn.

Ligamentum arteriosum

Fossa ovalis

Ligamentum venosum

Ligamentum teres

Lateral umbilical ligaments

will have laid down fat in brown adipose tissue and can utilize this for heat production without shivering. Preterm babies have less brown fat and may become hypothermic.

Because of the instability of temperature control, neonates should be wrapped properly in cold environments, but in hot environments too much wrapping should be avoided.

PERINATAL HYPOXIA

Any condition occurring during late pregnancy or labour that reduces the oxygen available to the fetus will predispose it to cardiorespiratory and neurological depression at birth. These conditions have been mentioned when discussing the at-risk fetus in pregnancy and labour (see p. 152).

If severe fetal hypoxia develops in pregnancy, the fetus may die in utero or may be born with acidaemia and hypercapnia as well as hypoxia (asphyxia). A blood pH of less than 7.10 may lead to pulmonary vasoconstriction, which further impairs gas exchange. Hypoxia increases the base deficit and blood lactate level. Both of these changes increase the risk to the fetus of neurological damage. In such cases, resuscitation is urgently needed at birth.

The severity of cardiorespiratory and neurological depression around the time of birth can be assessed by the Apgar scoring system (Table 26.1) or by the pH and/or blood lactate of umbilical artery blood. Both are useful in managing the immediate problem but are relatively poor indicators of long-term outcome.

The basic resuscitation of the newborn is described on page 77 (see Fig. 8.15). The most important step in resuscitation is to initiate ventilation with intermittent positive-pressure respiration; current evidence suggests that ventilation using air (21% oxygen) should be the initial step for term babies, with oxygen being added only if hypoxia persists despite adequate ventilation. Initial ventilation should be with a mask and inflating device; failure to initiate spontaneous breathing within 2–5 minutes may require endotracheal intubation – but only if a person skilled in this technique is present. If the infant remains bradycardic (HR <60) despite adequate ventilation, the circulation should be supported by external cardiac massage (Fig. 26.2) and, possibly, endotracheal 1:10 000 adrenaline 0.3–1.0 mL/kg. Once the umbilical

Table 26.1 Apgar scoring method for evaluating the infant (from Apgar and associates)			
SIGN	**SCORE**		
	0	**1**	**2**
Colour	Blue; pale	Body pink; extremities blue	Completely pink
Respiratory effort	Absent	Weak cry; hypoventilation	Good, strong cry
Muscle tone	Limp	Some flexion of extremities	Active motion; extremities well flexed
Reflex irritability (response to stimulation of sole of foot)	No response	Grimace	Cry
Heart rate	Absent	Slow (<100)	Fast (>100)

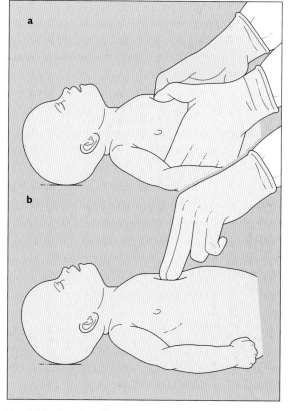

Fig. 26.2 Closed cardiac massage. Intermittent pressure is applied over the middle third of the sternum (which is pressed down about half an inch) with two fingers or thumbs. The heart is compressed between the rib cage and the vertebral column, and blood is expelled into the great vessel. For clarity, the endotracheal tube has been omitted in the drawing.

vein is cannulated a further 0.1–0.3 mL/kg dose of adrenaline is given, and if there is no response further doses of adrenaline 0.1–0.3 mL/kg can be given at 3–5-minute intervals.

A 5-minute Apgar of less than 6 should be followed by measurements of arterial blood gases and pH, and treatment given to adjust the findings if necessary.

Infants who have required advanced resuscitation or have prolonged cardiorespiratory depression should be closely observed in a special care nursery until it is clear that they have recovered or need continuing specialist care.

BIRTH INJURIES

With increasingly good obstetric care during childbirth, birth injuries are becoming less common and less severe. Only those injuries most likely to occur will be discussed. In all cases, the injury must be explained to the parents and the treatment and prognosis discussed.

Cranial injuries (Fig. 26.3)

Caput succedaneum

Caput succedaneum is caused by pressure on the fetal scalp when the head is being pushed deeply into the pelvis and the venous return from the scalp is impeded. The oedematous swelling and bruising is subcutaneous and can cover a large area of scalp. Treatment is not required; the swelling of the caput disappears rapidly and the bruising within a few days.

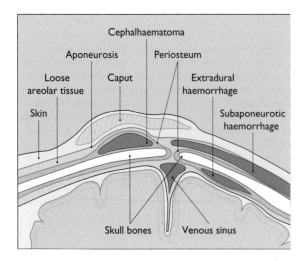

Fig. 26.3 Location of extracranial and extradural haemorrhages.

Cephalhaematoma

Cephalhaematomas may occur after a spontaneous vaginal delivery or following trauma from the obstetric forceps or the ventouse. The periosteum is sheared from the underlying parietal bone and subperiosteal haemorrhage occurs. The swelling is limited to the outline of the bone; initially it is tense, subsequently it is fluctuant and the rim may calcify. The haematoma remains for 2 weeks to 3 months and is slowly absorbed.

Subaponeurotic (subgaleal) haemorrhage

Subaponeurotic haemorrhage, while rare, occurs most commonly after a traumatic vacuum extraction (see p. 195–197) and may result in significant blood loss from the infant's circulation. Occasionally the bleeding is very rapid and life-threatening and requires urgent blood transfusion. Frequent observation for diffuse head swelling following vacuum extraction is mandatory.

Intracranial haemorrhage

Intracranial haemorrhage may be subarachnoid, subdural or intraventricular. Subarachnoid haemorrhage is common and may cause irritability and even convulsions over the first 2 days; it rarely has longstanding effects. Subdural haemorrhage can follow the misapplication of forceps; in severe cases the infant may be shocked and show little response to resuscitation. Intraventricular haemorrhage is found most often in preterm infants; it is diagnosed by ultrasound examinations, which should be performed routinely on very preterm infants.

Nerve injuries

Most nerve injuries involve the face (facial palsy) or the brachial plexus, and usually follow a forceps delivery, shoulder dystocia or a difficult breech birth.

Facial palsy

Facial palsy is a lower motor neurone disorder with paresis or paralysis of the facial nerve and inability to close the eye on the affected side. The lesion usually resolves spontaneously within 2–3 weeks.

Brachial palsies

These are due to nerve damage, usually following difficulty delivering a shoulder or the aftercoming head of a breech. In most cases the nerve sheath is torn and the nerve is compressed by haemorrhage and oedema, but its integrity is preserved. *Erb's palsy* is due to compression of the fibres of C5 and C6. The infant's arm hangs limply by its side. Most recover within a few weeks. *Klumpke's paralysis* is rare and it occurs when nerves C7 and C8 are affected.

The infant has a paralysed arm, with wrist drop and flaccid paralysis of the hand muscles. The prognosis is worse than that following Erb's palsy. Nerve injuries are best referred to neurology or plastic surgery clinics that specialize in their management.

Bone and muscle injuries

A fractured clavicle or, less commonly, humerus most often results from the interventions used by the accoucheur when faced with a severe shoulder dystocia. They may also occur following a breech extraction, and in addition the femur may be damaged. Injury to the sternomastoid muscle, due to a haematoma, may occur following a difficult delivery. It should be looked for after any difficult delivery as, unless treated by stretching the muscle, permanent shortening may result.

RESPIRATORY DISORDERS

Transient respiratory distress

There are a number of causes of transient respiratory distress; most commonly there may be some retained lung fluid – the 'wet-lung' syndrome; other causes include hypothermia, acidosis and polycythaemia; all tend to resolve spontaneously over a few hours or 2–3 days, but occasionally may be more severe and contribute to the development of hyaline membrane disease.

Hyaline membrane disease (HMD)

HMD is almost universally a problem of premature infants; it is uncommon if the baby is 35 weeks' gestation or more; hypoxia, hypothermia and maternal diabetes are predisposing factors.

HMD is caused by a relative lack of surfactant in the alveoli. Surfactant assists the stability of the lung after birth and lowers the surface tension in the alveoli, ensuring a normal residual volume of air and the capacity for gas exchange. In the absence of surfactant, the alveoli become airless at the end of each breath and their ability to expand against the forces of surface tension is decreased, leading to poor oxygen exchange.

Pneumonia

Pneumonia may be initially difficult to distinguish from other causes of respiratory distress so all babies with respiratory distress must have infection considered as a cause. Several different organisms may cause neonatal pneumonia, but group B streptococcus (see p. 137) may cause rapid deterioration and requires early treatment. *Listeria monocytogenes* is prevalent in some communities. Aspiration of meconium causes a chemical pneumonitis that can be life-threatening.

Other causes of respiratory distress

Other rarer causes include upper airway obstruction such as choanal atresia, Pierre Robin syndrome or laryngeal anomalies; conditions impeding lung expansion include pneumothorax, diaphragmatic hernia and rare musculo-skeletal anomalies.

Diagnosis of respiratory distress

The infant's respiratory rate increases, with nasal flaring, expiratory grunting and sternal and/or intercostal retraction. The infant may be cyanosed and tachycardic. The diagnosis is aided by radiology; HMD shows characteristic frosted-glass shadowing, but this may be similar in pneumonia. 'Wet-lung' has clearer lung fields with perihilar streaks of fluid. Investigations to exclude infection should be performed in all babies in which the respiratory distress is not clearly transient.

Management

A paediatrician should be consulted and the infant admitted to a neonatal special or intensive care nursery. The principles of treatment are:

- To keep the infant warm in an incubator adjusted to the neutral thermal range
- To provide oxygen to obtain an oxygen saturation of 90–94% by continuous pulse oximetry monitoring, or a tension of 50–80 mmHg by blood gases monitoring; to avoid retinal damage from the uncontrolled use of oxygen
- To provide assisted ventilation if needed
- To give intravenous antibiotics unless infection can be excluded as the cause
- To ensure that the baby is adequately hydrated and nourished by giving an intravenous infusion of a glucose electrolyte solution
- The use of continuous positive airway pressure (CPAP) to maintain lung volume
- To give exogenous surfactant in cases of HMD that require mechanical ventilation. The installation of surfactant into the infant's trachea reduces the severity of the HMD, reduces its complications such as pneumothorax, and halves the mortality.

NEONATAL INFECTIONS

Infections occurring during pregnancy that affect the fetus are discussed in Chapter 17. Infection may be acquired during labour, particularly if the membranes have been ruptured for a long time, or from vaginal colonisation by group B streptococci (GBS) (see p. 137). Acquired GBS infection may cause rapid onset of septicaemia, pneumonia ± meningitis within hours of birth.

Infections occurring after birth include:

- *Candida* spp. that infect the infant's mouth, white patches being formed
- Staphylococcal infections which present as skin pustules, periumbilical infection or blepharoconjunctivitis
- *Neisseria gonorrhoeae*, causing early conjunctivitis, requiring systemic penicillin
- *Chlamydia trachomatis*, which may cause conjunctivitis 1–3 weeks after birth, or pneumonia 3 weeks later
- *Escherichia coli* infections causing gastroenteritis, urinary tract infection (which is difficult to diagnose) or meningitis
- Herpes simplex should always be considered when neonatal meningitis is suspected.

The signs of neonatal infection may be non-specific, with lethargy, poor temperature control (including hypothermia as well as fever), poor feeding, vomiting and/or compromised perfusion. Any infant suspected of having infection requires a blood culture, blood picture examination and possibly non-specific infection marker (e.g. C-reactive protein); if the diagnosis remains unclear collection of a urine specimen (by suprapubic aspiration), a chest X-ray and a lumbar puncture to exclude meningitis should be performed.

Treatment consists of giving the appropriate antibiotic, depending on local bacterial sensitivities and experience. Early treatment is of the utmost importance to minimize the risk of death or long-term sequelae. Care must be taken to prevent cross-infection by ensuring that the staff practise infection control measures, especially hand hygiene.

JAUNDICE

Over half (50–60%) of all babies will have visibly detectable jaundice, but most will be physiological in origin requiring neither investigation nor treatment. Any doubts about the severity of the jaundice requires a serum bilirubin (SBR) estimation. In a term baby an SBR of >250 μmol/L requires further investigation and possible treatment. Likewise for any jaundice appearing in the first 24 hours of life.

Jaundice is further considered on page 216.

INFANTS OF DIABETIC MOTHERS

Babies born to mothers with diabetes have a range of special issues, and are discussed on pages 132–134.

CONGENITAL MALFORMATIONS

Congenital malformations affect up to 3.5% of all infants. In about 2% of all infants such defects are major (Table 26.2). Many of the more severe structural abnormalities are now diagnosed antenatally during the 18-week morphology

Table 26.2 Order of prevalence of 28 selected birth defects: Victoria, Australia 2005–6		
DEFECT	**N/10 000**	**1 IN *N* BIRTHS & TOPS†**
Hypospadias*	74	135
Obstructive defects of renal pelvis	40	250
Ventricular septal defect	32.2	311
Trisomy 21	29.5	339
Developmental dysplasia of hip	27.5	364
Trisomy 18	8.4	1190
Hydrocephalus	8.1	1235
Cleft palate	8.0	1250
Cystic kidney	6.8	1471
Renal agenesis/ dysgenesis	6.6	1515
Transposition of great vessels	6.3	1587
Spina bifida	6.0	1667
Cleft lip and palate	5.5	1818
Anencephaly	5.5	1818
Coarctation of aorta	4.9	2041
Limb reduction defects	4.8	2083
Hypoplastic left heart syndrome	4.5	2222
Anorectal atresia and/or stenosis	4.4	2273

Table 26.2 Order of prevalence of 28 selected birth defects: Victoria, Australia 2005–6—cont'd		
DEFECT	**N/10 000**	**1 IN _N_ BIRTHS & TOPS†**
Trisomy 13	3.9	2564
Cleft lip	3.9	2564
Oesophageal atresia and/or stenosis	3.8	2632
Tetralogy of Fallot	3.7	2703
Exomphalos	3.1	3226
Intestinal atresia and/or stenosis	3.2	3125
Diaphragmatic hernia	2.8	3571
Gastroschisis	2.3	4348
Microcephalus	1.8	5556
Encephalocele	1.2	8333

*Per male babies. From Riley M & Halliday J, _Birth Defects in Victoria 2005–2006_, Victorian Perinatal Data Collection Unit, Victorian Government Department of Human Services, Melbourne, 2008, with permission.

†Terminations of pregnancies.

explaining the malformation and the prognosis calmly and sympathetically. Most parents go through a grieving period. They may express anger and guilt, questioning whether anything they did or did not do during the pregnancy caused the malformation. Most appreciate counselling sessions.

The major malformations are described below.

Central nervous system defects

Anencephaly (Fig. 26.4) and spina bifida (Fig. 26.5) can be diagnosed in pregnancy, as described on page 43. Hydrocephalus can be diagnosed in the second half of pregnancy by ultrasound scanning, but may only be noticed when delivery is difficult.

Cardiovascular defects

Most major cardiovascular defects are diagnosed before birth. Presentation at or following birth may be from persisting cyanosis or the presence of a murmur; even loud murmurs may not be present at birth, but appear as the differential pressure between the systemic and pulmonary circulations changes; thus reassessment should be made before the infant is discharged from hospital. Likewise some murmurs are benign. Late presentations – often after discharge home – may occur when the ductus arteriosus finally closes. These problems require urgent referral to a paediatric cardiologist. The immediate management of both early and late presentations is supportive, but may also involve the infusion of prostaglandin E_1 to maintain patency of the ductus arteriosus prior to transfer to the cardiac facility.

Cleft lip and palate

A _cleft lip_ is obvious; the psychological impact on the family should not be underestimated. Early referral to a plastic surgeon is essential for planning treatment and giving the

ultrasound scan, which gives the opportunity for counselling and discussion of the likely prognosis. When the diagnosis has been established the doctor should talk with the parents,

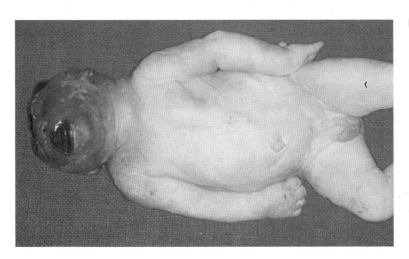

Fig. 26.4 Anencephaly.

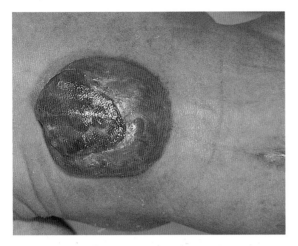

Fig. 26.5 Spina bifida.

parents a clear view of what is likely to be a good outcome. Some but not all babies with cleft lip can breastfeed.

A *cleft palate* may easily be missed initially unless specific examination is performed. Virtually all have feeding problems at the breast and require feeding with special techniques, preferably with expressed breast milk. Again early plastic surgery referral is essential. Results are generally good but there may occasionally be long-term feeding and speech issues.

Gastrointestinal defects

Oesophageal atresia should be considered in the babies of women who had polyhydramnios. A size 10 catheter should be passed through the mouth down the oesophagus, and an ultrasound examination made. Oral feeding should not be started until the condition has been excluded. Up to 50% of these babies have other congenital anomalies, and consequently need detailed assessment.

Duodenal stenosis or *atresia* should be suspected if early vomiting (usually bile-stained) occurs. Bile-stained vomiting is also associated with *malrotation* of the gut and thus should be investigated urgently. There is an association of duodenal atresia with Down syndrome.

Lower bowel obstructions are more likely to present with abdominal distension, failure to pass meconium and later-onset vomiting. Important causes include *Hirschsprung's disease* and *rectal/anal atresia*. Imperforate anus should be excluded at the initial examination.

Abdominal wall defects

Defects involving the umbilicus (*exomphalos*) and peri-umbilicus (*gastroschisis*), usually diagnosed antenatally, are obvious at birth. Exomphalos is often associated with other anomalies, including chromosomal, and gastroschisis may be associated with intra-uterine growth restriction

and bowel atresias but not with other anomalies. Optimal management is delivery in a hospital in which early surgical closure can be performed. The immediate care after birth is to cover the exposed intestine with clean plastic cling-wrap to decrease heat and fluid loss while awaiting transfer for surgery; it is vital to minimize tension on the mesenteric vessels.

Musculoskeletal defects

Diaphragmatic hernia affects 1 in 4000 babies. This is often detected during a routine antenatal ultrasound examination, or because of the neonate's failure to respond to resuscitation. Although there have been experimental attempts to repair the hernia antenatally the results are not reliable enough for this to be offered as an option. Survival post-surgery is dependent on the degree of lung hypoplasia.

The most common skeletal disorder is *talipes* – either equinovarus (the foot is turned in and points down) or calcaneovalgus (the foot is turned out and points up). It is important to distinguish between postural talipes, in which a normal position can be achieved through gentle manipulation, and fixed talipes which requires orthopaedic intervention by splints or plasters.

Developmental dysplasia of the hip (DDH) (including congenital dislocation) is characterized by an anteverted femoral head and neck and a shallow acetabulum, from which the femoral head may be partially or completely displaced. Between 1 and 3% of neonates show evidence of instability of the hip at birth, but in most cases this resolves spontaneously within a week or two. It is more common in females, in breech presentations and where there is a family history of DDH. In a few infants (1.5 per 1000) the defect persists. Examination of the newborn for congenital hip dislocation is described in Box 9.1, page 87. Any suspicion of congenital dislocation or subluxation of the hip is referred for an ultrasound examination; if confirmed, treatment is placement of the hips in abduction under specialist orthopaedic supervision.

Urogenital defects

Undescended testicles (cryptorchidism) – in 2% of boys at term and 20% of preterm boys one or both testes will have failed to descend into the scrotum. By the first birthday less than 1% remain undescended. Failure to descend by 6 months of age should prompt referral to a paediatric surgeon because of the increased risk of impaired spermatogenesis and testicular cancer in later life if the testicle remains undescended.

Hypospadias is a defect of closure of the urethra in males, with the opening of the urethra being at a variable point along the underside of the penis. Early referral to a paediatric urologist is required; under no circumstances should circumcision be performed, for the residual foreskin is required for the repair of the urethral defect.

Renal pelvis dilatation may be seen on antenatal ultrasound scans. While many of these resolve spontaneously postnatally, it is vital that all have paediatric follow-up to exclude persistent obstruction due to pelvi-ureteric stenosis.

Urethral valves may present in utero with oligohydramnios due to severe urethral obstruction; but less severe obstruction may present postnatally with poor urine stream, enlarged bladder and/or urine infection. Urgent referral to a paediatric urologist is mandatory.

Atresia of the kidneys is rare and fatal, presenting antenatally with oligohydramnios.

Ectopia vesicae due to defective cloacal closure is also very rare and requires complex surgical repair, with variable results depending on the extent of the defect.

Skin

Naevus flammeus occurs characteristically as a V-shaped red mark on the forehead, usually accompanied by a similar marking on the nape of the neck. Very commonly they are seen as red blemishes at the inner ends of the upper eyelids, sometimes on the nose and upper lip. The parents need to be reassured that these are normal variants, are not due to trauma and that they will regress over the next few months without treatment. Strawberry marks are generally not present at birth, appearing as tiny red dots in the first weeks of life, at which stage they can be treated by laser. Otherwise they may grow to a variable size over the first 6–12 months, following which they regress spontaneously over 2–5 years. Other angiomata include port wine stains, which tend to be permanent, although some may be amenable to laser treatment. Those on the forehead may be associated with underlying angiomatous malformation on the brain surface. Mongolian blue spots are patches of slate-blue discoloration over the sacrum or lower spine; they occur particularly in Asian infants. They have no clinical significance.

Down syndrome (Trisomy 21)

Down syndrome is the most common genetic defect. The infant may have slanting eyes with epicanthic folds, short hands, small fingers, simian creases of the palms and increased spacing between the first and second toes; the head is flattened at the back, the neck short and webbed, (Fig. 26.6). Generalized hypotonia is a characteristic finding. Most Down syndrome children have a lower than average cognitive ability, often ranging from mild to moderate impairment; a small number have severe to profound mental disability. There may be associated congenital anomalies – most commonly cardiac or gastrointestinal, but any system may be involved.

The incidence of Down syndrome increases with the age of the mother (Fig. 26.7). As mentioned in Chapter 6 (p. 42), Down syndrome can now be diagnosed by routine screening in over 80% of cases in early pregnancy, and termination offered.

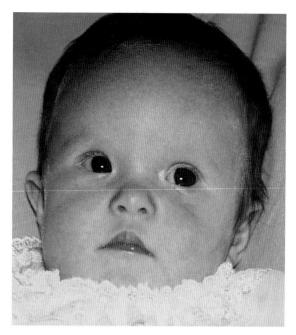

Fig. 26.6 Down syndrome.

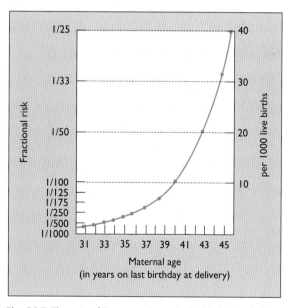

Fig. 26.7 The rate of Down syndrome in live births in relation to maternal age.

Open and honest communication with the parents from the outset is vital. Most communities have active Down syndrome support groups and specialist health professional programmes. Early referral should be made.

Table 26.3 Risks of recurrence of some congenital defects

DISORDER		RISK (%)	
	Incidence (per 100 births)	Normal parent having a second affected child	Affected parent having an affected child
Down syndrome	0.2	1	33
Anencephaly	0.2	2	–
Spina bifida	0.3	4	5
Cleft palate	0.04	2	7
Cleft lip and palate	0.1	4	4
Congenital heart disease	0.6	2	2

Risk of recurrence of congenital abnormalities

A question of great concern to the parents of a congenitally affected baby is: 'What is the risk of our next baby being affected?' Available data are shown in Table 26.3.

METABOLIC DISORDERS

Cystic fibrosis, affecting one baby in 2000; congenital hypothyroidism (1 in 6000), and phenylketonuria (1 in 10 000) can be detected by filter paper tests on blood samples taken at 48–72 hours of life. Following the introduction of tandem mass spectrometry (TMS), the pattern of biochemical markers may help identify over 20 additional metabolic conditions, for example, medium chain acyl-coenzyme A dehydrogenase (MCAD) deficiency, homocystinuria and maple syrup urine disease.

MATERNAL INGESTION OF DRUGS AFFECTING THE FETUS

Pregnant women should avoid taking medications as far as possible, as many pharmaceutical agents cross the placenta and may affect the fetus adversely. If a drug is required, the doctor should read the product information document before prescribing it. In some countries, lists of drugs that should be avoided during pregnancy are obtainable from the health authorities.

CIRCUMCISION

Current advice in most developed regions is that this is not required for medical reasons. There is evidence of a small increased risk of urinary tract infection in uncircumcised boys, and acquisition of HIV infection has been shown to be more likely in uncircumcised male adults. Thus in regions with a high prevalence of HIV circumcision may be indicated. Unless required for cultural or religious reasons it should be delayed until the infant is 6 months old and should be performed under a local or a general anaesthetic.

Chapter | 27 |

The low-birthweight infant

DEFINITION OF LOW BIRTHWEIGHT

A low-birthweight (LBW) baby is arbitrarily defined as weighing less than 2500 g at birth. There are further subdivisions of weight into very low birthweight (VLBW) – weighing <1500 g and extremely low birthweight (ELBW) weighing <1000 g at birth.

Low birthweight may occur because the infant is premature, less than 37 weeks' gestation, or because the infant's intra-uterine growth has been restricted.

Intra-uterine growth restriction (IUGR) is defined as a birthweight of less than the 10th centile of the weights for babies at that gestational age. Similarly babies whose birthweight is greater than the 90th centile for weights for babies at that gestational age are defined as large for gestational age (LGA).

It follows that since at any given gestational age 10% of babies are SGA and 10% are LGA then only 80% are of a birthweight that is appropriate for gestational age (AGA).

Although the rate of prematurity varies between communities, a common rate in developed countries is 7%, (and that of post-maturity up to 1%). The relation between growth and gestation is illustrated in Figure 27.1, including approximate percentages of the various combinations of gestation and growth relative to the normal parameters. Note that by these definitions less than 75% of babies are born of 'normal' gestation and weight. Note also that some LBW infants may be both premature *and* IUGR.

The growth chart illustrated in Figure 27.1 is from an Australian community. It is not necessarily applicable to all communities because of different genetic growth potentials; for instance the birthweights in a population of some Pacific Island groups would show higher growth centiles and some Indian populations would show lower centiles.

CAUSES OF LOW BIRTHWEIGHT

As stated above, low birthweight may occur because the infant is premature – less than 37 weeks' gestation – or because the infant's intrauterine growth has been restricted.

Causes and prevention of prematurity are discussed in Chapter 19, with a summary of causes given in Table 19.1.

The intra-uterine growth of the fetus depends on its inherited growth potential and the effectiveness of the support to its growth provided by the uteroplacental environment. The latter is affected by the presence or absence of maternal disease. The causes of IUGR can be classified according to maternal, placental and fetal causes, and are outlined in Box 27.1. In many cases no precise factor has been identified.

Data are available from several developed countries which show the proportion of babies who are of low birthweight, their perinatal mortality, and the survival of those babies born alive. These data obscure the fact that low-birthweight babies comprise two populations: preterm (premature) babies and small-for-gestational age (SGA) babies.

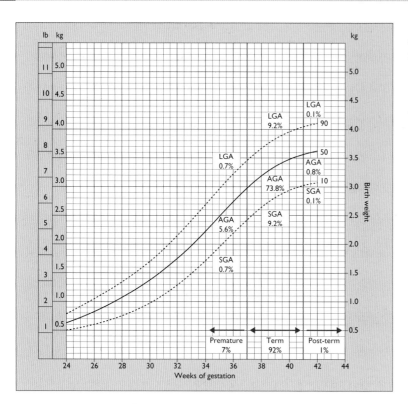

Fig. 27.1 Birthweight distribution versus gestation period. Dotted lines show the 10th and 90th centiles.

Box 27.1 Risk factors for intrauterine growth restriction

Maternal

Maternal age <17 or >35
Low socio-economic status
Cigarette smoking
Excessive alcohol consumption
High altitude
Malnutrition
Maternal disease – e.g. renal, cardiac, diabetes with microvascular disease
Antiphospholipid syndrome
Severe maternal anaemia

Placental

Hypertensive diseases of pregnancy
Site of implantation
Antepartum haemorrhage
Multiple pregnancy

Fetal

Chromosomal abnormalities
Congenital defects and dysmorphic syndromes
Intra-uterine infection

PROBLEMS OF PREMATURE AND GROWTH-RESTRICTED INFANTS

Distinction needs to be made between the problems of the two groups of infants. In *premature* infants, but not necessarily in IUGR infants, all organ systems are immature, giving rise to a variety of potential problems, including:

- Lack of respiratory drive at birth, with increased need for resuscitation
- Difficulties with temperature maintenance
- Respiratory distress syndrome (hyaline membrane disease)
- Immature feeding, with the potential need for tube feeding or intravenous nutrition, and the risk of gastro-oesophageal reflux and/or aspiration of feeds due to immature gag reflex
- Metabolic instability, especially of glucose, but also calcium, magnesium and sodium
- Jaundice of prematurity, with a risk of kernicterus at lower levels of bilirubin than is expected in a term baby
- Apnoea
- Increased susceptibility to infection
- Potential surgical problems – inguinal and persistent umbilical hernias and undescended testicles.

VLBW and ELBW infants are also at risk of persistent patency of the ductus arteriosus, intraventricular haemorrhage (IVH) and its complications, retinopathy of prematurity (ROP), necrotizing enterocolitis (NEC), bronchopulmonary dysplasia (BPD), anaemia and electrolyte disturbances due to renal immaturity.

IUGR infants have a different set of problems, but if they are also premature they also share the problems listed above. Specific problems of the IUGR infant include:

- Perinatal hypoxia–ischaemia – especially those whose IUGR is caused by placental compromise (the most common reason for IUGR)
- Hypothermia – although the neural control may be mature, the lack of subcutaneous insulation and lack of brown fat for heat generation (see Ch. 26) leads to heat loss
- Hypoglycaemia – due to lack of glycogen stores
- Other metabolic problems – hypocalcaemia and hypomagnesaemia – possibly related to the perinatal hypoxia–ischaemia rather that the IUGR itself
- Respiratory distress – but not respiratory distress syndrome (hyaline membrane disease). This may be due to the increased risk of meconium aspiration, to polycythaemia or, rarely but of great concern, pulmonary haemorrhage
- Polycythaemia, causing not only respiratory distress, but potential neurological damage, jaundice and/or renal vein thrombosis
- Increased risk of infection; intra-uterine infection may have caused the IUGR, but these infants are also susceptible to extra-uterine infection
- Congenital malformations.

MANAGEMENT OF PREMATURE AND GROWTH-RESTRICTED INFANTS

The care of these infants should be conducted by a paediatrician with the resources available in a neonatal special care nursery (SCN – often called a special care baby unit – SCBU). Most VLBW infants and *all* ELBW require the care of a specialist neonatal multidisciplinary team in a neonatal intensive care unit (NICU). As mentioned in Chapter 19, a woman who goes into labour before the 36th week of pregnancy should, if possible, be transferred to a hospital with an SCN. If delivery is required before the completion of 32 weeks (in some regions this may be a higher gestation) all attempts should be made to transfer the mother for delivery at a hospital with an NICU.

Key points in the management include:

- Attendance of a paediatrician at the delivery to ensure optimal transition to extra-uterine life, and to provide resuscitation as required to minimize hypoxia–ischaemia. If possible the paediatrician should see the parents prior to the delivery to discuss the likely course of events and possible outcomes.
- Thermal stability maintenance, if necessary by the use of a radiant warmer or closed incubator providing a neutral thermal environment.

- Monitoring of vital signs.
- Management of respiratory distress including the administration of oxygen and monitoring oxygen saturation by pulse oximetry.
- Prevention and treatment of infection – careful attention to hand-washing before handling a baby is the most important preventive measure. Infants suspected of infection and all those with respiratory distress that is not quickly and clearly settling should have investigations for infection performed and antibiotics started immediately.
- Early nutrition is important to prevent hypoglycaemia and catabolism. If the baby does not have the ability safely to suck and swallow a feed, then tube feeding or intravenous nutrition may be required. While all available breast milk should be used, this is an instance in which special premature baby formulae may have a place until the mother's milk is established. The baby is fed by tube, cup or spoon, and is gradually introduced to the breast. Vitamin supplements are given with or after feeding.
- Observation and testing as indicated for jaundice, with phototherapy according to local protocol.

MORTALITY AND MORBIDITY OF LOW-BIRTHWEIGHT INFANTS

The birthweight and gestational age of the infant are the greatest predictors of morbidity and mortality. Those at greatest risk of complications and of long-term morbidity are the VLBW babies (<1500 g), and at even higher risk are the ELBW babies (birthweight <1000 g).

Low-birthweight infants contribute 70% of early neonatal deaths; the smaller and less mature the infant, the less its chance of survival (Table 27.1). The survival rates depend on the place of birth. Few infants of less than 24 weeks' gestation survive; neonatal survival of live births at 24–25 weeks' gestation is 45%, 78% at 26–27 weeks', 90% at 28–31 weeks', and over 99% at 32 weeks' and above (Victoria, Australia, 2006).

The morbidity of the surviving infants has decreased in recent years; the highest morbidity is among infants whose gestational age is less than 27 weeks and whose birthweight is 750 g or less. An Australian study of outcome at 2 years of age of 168 surviving infants (a survival rate of 73%) who were born with birthweights less than 1000 g showed that 51% had no disability, 23% a mild disability, 13% a moderate and 14% a severe disability, 11% had cerebral palsy, 2% were blind and 2% were deaf. For those born 20 years earlier the survival rate was 25%; disability rates were mild 33%, moderate 13% and severe 15%, cerebral palsy 14%, blindness 7% and deafness 5% (Table 27.2).

Table 27.1 Perinatal mortality related to birthweight: Queensland, Australia

BIRTHWEIGHT (g)	TOTAL BIRTHS	FETAL DEATH RATE (PER 1000)	NEONATAL DEATH RATE (PER 1000)	PERINATAL MORTALITY RATE (PER 1000)	SURVIVORS (%)
<500	385	735	931	982	1.8
500–749	421	397	606	762	23.8
750–999	405	244	141	351	64.9
1000–1499	1013	92.8	44.4	137	86.3
1500–1999	2002	41.5	17.5	58.9	94.1
2000–2499	5526	13.2	7.1	20.4	98.0
2500–2999	21 356	4.7	2.4	7.1	99.3
3000–3499	51 849	1.5	1.2	2.7	99.7
3500–3999	44 410	1.0	0.7	1.7	99.8
4000–4999	14 642	1.1	0.8	1.8	99.8
>4500	2524	2.4	1.6	4.0	99.6
Total	144 533	7.3	4.0	11.3	98.9

Table 27.2 Gestational age and perinatal mortality: Victoria, Australia 2006

GESTATIONAL AGE (WEEKS)	BIRTHS		STILLBIRTHS			NEONATAL DEATHS			SURVIVORS
	n	%	n	%	Rate/1000	n	%	Rate/1000	%
20–21	165	0.2	117	25.6	709.0	48	21.1	1000	0
22–23	143	0.2	84	18.4	587.4	57	25.1	966.1	1.4
24–25	119	0.2	36	7.9	302.5	30	13.2	361.4	44.5
26–27	153	0.2	21	4.6	137.3	12	5.3	90.9	78.4
28–31	561	0.8	40	8.8	71.3	18	7.9	34.5	89.7
32–36	4395	6.3	65	14.2	14.8	26	11.5	6.0	97.9
37–41	63 185	90.5	94	20.6	1.5	35	15.4	0.6	99.8
≥42	963	1.4	0	0	0	1	0.4	1.0	99.9
Total	69 686	100	457	100	6.6	227	100	3.3	99.0

Chapter | **28** |

Disorders of menstruation

Menstruation is normal if it occurs at intervals of 22–35 days (from day 1 of menstruation to the onset of the next menstrual period), as mentioned in Chapter 1; if the duration of the bleeding is less than 7 days; and if the menstrual blood loss is less than 80 mL. It was also noted that menstrual discharge consists of tissue fluid (20–40% of the total discharge), blood (50–80%), and fragments of the endometrium. However, to the woman menstrual discharge looks like blood and is so reported.

By convention, the notation of menstruation and its disturbances is written as, for example, 5/28. This indicates that the woman bled for 5 days and that menstruation occurred at an interval of 28 days. The quantity of menstrual loss is entered as slight, normal or heavy.

Disorders of menstruation occur most commonly at each extreme of the reproductive years, that is, under the age of 19 and over the age of 39. The disorder may relate to the length of the menstrual cycle, or to the amount and duration of the menstrual loss. A woman may have both disturbances.

DEFINITIONS

Changes in the length of the menstrual cycle

Menstruation may occur at intervals longer than 35 days, when it is termed oligomenorrhoea; if menstruation does not occur for more than 3 months (in the absence of pregnancy) a diagnosis of secondary amenorrhoea is made. Primary amenorrhoea is diagnosed if menstruation has not commenced by the age of 16 years. Menstruation may also occur at intervals of less than 21 days, when it is given the term epimenorrhoea or polymenorrhoea.

Changes in the amount of menstrual loss

The quantity of menstrual discharge may vary, without altering the cyclicity of menstruation. Scanty or light menstrual discharge is termed hypomenorrhoea; heavy 'bleeding' is termed menorrhagia. In menorrhagia there may be an excessive amount of blood lost, or the apparently heavy bleeding may be due to an increased loss of tissue fluid.

Menorrhagia may occur in association with an organic condition in the uterus, or in the absence of any detectable uterine abnormality. In this case it is termed dysfunctional uterine bleeding.

Disturbances in cyclicity and amount of menstrual loss

In this disturbance the cyclicity of menstruation is lost, bleeding occurring at irregular intervals and the quantity of menstrual loss varying considerably. This pattern is termed metrorrhagia. Generally it indicates a local condition in the uterus and mandates investigation.

AMENORRHOEA AND OLIGOMENORRHOEA

Primary amenorrhoea

Primary amenorrhoea (affecting 5% of amenorrhoeic women) may be due to a genetic defect, such as gonadal dysgenesis, in which case the secondary sexual

characteristics will not have developed. It may be due to a Müllerian duct abnormality, such as an absent uterus, vaginal agenesis, a transverse vaginal septum or an imperforate hymen. In the last three causes, menstruation may occur but the menstrual discharge cannot escape from the genital tract. The condition is cryptomenorrhoea rather than amenorrhoea. Rarely testicular feminization is the cause.

In many cases, however, no abnormality is found and the young woman may be expected to menstruate in time. Some of these women have an eating disorder or exercise excessively. If an adolescent girl has not started menstruating by the age of 17, investigations should be made as described on page 321.

Secondary amenorrhoea

The most common cause of secondary amenorrhoea is pregnancy, but the condition may occur during the reproductive years for a variety of reasons. Figure 28.1 and Table 28.1 show the most common causes of amenorrhoea and their frequency. Only these causes will be discussed in this chapter.

As noted in Chapter 1, normal menstruation depends on a normal uterus and vagina, and on the reciprocal interaction between hormones released from the hypothalamus (gonadotrophin-releasing hormones), the pituitary

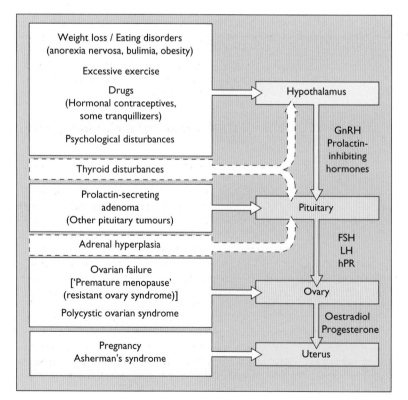

Fig. 28.1 The aetiology of secondary amenorrhoea.

Table 28.1 Causes of secondary amenorrhea

CAUSE	INCIDENCE (%)
Weight loss, low body weight, exercise	20–40
Polycystic ovarian syndrome	15–30
Pituitary insensitivity (post-pill)	10–20
Hyperprolactinaemia	10–20
Primary ovarian failure	5–10
Asherman's syndrome	1–2
Hypothyroidism	1–2

(the gonadotrophins – follicle-stimulating hormone (FSH) and luteinizing hormone (LH)) and the ovaries (oestrogen and progesterone).

Investigation of secondary amenorrhoea

Unless organic disease is suspected, or the woman is desperately seeking relief from infertility, most experts would not investigate amenorrhoea until it has lasted for 6–12 months, as most women start menstruating during this time.

When investigation is indicated, a careful history is essential in which the doctor inquires about the woman's general health, and seeks to determine whether she has an eating disorder or exercises excessively, or if any medical or psychiatric condition is present. A physical examination, including a vaginal examination, follows and in certain cases a pelvic ultrasound examination may be performed. If these examinations reveal no definite diagnosis, the following tests are ordered:

- Hormone assays
  - FSH and LH. An FSH level above the normal range of the laboratory, confirmed by repeating the measurement, indicates primary ovarian failure.
  - Prolactin (hPr). A raised hPr level on two or more occasions indicates hyperprolactinaemia.
  - Thyroid-stimulating hormone (TSH) and serum free T.
  - Oestradiol 17β. This may be measured or a 'progestogen stimulation test' made.
- Progestogen stimulation test. This seeks to determine whether the uterus responds to progestogen withdrawal. Progestogens will only provoke bleeding if there is sufficient circulating oestradiol (>150 pmol/L). The test determines whether the endometrium will respond and indirectly determines that the oestradiol is above a critical level. Medroxyprogesterone acetate 5 mg is given daily for 5 days. If menstrual bleeding occurs within

7 days the test is positive, and clomifene is likely to induce ovulation.
- X-ray of the pituitary fossa, MRI, or a CT scan if the hPr level is raised, to exclude the presence of a pituitary tumour.

The purpose of the investigations is to exclude organic disease (for example a prolactin-secreting microadenoma or hypothyroidism) and to treat anovulation as a cause of infertility. If organic disease is not detected and infertility is not a problem, amenorrhoea does not represent a danger to the woman, but because low oestrogen levels may lead to bone loss, after 6 months of amenorrhoea hormone replacement treatment (see p. 325) should be advised.

The sequence of investigations is shown in Figure 28.2.

More common causes of amenorrhoea

Weight loss

Women who have an eating disorder, particularly anorexia nervosa, cease to menstruate, as do some women who are compulsive exercisers. Amenorrhoea can occur in obese and overweight women who lose weight rapidly. The cause is a failure of the hypothalamus to release sufficient gonadotrophin-releasing hormone (GnRH) to initiate the release of gonadotrophins, and in consequence only a small quantity of oestrogen is secreted by the ovaries. If this persists for more than 6 months, bone loss may occur at a time when bone formation is reaching its peak. A consequence of this is a greater risk of osteoporosis in later life. Even during the recovery phase menstruation may not occur for several months, which may aggravate the problem.

Hyperprolactinaemia and prolactin-secreting tumours

Prolactin secretion by the pituitary gland is inhibited under normal conditions by dopamine released from the hypothalamus. In certain circumstances, this control is diminished. Examples are hypothyroidism and the administration of dopamine-depleting agents or dopamine receptor-blocking agents. A more common cause of hyperprolactinaemia is a microadenoma of the pituitary gland. In these cases, the increased circulating levels of prolactin act directly on the hypothalamus to reduce the secretion of GnRH, which in turn prevents the FSH and LH rises needed for follicle development and ovulation.

The woman develops oestrogen deficiency, with menstrual disturbances (usually amenorrhoea), a dry vagina and, often, a reduction of her libido. If the hyperprolactinaemia persists, osteopenia and, perhaps, osteoporosis will result. In 30% of women inappropriate milk secretion (galactorrhoea) occurs.

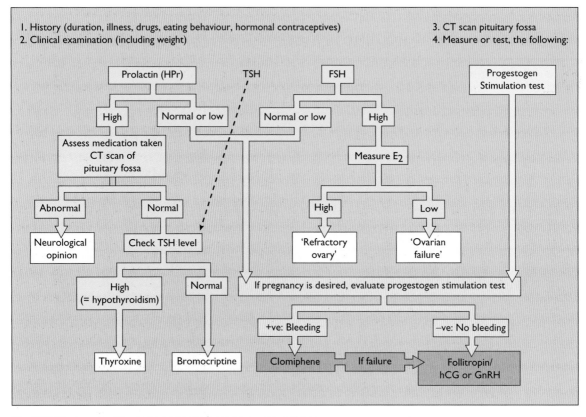

Fig. 28.2 The investigation and treatment of secondary amenorrhoea.

As hyperprolactinaemia accounts for 10–20% of cases of amenorrhoea, investigation is important. The diagnosis is made if a raised blood level of prolactin is found. If this is noted during investigation, a high-resolution CT scan of the pituitary is made to detect a prolactin-secreting tumour, although in most cases none is found. A micro-adenoma (<10 mm in diameter) is more common than a macroadenoma.

Treatment is needed if a macroadenoma is detected, or if the woman desires to become pregnant, but in all cases of hyperprolactinaemia careful follow-up is needed as some women with this condition, but no tumour, eventually develop one. Women who have functional hyper-prolactinaemia require assessment at 1–3-year intervals, when the level of prolactin in a blood sample is measured and a CT scan made. Women who have a microadenoma need to be assessed annually, but treatment is not required unless they are infertile or have marked symptoms of low circulating levels of oestradiol. In both these groups, if amenorrhoea persists for more than 6 months, as is likely, hormone replacement treatment should be offered to prevent bone loss and the development of osteoporosis.

If a macroadenoma is detected, treatment consists of prescribing a dopamine agonist, such as bromocriptine or cabergoline, in a dose that reduces the prolactin levels to the normal range and maintains them in this range. In most women the treatment causes the tumour to shrink.

Surgery is only indicated if bromocriptine treatment fails. Both during and after treatment, regular measurements of serum prolactin and an annual CT scan are mandatory.

A patient who has a macroadenoma should avoid becoming pregnant until the tumour has shrunk to lie completely within the pituitary fossa, as shown by a CT scan, as it may grow during pregnancy.

Hypothalamopituitary insensitivity: hypothalamic amenorrhoea

In about one-third of cases of amenorrhoea, hypothalamo-pituitary insensitivity is postulated. Many of these cases, coincidentally, follow the use of oral contraceptives, but eating disorders may also be involved, as may psychosomatic factors (for example change of work, marital disharmony or separation). Severe depression or acute or chronic illness may be factors.

Treatment of hypothalamic amenorrhoea

If the amenorrhoea has persisted for 9–12 months and anovulation is the only or the main cause of the couple's infertility, treatment should be offered. Women whose body weight is low (body mass index (BMI) <19) or who are compulsive exercisers should be persuaded to change their behaviour and try to obtain a body weight within the normal range for women (BMI 19.0–24.9) before starting drug treatment. The reasons are that these women are at greater risk of developing the ovarian hyperstimulation syndrome and, if they achieve a pregnancy, have a greater risk of miscarriage and delivering prematurely and a growth-restricted infant.

Clomifene is an antioestrogen which may sometimes act as a weak oestrogen. It acts by binding to oestrogen receptors in target cells, thereby preventing oestradiol binding to them. Transferred to the cell nucleus, it renders the cells relatively insensitive to the effects of endogenous oestradiol. This inhibits the negative feedback with the release of GnRH and, subsequently, FSH and LH. The regimen for clomifene use is shown in Table 28.2. Clomifene will induce ovulation in over 80% of women who have hypothalamic amenorrhoea, particularly if the progestogen test is positive, and should be chosen first.

Should anovulation persist in spite of the clomifene regimen, the patient should be referred to an infertility specialist, as laboratory control is needed if other drugs regimens are used. The regimens are follitropin (recombinant FSH: Puregon and Gonal-F) and human chorionic gonadotrophin (hCG, Pregnyl, Profasi).

Using these treatments about 90% of women with amenorrhoea and 40% of women with oligomenorrhoea will ovulate, and 70% and 25% will conceive. A number of women continue to ovulate after the treatments have ceased and become pregnant.

Polycystic ovarian syndrome (PCOS)

PCOS is the most common cause of anovulatory infertility, affecting around 6–10% of premenopausal women. The diagnosis of PCOS is dependent on the exclusion of other causes of androgen excess (pituitary or adrenal disorders) and with the presence of 12 or more primordial ovarian follicles (Fig. 28.3). Obesity is a common feature and its presence extenuates the physical and biochemical abnormalities. Polycystic ovaries are present in 20% of normal females many of whom have androgen levels within the normal range and have regular menses.

The aetiology of PCOS has not been resolved but there is increasing evidence of a genetic basis with in utero androgen 'programming' of the fetal ovary during ovarian development and oogenesis. Insulin resistance is present in most women with PCOS. Insulin activates the biosynthesis of ovarian androgens, synergistically with LH. In addition it increases free androgen index by suppressing hepatic synthesis of sex hormone-binding globulin and by stimulation of adrenal androgen secretion.

Treatment depends on the presenting symptoms and on the wishes of the woman (Box 28.1). If there are no symptoms no treatment is indicated. Lifestyle changes should be encouraged, and obese women persuaded to seek help from an experienced dietitian. If the woman wishes to conceive then metformin, which acts by reducing hepatic glucose production and increasing peripheral tissue sensitivity, and or/clomifene (see above), can be used to induce ovulation. They should be screened for glucose intolerance preferably before conception and certainly during early pregnancy.

Table 28.2 Therapeutic regimen using clomifene to induce ovulation

STAGE	MONTH	DOSE
1	1	Clomifene 50 mg daily for 5 days
2	2	Clomifene 100 mg daily for 5 days
3	3	Clomifene 150 mg daily for 5 days
4	4	Clomifene 200 mg daily for 5 days
5	6–8	No treatment
6	9	Clomifene 100 mg daily for 5 days + hCG 5000 IU 7 days later
7	10	Clomifene 150 mg daily for 5 days + hCG 5000 IU 7 days later

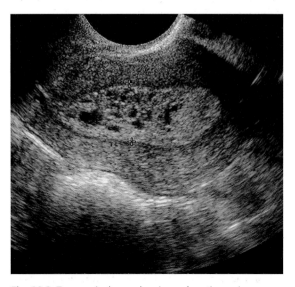

Fig. 28.3 Transvaginal scan showing polycystic ovaries.

Diagnosis (Rotterdam criteria)

At least two of:
1. Oligomenorrhoea or anovulation
2. Clinical or biochemical androgen excess
3. Polycystic ovaries

Treatment

Depends on the presenting symptoms, past history, underlying cause and the wishes of the woman.

General counselling

Improving lifestyle and health, with particular attention to current eating behaviour and exercise; if an eating disorder is still present treatment should be continued. Counselling about increased time needed for spontaneous pregnancy and increased rate of miscarriage and assisted conception.

Useful medications

- Oral contraception (monophasic). Reduces further 'cyst' formation, acne, lowers androgens.
- Spironolactone. Blocks androgen effects on the body, slightly improves insulin resistance.
- Metformin. An oral hypoglycaemic agent that improves insulin resistance, assists weight reduction, improves fertility, reduces miscarriage. It may decrease endometrial cancer and onset of diabetes.
- Clomifene. Most effective for inducing ovulation.

Acne and hirsutism

Laser for permanent removal of hair and treatment appropriate for acne should be discussed.

Obesity

Weight gain is easy and weight loss difficult if the liver cells are resistant but the fat cells are not resistant to insulin. The high level of insulin in the blood will cause the uptake of fat into fat cells at a rapid rate. Metformin in conjunction with a sensible diet and exercise will aid weight loss.

Women with PCOS should be followed up, as over 20% will be found to have, or will develop, impaired glucose tolerance or diabetes. They also have an increased risk of developing endometrial carcinoma if the anovulation persists for a number of years.

Uterine abnormalities

Surgical removal of the uterus, endometrial ablation or radiation result in amenorrhoea. Excessive curettage (particularly following an abortion or postpartum) may act in the same way as endometrial ablation, producing amenorrhoea by removing the basal endometrial layer and permitting synechiae to form (Asherman's syndrome). The diagnosis is made by hysteroscopy, transvaginal ultrasound scanning, or from a hysterogram.

Primary gonadal (ovarian) failure

In most cases the cause of primary ovarian failure is unknown. In this condition the ovarian follicles disappear before the age of 40, and the woman undergoes a premature menopause. In other women the follicles persist but the woman develops autoantibodies that mask the gonadotrophin receptors in the ovaries, with the result that the gonadotrophins can no longer bind to them. These women may have a premature menopause, but inexplicably, some months or years later the woman ovulates and menstruates – the 'resistant ovarian syndrome'. Treatment consists of providing hormone replacement to control menopausal symptoms and to prevent bone loss and cardiovascular sequelae (see p. 324). If the woman wishes to have a child, she may enter an assisted conception programme and receive a donor ovum.

MENORRHAGIA

Menorrhagia may have an organic cause, but in many instances is dysfunctional; in other words, menorrhagia is due to an alteration in the endocrine or local endometrial control of menstruation (see pp. 11–12). Ovulation has often occurred, but not always. Organic causes include uterine myomata, particularly if the myoma is intramural or submucous and distorts the endometrial cavity; diffuse adenomyosis; endometrial polyps and, rarely, chronic pelvic infection (pelvic inflammatory disease); a blood dyscrasia; and hypothyroidism. If the clinician thinks hypothyroidism is a possible diagnosis, TSH and free T_4 levels should be measured. Treatment in these cases is directed to the cause.

Investigation

A careful history and a physical examination should be carried out and, from these, specific laboratory tests ordered. These include a full blood picture, including a coagulation screen if indicated.

These tests may be sufficient to reach a diagnosis, but if the woman is over 35 it is usual to investigate further. The additional tests are transvaginal ultrasound scanning hysteroscopy and endometrial biopsy, and endometrial sampling.

Transvaginal ultrasound

This is the least invasive method of imaging the uterine cavity. The presence of submucous myomata can be detected and the width of the endometrium measured.

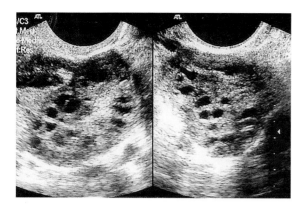

Fig. 28.4 Transvaginal scan showing thickened cystic endometrium measuring 1.41 cm, indicative of endometrial hyperplasia.

An endometrium more than 5 mm wide in a postmenopausal woman indicates the need for curettage to exclude endometrial pathology (Fig. 28.4).

Hysteroscopy

Using a hysteroscope, the uterine cavity can be inspected and abnormalities, such as endometrial polyps (Fig. 28.5) or submucous fibroids, can be detected and often removed. In addition, an endometrial sample can be taken for histological examination. Hysteroscopy is an office procedure that can be performed either with or without a local anaesthetic.

Hysteroscopy provides a clearer picture of the interior of the uterus and makes the diagnosis clearer than diagnostic curettage under anaesthesia, which it has replaced.

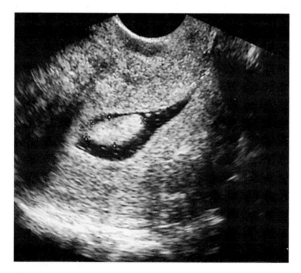

Fig. 28.5 Transvaginal scan demonstrating a 2 cm endometrial polyp.

In several large studies hysteroscopy has shown that about 25% of women with menorrhagia or irregular menstruation have submucous myomata, usually projecting into the uterine cavity, and of these about 10% have endometrial polyps. Previously, these cases would have been identified as dysfunctional uterine bleeding. They can be treated at the time of hysteroscopic diagnosis by hysteroscopic resection.

Endometrial sampling (biopsy)

Endometrial sampling (biopsy) is carried out by introducing a narrow biopsy curette through the uterine cervix and obtaining a representative sample of the endometrium. The procedure can take place in the doctor's office.

There is now no place for a diagnostic curettage per se.

Diagnosis

If no organic cause for menorrhagia is found, a diagnosis of dysfunctional uterine bleeding is made. In these cases the immediate cause of the menorrhagia is thought to be that there is reduced vasoconstriction and a lack of platelet aggregation, hence the haemostatic plugs occluding the endometrial blood vessels are less effective in achieving haemostasis. These changes may reflect increased prostacyclin and prostaglandin E_2 secretion by the endometrium. Dysfunctional uterine bleeding is more common under the age of 19 and after the age of 39.

DYSFUNCTIONAL UTERINE BLEEDING

The importance of an accurate menstrual history cannot be overstated. If the patient agrees, and the bleeding is not too severe, or if she has not recorded a menstrual history herself, it is helpful if she records the duration of, the interval between, and the perceived amount of menstrual discharge for a 3-month period. The latter is difficult for a woman to measure and it is usually overestimated. Ideally, the actual blood loss should be determined (by collecting all pads and tampons and measuring the haemoglobin content by the alkaline haematin method), but this is not practicable except in a research programme. Certain clinical pointers help. These are the occurrence of 'flooding'; saturation of tampons or pads or changing pads every half-hour to 2 hours; the presence of large blood clots; and prolonged duration of the menstrual period.

Although dysfunctional uterine bleeding is usually regular the duration of the menstrual cycle may be increased, with the result that the menorrhagia occurs less frequently. In this group of cases, which are usually found at the extremes of the reproductive period, oestrogen secretion may be less than normal and is not opposed by progesterone. In other words, the bleeding is anovulatory. In other cases the unopposed oestrogen levels are high, resulting in an increased thickness of the endometrium and causing cystic hyperplasia (Fig. 28.6). The pathology of an endometrial sample may show simple (cystic) endometrial hyperplasia (Fig. 28.7); complex adenomatous hyperplasia (Fig. 28.8); simple hyperplasia with atypia or complex hyperplasia with atypia (Fig. 28.9). If the pathology shows atypical hyperplasia (the treatment is that described on p. 297) follow-up with further endometrial studies is mandatory (unless the woman chooses to have a hysterectomy), as between 10 and 25% of cases progress to endometrial carcinoma.

Fluctuations in the circulating levels of oestrogen tend to occur, resulting in a 'lack of support' for the endometrium and leading to cyclical, profuse bleeding. In other cases, the heavy bleeding occurs at shorter intervals, the cycle length being reduced. This is referred to as polymenorrhagia. The treatment of these variants is the same as that for dysfunctional uterine bleeding.

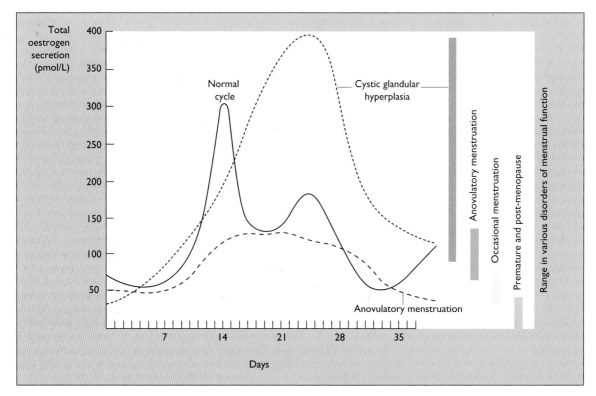

Fig. 28.6 Urinary oestrogen secretion in certain gynaecological conditions related to the menstrual cycle.

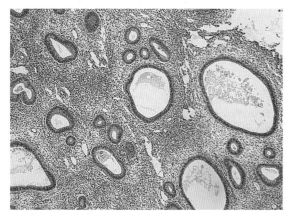

Fig. 28.7 Cystic endometrial hyperplasia.

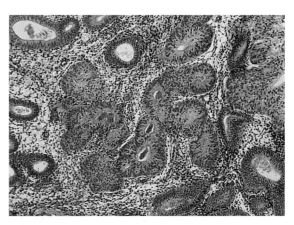

Fig. 28.8 Complex adenomatous hyperplasia.

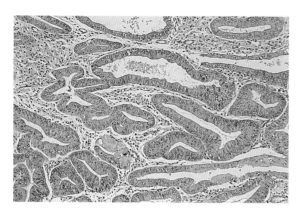

Fig. 28.9 Complex hyperplasia with atypia.

Treatment of dysfunctional uterine bleeding

Patients seen during a severe bleeding episode

In this situation treatment may be required urgently. Two methods are available: to perform curettage and to administer hormones. The hormones usually chosen are combined equine oestrogens (CEE), 25 mg given intravenously and repeated 6-hourly for two to three doses. CEE in this dosage may cause marked nausea in some women. Once CEE has stopped the bleeding, a progestogen must be given for 14 days to induce secretory change and then endometrial shedding. An alternative to CEE is to give 17-hydroxyprogesterone acetate 125–250 mg intramuscularly, or oral norethisterone 20–30 mg/day, in divided doses, for 4 days. If a progestogen is used, a withdrawal bleed may be expected 3–6 days later. This can be avoided if norethisterone (5–10 mg daily) is continued for 20 days.

Patients seen between bleeding episodes

In this situation several choices are available. They should be discussed with the woman, as her wishes and concerns should be addressed before treatment is instituted. The choices fall into two main groups: hormonal treatment and surgical treatment.

Medical treatment

The treatments of choice are:

- Tranexamic acid, an antifibrinolytic agent, reduces menstrual loss by 50%. The dose is 1 g 6-hourly for 5 days, commencing on the first day of menstruation.
- Nonsteroidal anti-inflammatory drugs (NSAIDs). These drugs inhibit prostaglandin synthesis and reduce both the volume of blood loss (by 20–30%) and the associated dysmenorrhoea. A widely used example is mefenamic acid, which is taken in a dose of 500 mg 8-hourly, if possible commencing 4 days before menstruation.
- Levonorgestrel intra-uterine device (Mirena) This device releases 20 mg of levonorgestrel a day and is effective for 5 years. As well as regulating the menorrhagia it is an effective contraceptive. In 90% of women the menorrhagia is cured within 3 months.
- Oral contraceptives. If the bleeding is not too severe, a monophasic progestogen-dominant hormonal contraceptive may be used.

Note that the use of cyclical progesterone therapy, especially in the luteal phase, is not effective.

Surgical treatment

Curettage

Before the availability of hormones, or the newer surgical treatments, curettage was the only treatment of menorrhagia, apart from hysterectomy. Curettage controls heavy bleeding for a short time but there is usually a recurrence in 4–6 months. For this reason, it was replaced by medical treatment or endometrial ablation.

Endometrial ablation

The concept of this procedure is that by ablating the basal layer of the endometrium, endometrial regeneration is prevented or reduced and the menorrhagia cured. Endometrial ablation should only be performed by a gynaecologist experienced in the technique, or the results will be poor and the woman may be at risk of severe complications. Before endometrial ablation is carried out the cavity of the uterus is inspected with a hysteroscope. Many gynaecologists prescribe danazol 200 mg two or three times a day for 4 weeks before the operation, or a GnRH analogue (for example depot leuprolide 7.5 mg, 4 weeks before the procedure) to reduce endometrial thickness. Endometrial ablation may be performed using 'roller ball' electrocoagulation, loop resection or laser, after distending and flushing the uterine cavity with a glycine mixture. If laser is chosen, the uterine cavity is continuously flushed with a sodium chloride infusion system. An alternative is to use radiofrequency-induced thermal endometrial ablation. In this method the uterine cavity is not distended with fluid.

The procedures are not without problems. In 1% of cases the uterine wall is perforated. Glycine and sodium chloride are absorbed into the vascular system and may cause fluid overload, pulmonary oedema and hyponatraemia.

These different methods produce similar results: 30–60% of women become amenorrhoeic, 35–60% become hypomenorrhoeic, and the remaining 5–15% require a repeat of the procedure or a hysterectomy. Interviewed up to 2 years after the procedure, three-quarters of women express satisfaction, the remainder complaining of persistent menstruation, dysmenorrhoea or pelvic pain.

The benefits of endometrial ablation are that it is less invasive and painful than hysterectomy, the woman is in hospital for 1–2 days rather than 7–10 days, and it is less expensive. The woman should be convalescent for 7–14 days.

Hysterectomy

Although there is no argument that hysterectomy is an appropriate operation in many cases of uterine fibroids, adenomyosis, advanced endometriosis, uterine malignancy and in some cases of pelvic infection, its position in the treatment of dysfunctional uterine bleeding is not so clear. Many women welcome hysterectomy for the relief of a distressing symptom, whereas other prefer to keep organs related to reproduction (ovaries and uterus). A woman must have the opportunity to discuss the choices for the treatment of menorrhagia, and be given time to consider the pros and cons of the operation, if hysterectomy is recommended to her. There is rarely any need for an urgent hysterectomy and, once the operation has been recommended by a gynaecologist, it may be helpful for the woman to talk with her general practitioner about the benefits of and problems related to the operation. These matters are discussed further on page 233.

METRORRHAGIA

In metrorrhagia the bleeding is irregular in quantity, acyclical in character, and often prolonged. The condition is usually due to pathology in the uterus or other internal genital organs. Its presence demands that the doctor investigate further. The investigations include hysteroscopy and/or endometrial biopsy. Treatment is directed to the underlying cause. Hysterectomy is often appropriate.

OTHER DISTURBANCES OF MENSTRUATION

In some women the duration of the cycle is shortened to less than 21 days (polymenorrhoea). Most women have no concerns about this, but if the change is annoying the menstrual period can be regulated by prescribing an oral contraceptive.

Some women complain of slight menstrual staining occurring 2–3 days before or following the end of a normal menstrual period. Apart from being annoying, the condition has no sinister consequences, although some doctors believe that premenstrual staining is a sign of endometriosis. The woman should be reassured, but if she requests treatment, menstruation is usually regulated by prescribing oral contraceptives or norethisterone 2.5 mg from days 20–25 of the menstrual cycle for a few months.

Another concern of some women is that the amount of menstrual discharge has decreased. This condition, known as hypomenorrhoea, occurs most commonly in women taking oral contraceptives. The woman should be reassured that it has no abnormal consequences.

Chapter | **29** |

Psychological and physical disorders of the menstrual cycle

MOOD AND PHYSICAL SYMPTOMS IN THE MENSTRUAL CYCLE

In the proliferative phase of the menstrual cycle few problems occur. Some women experience lower abdominal pain, which is unilateral and occurs at the time of ovulation. The pain is usually not severe and lasts for 12 hours or less. The condition is called mittelschmerz. It indicates that ovulation has occurred, but investigations show no intra-abdominal pathology. If mittelschmerz is recurrent and distressing, relief can be obtained if the woman takes a hormonal contraceptive.

Most women in the reproductive years experience some psychological (negative mood) or physical symptoms in the luteal phase of the menstrual cycle. The symptoms vary in character and tend to become worse as menstruation approaches. They do not occur in every cycle, and may vary in intensity in different cycles. A few women have severe mood and physical symptoms; a diagnosis of premenstrual syndrome (PMS) or premenstrual dysphoric disorder is made in these cases.

PREMENSTRUAL SYNDROME

Premenstrual syndrome (premenstrual dysphoric disorder)

In 5–15% of women, who are usually aged in their late 20s or early 30s (range 20–40), the negative mood and physical changes occurring in the luteal phase are sufficiently severe to affect day-to-day living and social and personal relationships, particularly with partners and children, most or all months. With the onset of menstruation, or during it, the symptoms disappear. During the postmenstrual period, for at least a week the woman feels well, sometimes euphoric, but with – or soon after – ovulation the symptoms reappear.

The symptoms vary in character and in severity in different menstrual cycles, but there is always a symptom-free interval of at least 1 week. The mood changes tend to cluster together and are described as irritable, depressive, anxious and tense, with mood swings and feelings of being out of control, fatigued and lacking motivation. Different women will describe slightly different symptoms as the most problematic. This may depend on the woman's country of birth and her current lifestyle and stresses.

The same symptoms can be reported by women taking oral contraception just before and during the pill-free week; the symptoms are usually mild.

Diagnosis of PMS

The diagnosis of PMS is made after evaluating the periodicity of the physical and mood symptoms, ascertaining that there is a symptom-free period after menstruation, and ensuring that the symptoms cannot be explained by some other illness. Other illnesses can be exacerbated during the luteal phase of the menstrual cycle, and this can lead to inaccuracies in the diagnosis. The suspected diagnosis should be confirmed by asking the woman to complete a daily record of symptoms over three menstrual cycles (Fig. 29.1). As well as establishing a firm diagnosis, the value of the daily record is that the woman develops an insight into her symptoms and is encouraged by the fact that the medical practitioner has an interest in her problems.

Aetiology of PMS

The aetiology of PMS is unknown (Box 29.1). It is reported to be more severe if the woman is under stress. There may be a genetic component, but the current theory is that PMS is multifactorial. One underlying abnormality may be a fluctuation in the levels of oestradiol in the luteal phase, which may cause the symptoms directly or by decreasing brain serotonin activity. A problem in accepting this theory is that no consistent fluctuations have been detected with daily monitoring. PMS does not occur if the ovaries are absent.

Management of PMS

The importance of obtaining a thorough history and an ongoing therapeutic relationship with the woman cannot be overestimated. Once this has been established, explanation and counselling will be accepted. The woman's lifestyle should be explored and suggestions made to reduce stress. The predominant symptoms should be identified from the completed charts and treatment directed to specific problems, for example regular 'normal' eating during the follicular phase may prevent overeating or binge eating premenstrually.

Many medications and 'natural cures' including evening primrose oil, Chinese herbal medications and progesterone have been tried, but in spite of enthusiastic reports Cochrane reviews have not demonstrated that they are more effective than placebo.

Three approaches have been suggested for women who have severe, intractable PMS. The first is to prescribe a hormonal contraceptive. The pill (monophasic pill) has been prescribed for some years, with varying rates of success in relieving PMS. Some women suffering severe symptoms find they 'react badly' to the pill, whereas others find relief, particularly if the active tablets are taken continuously (pill-free week excluded). Transdermal oestrogen patches or an oestrogen implant suit some women better. In these cases the woman has to be protected from the development of endometrial carcinoma due to the presence of unopposed oestrogen, and a progestogen is prescribed cyclically. During the period when the progestogen is taken symptoms of PMS may recur, and so continuous progestogen may be preferred. The second approach is to prescribe a selective serotonin reuptake inhibitor (SSRI) in the lowest dose available, either continuously or during the luteal phase. The mode of action of SSRIs in relieving symptoms of PMS is unknown but has been shown to be highly effective in reducing the physical, functional and behavioural symptoms of moderate to severe PMS. The third approach is radical and not recommended, being either to suppress ovarian activity with gonadotrophin-releasing hormone agonists or to perform a bilateral oophorectomy (and total hysterectomy).

FUNCTIONAL BOWEL DISEASE

Irritable bowel syndrome

Symptoms of irritable bowel syndrome (IBS) and other disorders of gastrointestinal function may be exacerbated premenstrually. IBS affects 14–24% of women, although a clinical diagnosis is made in only 1–2% of the population. A patient with IBS may complain of abdominal pain associated with a change in bowel habit (diarrhoea, constipation, or alternating between the two), and symptoms of abdominal bloating, passage of mucus, and feelings of incomplete evacuation. It is currently believed that IBS and other disorders of gastrointestinal function result from an interplay of altered gut motility, increased sensitivity of the intestine or colon, and psychosocial factors. Food intake and prior gastrointestinal infection may also play a role. Diagnosis is based on a positive symptom diagnosis, and investigations should be made to exclude organic disease, particularly in the elderly. Treatment, although often unsatisfactory, is tailored to reduce the dominant symptom: dietary fibre for constipation; opioid agents for diarrhoea; and low-dose antidepressants or infrequent use of antispasmodics for pain. Psychotherapy and hypnotherapy have not been shown in Cochrane reviews to be of definitive benefit. The patient needs reassurance that she is not suffering from cancer or a serious bowel disease, and extensive investigations or referrals are not usually warranted.

CHRONIC PELVIC PAIN

A few women complain of chronic pain in the lower abdomen and pelvis which fluctuates in intensity and tends to increase in the premenstruum. It may occur on either

Month---------------------------   Name---------------------------

Date	Mood					Performance					Vaginal discharge			Menses			Abdominal symptoms		
	Happy, calm, worthwhile, friendly, easygoing		Sad, tense, hopeless, uptight, irritable, angry, withdrawn			Excellent, alert, decisive		Poor, confused, indecisive									Bloating, sensation of weight gain		
	0	1	2	3	4	0	1	2	3	4	0	1	2	0	1	2	0	1	2
1	○	○	○	○	○	○	○	○	○	○	○	○	○	○	○	○	○	○	○
2	○	○	○	○	○	○	○	○	○	○	○	○	○	○	○	○	○	○	○
3	○	○	○	○	○	○	○	○	○	○	○	○	○	○	○	○	○	○	○
4	○	○	○	○	○	○	○	○	○	○	○	○	○	○	○	○	○	○	○
5	○	○	○	○	○	○	○	○	○	○	○	○	○	○	○	○	○	○	○
6	○	○	○	○	○	○	○	○	○	○	○	○	○	○	○	○	○	○	○
7	○	○	○	○	○	○	○	○	○	○	○	○	○	○	○	○	○	○	○
8	○	○	○	○	○	○	○	○	○	○	○	○	○	○	○	○	○	○	○
9	○	○	○	○	○	○	○	○	○	○	○	○	○	○	○	○	○	○	○
10	○	○	○	○	○	○	○	○	○	○	○	○	○	○	○	○	○	○	○
11	○	○	○	○	○	○	○	○	○	○	○	○	○	○	○	○	○	○	○
12	○	○	○	○	○	○	○	○	○	○	○	○	○	○	○	○	○	○	○
13	○	○	○	○	○	○	○	○	○	○	○	○	○	○	○	○	○	○	○
14	○	○	○	○	○	○	○	○	○	○	○	○	○	○	○	○	○	○	○
15	○	○	○	○	○	○	○	○	○	○	○	○	○	○	○	○	○	○	○
16	○	○	○	○	○	○	○	○	○	○	○	○	○	○	○	○	○	○	○
17	○	○	○	○	○	○	○	○	○	○	○	○	○	○	○	○	○	○	○
18	○	○	○	○	○	○	○	○	○	○	○	○	○	○	○	○	○	○	○
19	○	○	○	○	○	○	○	○	○	○	○	○	○	○	○	○	○	○	○
20	○	○	○	○	○	○	○	○	○	○	○	○	○	○	○	○	○	○	○
21	○	○	○	○	○	○	○	○	○	○	○	○	○	○	○	○	○	○	○
22	○	○	○	○	○	○	○	○	○	○	○	○	○	○	○	○	○	○	○
23	○	○	○	○	○	○	○	○	○	○	○	○	○	○	○	○	○	○	○
24	○	○	○	○	○	○	○	○	○	○	○	○	○	○	○	○	○	○	○
25	○	○	○	○	○	○	○	○	○	○	○	○	○	○	○	○	○	○	○
26	○	○	○	○	○	○	○	○	○	○	○	○	○	○	○	○	○	○	○
27	○	○	○	○	○	○	○	○	○	○	○	○	○	○	○	○	○	○	○
28	○	○	○	○	○	○	○	○	○	○	○	○	○	○	○	○	○	○	○
29	○	○	○	○	○	○	○	○	○	○	○	○	○	○	○	○	○	○	○
30	○	○	○	○	○	○	○	○	○	○	○	○	○	○	○	○	○	○	○
31	○	○	○	○	○	○	○	○	○	○	○	○	○	○	○	○	○	○	○

Date	Breast symptoms			Appetite			PMS			Impact of PMS			Instructions for completing the diary
	Swelling, pain, tenderness			Increased appetite, craving for certain foods			Patient's diagnosis			Effect on work, relationships or social activity			1 Fill in the diary every night before retiring to bed. Leave blank if you forgot to fill it in before retiring.
	0	1	2	0	1	2	0	1	2	0	1	2	
1	○	○	○	○	○	○	○	○	○	○	○	○	2 For each symptom, place a mark in the circle which best corresponds to the degree of severity of that symptom experienced that day.
2	○	○	○	○	○	○	○	○	○	○	○	○	
3	○	○	○	○	○	○	○	○	○	○	○	○	
4	○	○	○	○	○	○	○	○	○	○	○	○	
5	○	○	○	○	○	○	○	○	○	○	○	○	
6	○	○	○	○	○	○	○	○	○	○	○	○	3 When the diary has been completed for the month, turn the page on its side and join up the marks to obtain a graph for each symptom.
7	○	○	○	○	○	○	○	○	○	○	○	○	
8	○	○	○	○	○	○	○	○	○	○	○	○	
9	○	○	○	○	○	○	○	○	○	○	○	○	
10	○	○	○	○	○	○	○	○	○	○	○	○	4 The diary should be kept for two or three menstrual cycles.
11	○	○	○	○	○	○	○	○	○	○	○	○	
12	○	○	○	○	○	○	○	○	○	○	○	○	
13	○	○	○	○	○	○	○	○	○	○	○	○	
14	○	○	○	○	○	○	○	○	○	○	○	○	
15	○	○	○	○	○	○	○	○	○	○	○	○	For mood and performance 0 = best 2 = average/usual; 4 = worst.
16	○	○	○	○	○	○	○	○	○	○	○	○	For symptoms (i.e. all other boxes):
17	○	○	○	○	○	○	○	○	○	○	○	○	0 = absent;
18	○	○	○	○	○	○	○	○	○	○	○	○	1 = present; 2 = severe.
19	○	○	○	○	○	○	○	○	○	○	○	○	
20	○	○	○	○	○	○	○	○	○	○	○	○	
21	○	○	○	○	○	○	○	○	○	○	○	○	
22	○	○	○	○	○	○	○	○	○	○	○	○	
23	○	○	○	○	○	○	○	○	○	○	○	○	
24	○	○	○	○	○	○	○	○	○	○	○	○	
25	○	○	○	○	○	○	○	○	○	○	○	○	
26	○	○	○	○	○	○	○	○	○	○	○	○	
27	○	○	○	○	○	○	○	○	○	○	○	○	
28	○	○	○	○	○	○	○	○	○	○	○	○	
29	○	○	○	○	○	○	○	○	○	○	○	○	
30	○	○	○	○	○	○	○	○	○	○	○	○	
31	○	○	○	○	○	○	○	○	○	○	○	○	

Fig. 29.1 Menstrual history diary.

Box 29.1 PMS summary

What is PMS?	Negative mood and physical symptoms commencing after ovulation and resolving during the luteal phase of the menstrual cycle. There must be at least 7 days free of symptoms each month and the symptoms must be of sufficient severity to affect the woman's lifestyle
Aetiology	Unknown
Prevalence	All women have cyclical changes in symptoms; 5–15% of women in their 20s and 30s have moderate to severe symptoms
Diagnosis	By history and examination, daily diary, and excluding other causes for the symptoms
Symptoms	**Mood**: irritability, depression, sadness, fatigue, labile mood, anxious, tense **Physical symptoms**: breast swelling and soreness, abdominal swelling and discomfort, headache and backache and increased appetite
Management	Taking a very good medical and psychosocial history and discussing management with the woman **Psychological**: cognitive behavioural therapy to help the woman understand her symptoms and make changes to reduce stress and the factors exacerbating her symptoms. Keeping a daily diary to help understand the symptoms and their changing severity each month assists both diagnosis and management **Hormonal**: oral contraception or continuous low-dose oestrogen and progestogen **Other medication**: SSRIs, lowest dose available continuously or during luteal phase **Surgical**: removal of the ovaries is of theoretical interest only
Outcome	Unknown

episodes of 'pelvic inflammatory disease' which have been diagnosed on clinical findings rather than by laparoscopy, and she may have had episodes of pelvic surgery.

The diagnosis is made after excluding organic causes of chronic pelvic pain, such as adenomyosis, endometriosis and pelvic inflammatory disease, which are present in about one-third of cases. This indicates that laparoscopy is mandatory to make a diagnosis. The procedure should be made during menstruation to disclose endometriotic lesions deep in the cul-de-sac when the lesion is most likely to be seen. Two studies in the USA showed that over half of the women who had chronic pelvic pain had been severely sexually abused (penetration or other contact with the patient's vagina or anus) before the age of 15, and 42% had also been physically abused. These issues are worth exploring.

In some cases chronic pelvic pain is associated with an ovarian remnant that was left behind after hysterectomy and bilateral oophorectomy.

Treatment

The investigations themselves may constitute a form of treatment, as in one study of 60 women in whom laparoscopy showed no pathology, 90% of the patients assessed 6 months later said that, since the laparoscopy, they had no pelvic pain or that there was much less pain.

The woman's psychological, marital and psychosexual problems need to be explored and supportive psychotherapy offered. Referral to a pain clinic may be useful. If the woman asks for medications, medroxyprogesterone 30 mg/day may be prescribed. An alternative is to prescribe danazol 200 mg three times daily for 2–3 months, although the side-effects may deter the woman from taking this treatment. Antidepressant medication, particularly selective serotonin reuptake inhibitors (SSRIs), may help some women.

DYSMENORRHOEA

Dysmenorrhoea means painful menstruation. Two types are described: primary, or spasmodic dysmenorrhoea, and secondary dysmenorrhoea.

Primary dysmenorrhoea

This form usually starts 2–3 years after the menarche and is maximal between the ages of 15 and 25. It decreases with age and usually ceases after childbirth. The crampy pains start during the 24 hours before menstruation and may last 24–36 hours, although they are only severe for the first 24 hours. The cramps are felt in the lower abdomen, but may radiate to the back or down the inner surface of the thighs. In severe cases vomiting or diarrhoea may accompany the cramps.

side of the abdomen and may be felt on different sides at different times. The woman may also complain of deep dyspareunia or a postcoital pelvic ache, which may last for 24 hours. The woman may have a history of several

Spasmodic dysmenorrhoea is experienced by 60–75% of young women. In three-quarters of affected women the cramps are minor or moderate in severity, but in 25% they are severe and incapacitating.

The aetiology of spasmodic dysmenorrhoea has now been clarified. When progesterone is secreted following ovulation, the luteinized endometrium is able to synthesize prostaglandins. If the balance between prostacyclin (which causes vasodilatation and myometrial relaxation), prostaglandin $F_{2\alpha}$ (which causes vasoconstriction and myometrial contraction) and prostaglandin E_2 (which causes myometrial contraction and vasodilatation) is disturbed, causing $PGF_{2\alpha}$ to predominate, myometrial ischaemia (uterine angina) and uterine hypercontractility occur. In addition, vasopressin is involved in dysmenorrhoea. Vasopressin increases prostaglandin synthesis and may act on the uterine arteries directly.

Treatment

Treatment consists of suppressing ovulation, by prescribing an oral contraceptive or by inhibition of prostaglandin synthesis by one of the prostaglandin synthetase inhibitors, mefenamic acid, ibuprofen, diclofenac sodium or naproxen. There appears to be little difference in their effectiveness.

- Oral contraceptives may be preferred by a woman who is sexually active, as the pill will protect her against an unwanted pregnancy as well as relieving the dysmenorrhoea.
- Nonsteroidal anti-inflammatory drugs (NSAIDs) may be preferred by women who do not wish to use hormones and prefer to take medication for as short a time as possible. The chosen medication is taken at the first sign of pain and continued for up to 5 days.

Dysmenorrhoea is relieved in 95% of cases, whether oral contraceptives or NSAIDs are chosen. If the chosen treatment fails to relieve the dysmenorrhoea, an alternative can be tried.

Secondary dysmenorrhoea

Secondary, or acquired, dysmenorrhoea is unusual before the age of 25 and uncommon before the age of 30. In most cases the underlying cause is either endometriosis or pelvic inflammatory disease. Typically, the cramps start 2 or more days prior to menstruation, and the pain increases in severity until late menstruation, when it peaks, taking 2 or more days to cease. The management is that of the primary condition.

EATING AND EXERCISE DISORDERS

The presence of an eating or exercise disorder may have profound effects on the health and wellbeing of a woman throughout her reproductive life and on the development of her child. The aim of this section is not to describe in detail eating and exercise disorders but to alert the medical practitioner to the need to ask a few questions about a woman's body weight (BMI) and her eating and exercise behaviour. Eating and exercise problems are associated with delayed menarche, secondary amenorrhoea, infertility, miscarriage, low-birthweight (premature and growth-restricted) babies, postpartum depression, pelvic pain and irritable bowel, sexual problems and polycystic ovarian syndrome and osteoporosis. The doctor is easily alerted to the possibility of a disorder if women are very thin or obese, but many disordered women have a body weight in the normal range. Most gynaecological and obstetric problems are reversed if the woman seeks help and recovers from her eating disorder. Some women may not be aware they have an eating or exercise problem, and may need encouragement to talk about their behaviour and possible treatments. Other women who are aware that their behaviour and thinking are disordered may prefer to seek alternative remedies and undergo assisted conception or medications for their medical complications; these women need careful and regular medical monitoring.

PSYCHOLOGICAL SYMPTOMS AFTER HYSTERECTOMY AND OOPHORECTOMY

In recent years the frequency of hysterectomy has fallen as other methods of treatment for conditions previously treated by hysterectomy have been developed. The effects of the operation depend on the condition that led to the hysterectomy, and the woman's knowledge and attitude to hysterectomy. Some women recover quickly, others are mildly or moderately incapacitated for up to 3 months. One-third of women take 3 months to recover fully from the operation, and 20% take longer. Five to ten per cent of women feel well generally but have bowel or bladder symptoms, particularly genuine stress incontinence, which may persist for months.

Although most gynaecologists choose total hysterectomy so that cervical cancer will not develop, there is a small trend back to subtotal hysterectomy in selected cases. The reasons for this are:

- The operation is less dangerous as the ureters are avoided.
- The sequelae of bowel and bladder symptoms occur less frequently.
- The woman's sexual response, sexual enjoyment and orgasm are less negatively affected.
- The risk of developing cervical cancer is very small if a woman has had regular cervical smears which have always been normal and she continues to have regular smears. If any cervical cell abnormality is detected it

will be early, and conization or other local treatment can be offered.

Most women understand and respond well to removal of an organ that is 'diseased' or dysfunctional. They do not necessarily agree with the removal of reproductive organs for prophylactic reasons, or which could be preserved if another treatment is equally as effective.

Hysterectomy

Some women after hysterectomy become anxious and distressed. This is more likely to occur if the woman believes that her body image, her femininity and her sexual attractiveness are reduced. Such anxiety follows misconceptions about hysterectomy, including notions that:

- A woman will be unable to have or enjoy sexual intercourse because her vagina will be shorter.
- She will become obese.
- She will be severely depressed after the operation.
- She will become postmenopausal.

The patient should be reassured about the first two misconceptions before the operation takes place. The third misconception is untrue. There is no evidence that hysterectomy increases clinical depression, unless the woman had a history of depression prior to surgery. The fourth misconception is only likely to be true if she has her ovaries removed at the operation, or if the surgeon has damaged the ovarian blood supply.

Oophorectomy

Some women after loss of their ovaries will also feel incomplete as a woman, a loss of femininity and of sexual interest. Her feelings can be intense if she did not feel she had a chance to discuss this with her doctor, and was unaware she would need to take hormone replacement for the symptoms of menopause.

The question of bilateral oophorectomy of normal ovaries at the time of hysterectomy is contentious. Ovarian extirpation is not usually carried out in women under 45, but some gynaecologists perform it in older women. Their reasons are, first, that if the ovaries are left, 1 in 1000 women will develop ovarian cancer, and second, the ovaries have no function after the menopause (although they do produce DHEA (dehydroepiandrosterone)). There are also data to the effect that up to 20% of women aged 40–45 experience ovarian failure within 3 years of hysterectomy.

Bilateral oophorectomy at the time of hysterectomy is associated with severe menopausal symptoms requiring hormone replacement treatment (see p. 325). Women may wish to try to avoid taking hormones and wait for the 'natural' menopause, when their symptoms may be less severe.

The woman should make her own decision, after discussion with her doctors and after she has had time to think it over and seek other advice if she wishes.

Hysterectomy is safe today, but as it is not without morbidity, alternative therapies should be considered.

To reduce the psychological and physical problems that may occur after hysterectomy, the attending doctors, whether specialists or GPs, must talk with the woman and her partner. The reason for the operation should be explained, its extent described, alternative treatments discussed, and problems that may arise mentioned. In most cases the woman should be given time to think about the discussion and to ask further questions, if she has any, before the operation is performed.

Chapter | **30** |

Human sexuality

In the past 50 years more people than ever before have been able to learn about human sexuality and the human sexual response. Discussion about human sexuality has become more open.

Sexual problems within a relationship are not uncommon, and women and men now feel able to seek advice about them. Often the first reference point is the person's general practitioner. General practitioners, like other people, have inhibitions about sexuality and a variety of values about sexual behaviour. These inhibitions and values are based on the person's religious beliefs and upbringing, and on values obtained from parents and colleagues. If a medical practitioner is uncomfortable discussing sexual problems with patients they should refer the patient to a colleague. If the medical practitioner feels able to treat sexual dysfunctions they should try to determine the patient's sexual values and try to solve the problem within that value system.

Sexual advice can only be given if the practitioner has some knowledge of sexuality and sexual behaviours.

SEXUALITY

Sexuality may be defined as the sum of a person's inherited characteristics, knowledge, experience, attitudes and behaviour as they relate to being female or male. Human sexuality is as much psychological as physical, and involves feelings as well as physicality. It includes communication with the other person and being open to and respecting their wishes. It also involves touching and exploring each other's bodies to learn the textures and surfaces, and the sight and smell of another person.

Sexuality includes the sexual drive, which is the sum of the desire to have sex and the ability to accomplish the act. Sexual drive varies considerably between people. In some, a low drive is due to constitutional factors such as ill health or advanced age. In others, low drive is due to a traumatic sexual experience in childhood or adolescence. Recently, more women are reporting that they have been sexually assaulted in childhood or early adolescence, and this can be the basis of a fear of sex and a low sexual drive.

During adult life the intensity of the sexual drive is maximal in the years up to the age of 40, and tends to lessen after this time, but there are considerable variations. Problems may arise if the sexual drive of two partners is markedly different.

HUMAN SEXUAL RESPONSE

The physiology of the human sexual response was not described until 1966, by Masters and Johnson. For descriptive purposes they divided the sexual response in women and men into five phases, although the distinction between each phase is often blurred and one phase tends to merge into the next provided the appropriate stimulation occurs.

The phases are:

- Sexual desire
- Sexual arousal or excitement
- Plateau
- Orgasm
- Resolution.

Care needs to be taken to not see these phases as directional, assuming orgasm to be the goal.

Sexual desire is stimulated by the thought, sight, touch or smell of another person. It may be suppressed, or merge into the arousal phase.

In the arousal phase, a man's penis becomes erect and a woman's vagina becomes lubricated. In this phase, sexual enjoyment is increased if the couple pleasure each other sexually by cuddling, stroking and exploring each other's body with fingers, tongue, lips and thighs. Arousal is increased further if the erogenous zones of the body, a woman's clitoral area, breasts and vulva and a man's penis and scrotum, are stimulated. A woman's breasts become larger due to engorgement with blood, and her nipples become erect. Her clitoris increases in width and becomes more sensitive to touch, and her labia and the lower part of her vagina become congested and softer and thicker. The subvaginal tissues become increasingly congested, and fluid transudes between the vaginal cells to increase lubrication.

During the following plateau phase, the sexual pleasure is intensified and the partners desire to have penile–vaginal, penile–oral or penile–anal penetration. The thrusting movement of the penis in the vagina, or its oral stimulation, causes an orgasm in the man, with the ejaculation of seminal fluid. In 90% of women the thrusting of the man's penis in her vagina indirectly, or the digital or oral stimulation of her clitoral area directly, leads to orgasm. Fifty per cent of sexually active women reach orgasm when the clitoral area is stimulated by finger or tongue; 25% reach orgasm during penile thrusting in the vagina; 15% of women can achieve multiple orgasms; and the remaining 10% are unable to achieve orgasm, although they may enjoy their partner's pleasure.

Orgasm provides an intense feeling of pleasure. During orgasm, the perineal muscles, the medial fibres of the levator ani and the sphincter ani muscles contract rhythmically and involuntarily, as do the muscles surrounding the vagina. Many other muscle groups, particularly those of the back, contract at the height of the orgasm, and a deep feeling of ecstasy (in its original sense) and relaxation follows.

In the resolution phase, both sexual partners are relaxed. In the initial moments the clitoris and the penis are exquisitely sensitive to touch, but this passes rapidly and the tissues of the lower genital tract, in both sexes, decongest, the penis becoming flaccid, the clitoris small and the woman's external genitals and vagina decongested.

The physiological basis of the observed changes during sexual response occurs in two parts. Both are mediated by psychic or physical sexual stimulation or, more usually, by both. Both parts can be inhibited by subconscious influences to a greater or lesser degree.

The phases of the sexual response up to orgasm are mediated by the parasympathetic nerves, which lead to vasodilatation and vasocongestion of the genital organs. In a man, this leads to an inflow of blood into the cavernous spaces of the penile cylinders and an inhibition of outflow from the cylinders. The result is an erection. In a woman, the changes lead to the development of congestive 'cushions' around the lower part of the vagina and to vaginal lubrication.

Failure of sexual arousal prevents these changes, with resulting erectile failure in a man, and general sexual dysfunction in a woman.

The second, orgasmic, phase is mediated by the sympathetic nerves, the stimulation of which leads to the clonic muscle contraction of the pelvic and other muscles. In a man these contractions lead to ejaculation, and in both sexes to the more general muscle contractions. The feeling of pleasure experienced by both sexes appears to have its origin in a 'sex centre' in the thalamic and limbic areas of the old cortex, which are closely related anatomically to the pleasure centres in the paleocortex. The messages that stimulate these centres are initiated from clitoral and vaginal stimulation in women and penile stimulation in men. Failure of the sympathetic element to proceed in an orderly fashion results in premature or restricted ejaculation in a man. Failure of the sensations invoked in the clitoris and vagina to be transmitted to the brain and interpreted as pleasurable is the reason for orgasm failing to occur in women.

SEXUAL DYSFUNCTIONS

Most sexual dysfunctions arise from a poor relationship with the partner, ignorance about sexuality and sexual technique, a low sexual drive, or performance anxiety. Additional factors are physical illness, the fear that sex will aggravate an existing illness, excessive alcohol use, or clinical depression and anxiety. All can appear to be lifelong, or occur after a time of 'normal' functioning. What is 'normal' for one woman may be 'disordered' for another.

As men and women age, changes occur in their sexual desire and sexual response. These are considered on page 324.

Women have four main sexual dysfunctions:
- Inhibited sexual desire
- Impairment of sexual arousal

Table 30.1 Sexual dysfunction

	CLINICAL SYNDROME	
	Male	Female
Inhibited sexual desire	No arousal	No arousal
Fear of sexual (genital) activity	Primary erectile failure (impotence)	Vaginismus
Impairment of sexual arousal Absence or inadequate vasocongestion* due to failure to respond to erotic stimulation because of anxiety, guilt, or fear of injury	Reduced libido and secondary erectile failure (impotence)	Reduced libido
Impairment or failure of orgasm. Extremely rapid, or absence of clonic rhythmic contractions of pelvic musculature due to inhibition of genital tactile or psychic erotic stimulation	Premature ejaculation Restricted ejaculation	Orgastic dysfunction

*In the male, penile erection; in the female, vaginal lubrication and perivaginal swelling.

Table 30.2 Prevalence of sexual disorders in the community*

	FEMALES (%)	MALES (%)
Inhibited sexual desire	up to 30	10–15
Impairment of sexual arousal	10–20	10–20
Failure to achieve orgasm	10–20	
Premature ejaculation		20–30
Dyspareunia	10–15	
Vaginismus	1–3	
Total sexual dysfunction	30–50	20–45
Total sexual dysfunction causing distress	9–15	

*Figures depend on age, presence of partner, medical, psychological and psychiatric status of the community studied.

- Failure to achieve orgasm
- Dyspareunia, including vaginismus.

Table 30.1 lists the sexual dysfunctions that occur in men and women. The approximate prevalences of these disorders are given in Table 30.2.

Inhibited sexual desire or hypoactive sexual desire disorder

Women with this disorder have little or no desire for sexual activity. Its prevalence is not known with any accuracy, but may be as high as 30%. Allied to this disorder is a failure to become sexually aroused, either by sexual fantasies or when sexually stimulated by the partner, and the woman may find sexual approaches distasteful. This may not mean that she will reject sexual advances by a partner, but that she will obtain little or no enjoyment from the contact.

Inhibited sexual desire, or inhibited sexual arousal, may have been present since puberty or may occur after some months or years of sexual activity. In the latter case it may be the manifestation of a deteriorating relationship or a sign of depression. If both partners have inhibited sexual desire a problem is not perceived, but if one has inhibited sexual desire and the other has a normal or raised desire, the problem becomes manifest. Inhibited sexual desire can be associated with a range of gynaecological conditions and treatments, and sexual desire can vary markedly during pregnancy and breastfeeding.

Impairment of sexual arousal or sexual arousal disorder

Sexual arousal disorder involves the inability to become sexually interested and aroused in the situations desired. This may be associated with poor technique, inadequate stimulation and relationship problems, resulting in inadequate lubrication or sensation. Lubrication may occur and be reported by her partner, but the woman may be unaware of the 'wetness'.

Failure to achieve orgasm (anorgasmia) or orgasmic disorder

Orgasm in women may be achieved during penile thrusting, but not usually simultaneously with the man's orgasm, or it may only be achieved if the woman's clitoral area is stimulated by finger or tongue. In both cases orgasm is reached and the woman cannot be considered to be anorgasmic. However, some women (and men) believe that unless a woman reaches orgasm during penile thrusting, preferably simultaneously with the man, she is sexually dysfunctional.

Sexual pain disorders, or dyspareunia and vaginismus

In most cases, when the woman is unable to accept a penis penetrating her vagina the problem is psychosomatic, the woman involuntarily tightening the muscles that surround the introitus and the lower third of the vagina. This is termed vaginismus, and in severe cases the woman is unable to accept an examiner's finger into her vagina, so marked is the muscle spasm. Vaginismus may be transient or permanent, and affects around 1% of women aged 15–50.

Although the woman is unable to have sexual intercourse, she may be able to enjoy masturbating her partner but avoids any contact with her own external genitals.

The cause of vaginismus lies in inadequate or faulty sex education, particularly in a belief that sex is 'dirty', or a fear based on ignorance that the penis may painfully damage the woman's body. Vaginismus can also be traced to a sexual assault during childhood, or to a painful, brutal early experience of intercourse, or traumatic childbirth.

Dyspareunia, or painful intercourse, is recurrent and persistent pain during or after intercourse. It usually has an organic component, at least when it commences. Examples are vulvovaginal infections, a painful episiotomy scar, atrophic vulvovaginitis, endometriosis, pelvic inflammatory disease, and ovarian cysts or tumours. Organic disorders must be excluded before the condition is ascribed to psychosomatic factors. These are usually found in cases of prolonged dyspareunia. The aetiology of psychogenic dyspareunia is unclear, but lack of sexual knowledge, guilt about sexuality, and childhood sexual assault have been postulated. The problem is aggravated when the woman fails to be aroused sexually and fails to lubricate.

General management strategies

The objectives of treatment are to alter an existing destructive attitude to sexuality; to reduce or resolve any underlying interpersonal sexual conflict, anxiety or fear; and to help a couple create an environment in which sexuality is perceived as a pleasurable experience. To achieve these objectives, the counsellor seeks to help the woman examine her attitudes to her sexuality and to discover what stimulates her sexually; to correct any false ideas or myths about sexuality; and to help her make her partner aware of her sexual feelings, needs and desires, so that they can better express their needs to each other.

The management of sexual dysfunctions in women begins with the medical practitioner obtaining a comprehensive general and sexual history. The general history should pay particular attention to physical illness and psychiatric problems such as depression. The sexual history must be obtained with great sensitivity. During the history, the medical practitioner explores the current relationship and seeks to find out the woman's attitudes to her body, to menstruation, and to her feelings about her sexuality.

Usually, the doctor needs to:

- Provide information about the female and male body
- Explore the patient's attitudes to her sexuality, sexual activities and responses
- Examine her relationships
- Reduce her anxiety
- Suggest strategies for helping the patient, such as giving permission and prescribing specific treatment, which may differ for different problems, as discussed later. Pelvic floor exercises (Kegel exercises) are a useful strategy for all women (see Ch. 39, p. 311).

The question of whether the partner should be involved depends on the sexual problem elucidated and, more particularly, on the patient's wishes.

Management of specific sexual problems

Although the general management of sexual problems is the same for all the sexual dysfunctions, the different categories of female sexual dysfunction require different strategies (Fig. 30.1).

Inhibited sexual desire

The most-used approach is to involve both partners when possible. The partners attend together and are helped to communicate better with each other, through words and actions. If they are poorly informed, the therapist helps them learn the anatomy and physiology of sexual intercourse. The main part of treatment is for the couple to perform a series of graded 'tasks' at short intervals over a period of weeks. The tasks are undertaken at home in a relaxed atmosphere. In the first stage, lasting 1 week, the couple set aside at least 30 minutes each day for nongenital pleasuring. The man fondles, caresses and massages his partner at her direction, avoiding her breasts and genitals, and responding if she says that she does not like a particular area being touched. The couple then change roles.

If the couple have made steady progress, they move to the second phase of genital pleasuring. In this phase they can touch, massage, kiss or lick each other's bodies and genitals. During the touching the active participant inquires: 'Do you like me touching you like this?', 'Does it feel good?' and 'How would you like me to do it?' After about 15 minutes they exchange roles.

The couple reach the third phase when they feel that they are confident that they have enjoyed the second

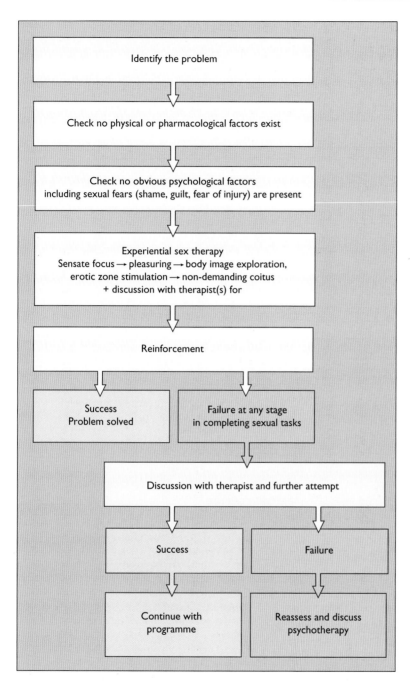

Fig. 30.1 Management of sexual problems.

phase. In the third phase, they proceed through the first two phases fairly quickly and then attempt sexual intercourse, preferably with the woman astride the man facing him so that she can introduce his penis into her vagina at her own speed.

The couple see the therapist at intervals so that their progress can be reviewed and any problems discussed.

Anorgasmia

If a woman wishes to increase her ability to achieve orgasm, or has never achieved orgasm, several techniques are available. Of these, masturbation has produced the most successes. Many young women have masturbated, but have felt guilty about it and have not reached orgasm. Others have never masturbated. Learning to achieve orgasm by masturbation often cures anorgasmia, but the woman needs to supplement this with discussion and counselling with a trained practitioner. For masturbation to be effective in achieving orgasm, the woman has to give herself time and privacy, and be able to fantasize, view or read erotic literature as she masturbates, using either her fingers or a vibrator.

Apareunia and dyspareunia

Any physical cause of these sexual dysfunctions must be identified, discussed with the woman and treated, if possible. If it is not, suggestions may be made about techniques with which the woman may better enjoy sex. For example, if she has a chronic pelvic infection she may find a different position for sexual intercourse more pleasurable. If sexual intercourse is painful whatever position the couple adopt, she may obtain sensual pleasure by body caressing and clitoral stimulation while giving her partner pleasure by oral sex or by stimulating his sexual organs.

If the woman has vaginismus, the therapist reinforces the general strategies discussed earlier by stressing that she is not 'small made' and that she can learn to relax her perineal muscles. She may be asked to try to insert a lubricated finger in her vagina, and given instructions to continue with the exercise at home. If her relationship with her partner is good, she may ask him to insert his finger. Once one finger is accepted, she progresses to the insertion of two and then three fingers or, if she prefers, a series of graded dilators. These steps require reinforcement and encouragement by the therapist, who should be visited weekly. Once she has introduced three fingers with comfort and without muscle spasm occurring, she may be ready to sit above her partner and to control his penis so that it touches the entrance to her vagina. In progressive steps, on different days, she inserts his penis into the entrance, then deeper into her vagina. When this is comfortable and accepted, she may move rhythmically with his penis deep in her vagina, and then permit him to thrust. Finally, having become confident that intercourse is painless, she will be able to have sexual intercourse with the man on top.

Evaluation of treatment outcomes

There is much confusion about treatment outcomes, as many of the patients seen have been selected and the data collection uncontrolled. There are no adequate studies of treatment and outcome.

OTHER SEXUAL PROBLEMS

Sexual abuse

Sexual abuse includes incest and rape, and in the medical literature the two terms are included in sexual abuse. It is defined as 'unlawful carnal knowledge of a woman without her consent by force, fear or fraud'. In over three-quarters of cases of rape the offender is known to the woman. Evidence has been published that between 8 and 13% of women are intimately abused by their partner during pregnancy, in addition to those who are 'battered' by their partner. Statistics about the prevalence of rape are difficult to obtain, as fewer than one-third of rapes are reported, but about one woman in 200 has been raped or suffered attempted rape in a year.

A woman who has been raped needs to be treated with great care and consideration when she presents to a medical practitioner. In most cases the woman attends a hospital or a 'rape crisis centre' where staff are trained to handle her emotional and physical problems.

The woman should be listened to sympathetically and non-judgementally as she tells her story. She should then be examined. It is important, during the examination, to explain what is being done and why. The presence of scratches or bruises on the woman's arms or body should be looked for, and the vulva examined for the presence of blood, bruising or seminal staining. A vaginal inspection is made and a vaginal smear taken to detect spermatozoa. The woman should be asked to return later, so that she can be tested to exclude gonorrhoea and so that serological tests can be made to exclude infection, particularly syphilis and HIV. If the rape took place at the time of ovulation, the woman should be given the choice of taking postcoital contraception – the 'morning after pill' – or asked to return if she fails to menstruate.

It is important to record all findings carefully.

Sexual abuse in childhood and adolescence

A particular group of females require special consideration. These are children and young women under the age of 16. Data from several western countries indicate that between 5 and 30% have been sexually abused, half of them repeatedly. In half of the girls only the breasts or genitals were touched or fondled, but in 20% the abuser made the girl practise fellatio, or forced her to have genital or anal intercourse. In over 40% of cases the abuser was a family member.

Although most of these young women overcome their disgust and fear as they grow older, women who have been sexually abused in childhood or adolescence are three times as likely to seek psychiatric help in adulthood and, if married, are more likely to be divorced. The reasons for seeking psychological and psychiatric help are many, and common problems are depression, chronic pelvic pain, eating disorders and sexual problems. Women presenting to a doctor with what are perceived as psychosocial problems should be questioned sensitively about any experience of sexual abuse and help offered.

Conception control

The availability of safe modern contraceptives has enabled women to avoid unwanted pregnancy, and couples to space their children. Spacing children to intervals of 2 or more years improves a woman's health.

Contraceptive choices now available permit the woman, or the couple, to choose the most appropriate contraceptive for their particular circumstances. Younger women usually prefer oral contraceptives or expect their male partners to use condoms, whereas older women are more inclined to choose the intrauterine device (IUCD) or a permanent method of birth control, such as tubal ligation or a vasectomy in her partner (Fig. 31.1).

Before choosing a particular contraceptive most people want to know its effectiveness in preventing pregnancy, its safety, and the side-effects associated with its use. A method of evaluating the effectiveness of the various contraceptive methods is the Pearl Index, which calculates the unintended pregnancy rate from the formula:

$$\frac{\text{The number of unintended pregnancies}}{\text{Total months of exposure to pregnancy}} \times 1200$$

The result is expressed as the failure rate per 100 woman years (HWY).

Table 31.1 shows the effectiveness of various contraceptive methods in preventing pregnancy.

Some women find it embarrassing to consult a medical practitioner about contraception and a sensitive doctor will do everything possible to diminish that embarrassment. The ability to listen to and to talk with the woman is of great importance.

The doctor should take a general history, a menstrual history and a sexual history in a non-judgemental way. With this information, the doctor will be better able to help the woman decide which method of contraception she would prefer.

A gynaecological examination should be made, although if the woman is teenaged and has not previously had a vaginal examination it can be deferred to a subsequent visit. If she has not had a Pap smear taken in the previous 2 years, the doctor should suggest that this be done, explaining how the smear is taken and the reason for it.

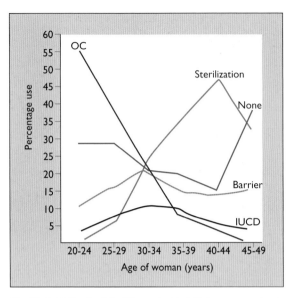

Fig. 31.1 Methods of fertility control in Britain.

Table 31.1 Ranking of contraceptive methods by rate of effectiveness

		FAILURE RATES PER 100 HWY
Group A	**Most effective**	
	Tubal ligation/ vasectomy	0.005–0.04
	Combined oral	0.005–0.30
	Continuous progesterone	0.07
Group B	**Highly effective**	
	IUCD	0.5–3.5
	Depot progestogen	1.5–2.3
	Diaphragm or condom	
	All users	4.0–7.0
	Highly motivated	1.5–3.0
	Periodic abstinence	
	All users	10.0–30.0
	Highly motivated	2.5–5.0
Group C	**Less effective**	
	Coitus interruptus	30.0–40.0
	Vaginal foam or cream	30.0–40.0
Group D	**Least effective**	
	Postcoital douche	45.0
	Prolonged breastfeeding	45.0

REVERSIBLE METHODS OF CONTRACEPTION USED BY THE COUPLE

Periodic abstinence

It is known that if a woman has a menstrual cycle of normal duration, ovulation occurs 14 ± 3 days before the start of her next menstruation. It is also known that pregnancy is most likely to occur if intercourse takes place in the 5 days before ovulation or on the day of ovulation. This interval is called the fertile period. This has led to the idea of periodic abstinence during the fertile period as a method of birth control.

The woman is taught to detect the presence of mucus at the vaginal entrance each morning (before any sexual arousal). Three types of mucus can be detected and, from this, the days on which sexual intercourse can take place can be calculated while to some extent avoiding the chance of an unwanted pregnancy (Fig. 31.2). The compliance of the man is essential if pregnancy is to be avoided.

Because of the difficulties in assessing the mucus and the need for the man to cooperate fully, the pregnancy rate varies from 10 to 30 per HWY for all couples, but for motivated couples it is 2.5–5.0 per HWY.

Coitus interruptus

Withdrawal, or coitus interruptus, is the oldest form of birth control apart from induced abortion. With the development of more modern contraceptives its frequency has declined, but it is still the preferred method in some sections of society. Its reliability for preventing pregnancy depends on the ability of the man to recognize the pre-ejaculatory phase and his agility in withdrawing his penis from the woman's vagina before ejaculation. Because of these constraints, the efficacy of coitus interruptus in preventing an unwanted pregnancy is rather low (see Table 31.1).

REVERSIBLE METHODS OF CONTRACEPTION USED BY MEN

Condom

Modern condoms, which are made of latex, prelubricated, and supplied in hermetically sealed aluminium sachets, are cheap, efficient and hardly noticeable to either partner. Their advantages are that they can be obtained from a variety of outlets without a doctor's prescription, and that they offer some protection against sexually transmitted diseases, including the human papilloma virus, chlamydia and the human immunodeficiency virus (HIV). The disadvantage of condoms is that many younger men refuse to use them in the belief that they reduce sexual pleasure and may burst during use.

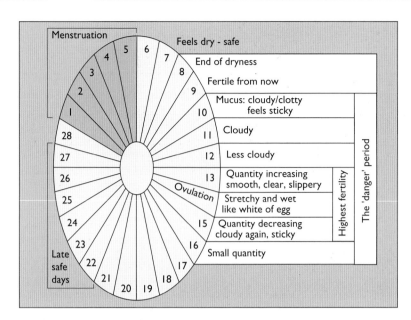

Fig. 31.2 Periodic abstinence: the mucus (ovulation) method.

The pregnancy rate following condom use relates to usage, to the way the condom is put on the penis, and how it is held on after penile detumescence. If consulted by a woman or her partner the doctor should explain how a condom should be used (Fig. 31.3).

REVERSIBLE METHODS OF CONTRACEPTION USED BY WOMEN

Women have more choices of reversible or temporary contraception than men. They may choose:

- Barrier methods – the vaginal diaphragm, the cervical cap
- Hormonal contraceptives – the pill, patches, injectables and implants
- The intra-uterine device (IUCD).

Barrier methods

Vaginal diaphragm and the cervical cap

The vaginal diaphragm and the cervical cap consist of a thin plastic or latex dome attached to a circular flat, coiled or arching spring rim. The vaginal diaphragm is easier to use than the cervical cap, as it fits diagonally across the vagina. The correct size of the diaphragm is determined by a medical practitioner examining the woman vaginally, by inserting the index and middle fingers as far as they will go into the posterior vaginal fornix and noting how far the index finger reaches behind the symphysis pubis. The diaphragm is made in sizes from 50 mm to 100 mm, in 5 mm steps. After measuring the vagina, the

doctor inserts a series of diaphragms or fitting rings until the most appropriate size is found.

Using a diaphragm or a cervical cap requires practice, and after teaching a woman how to use it (Fig. 31.4) many doctors ask the woman to learn the technique at home and return with the diaphragm or cap in place for checking.

When the woman is confident about the technique, she inserts the diaphragm each day or at any convenient time before sexual intercourse is anticipated. It should not be removed for cleaning until at least 6 hours after the last ejaculation. Some women choose to smear a nonoxynol-9 spermicidal cream around the rim, but whether this adds to the effectiveness of the diaphragm in preventing pregnancy is uncertain. It is known to destroy HIV to some extent, which is a benefit.

If a woman chooses a cervical cap she must have a healthy, short cervix. Fitting is carried out by a medical practitioner. The technique of insertion and removal is the same as that for the vaginal diaphragm.

Hormonal contraceptives

Hormonal contraceptives contain oestrogen and a progestogen (combined oral contraceptives) or progestogen alone. Oestrogen suppresses follicle-stimulating hormone (FSH) secretion and reduces luteinizing hormone (LH) secretion, and in this way prevents ovulation. The progestogen further suppresses LH release, alters the quality of the cervical mucus, rendering it less penetrable to sperm, and produces endometrial changes culminating in glandular exhaustion. Importantly, the progestogen also permits a withdrawal bleed, which is regular in onset, short in duration and light in amount.

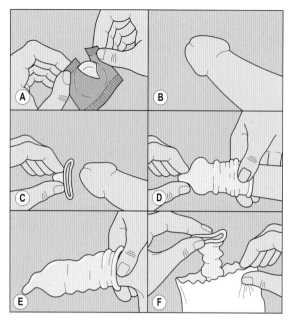

Fig. 31.3 Information for patients: how to use a condom, (A) Open the packet carefully, and do not unroll the condom before putting it on. (B) Semen can leak out soon after the penis becomes erect, prior to ejaculation. To prevent pregnancy or infection, the condom must be put on before any sexual contact takes place. (C) Ensure that the condom is the right way up. Squeeze the teat on the tip of the condom and hold it against the tip of the penis, (D), unroll the condom all the way to the base of the penis. (E) After ejaculation, the penis should be withdrawn before the erection is totally lost. When withdrawing, hold on to the condom. (F) Do not allow the condom or penis to come into contact with the woman's genital area, and carefully dispose of the condom.

Combined oral contraceptive (COC)

These formulations are chosen by most contraceptive users as they are effective in preventing pregnancy and are easy to take. Most types of currently available COCs contain less than 50 µg of ethinyl oestradiol per dose (one type contains mestranol, which is rapidly converted into ethinyl oestradiol), and one of several progestogens. These are called low-dose COCs.

The COCs prescribed are monophasic or triphasic. In the monophasic formulations the amount of oestrogen and progestogen is constant in each tablet throughout the cycle. The triphasic formulation tablets contain varying doses of both oestrogen and progestogen. The total progestogen in a cycle is less and the total oestrogen is more than in the monophasic formulations. The concept behind the development of the triphasic formulations was to reduce the effects of the pill on lipid metabolism. Oestrogen increases high-density lipoprotein cholesterol (HDL-c) and reduces low-density lipoprotein (LDL-c), and the first-generation progestogens decrease the level of

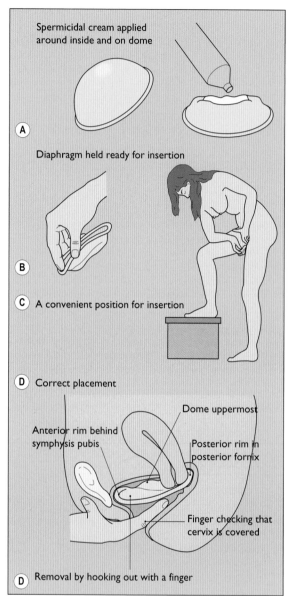

Spermicidal cream applied around inside and on dome

(A)

Diaphragm held ready for insertion

(B)

(C) A convenient position for insertion

(D) Correct placement

Dome uppermost

Anterior rim behind symphysis pubis

Posterior rim in posterior fornix

Finger checking that cervix is covered

(D) Removal by hooking out with a finger

Fig. 31.4 The use of the vaginal diaphragm.

HDL-c. Combined, as in the pill, total cholesterol is not increased but HDL-c is reduced slightly (compared with oestrogen alone), the decrease being related to the total dose of progestogen. The triphasic formulations reduce the total quantity of progestogen given in a cycle, and thus reduce the decrease in the circulating levels of HDL-c.

Oral contraceptives containing the newer (second-generation) progestogens, such as desogestrel and gestodene, and drospirenone, a spironolactone analogue, do not reduce HDL-c and thus can be given in a monophasic preparation. They are replacing the older COCs.

Until recently COCs were prescribed and prepared in packs with 21 days of active hormones to be followed by 7 days of placebo tablets during which time a 'withdrawal bleed' occurs. Newer formulations are reducing the length of the placebo phase to reduce bleeding and the premenstrual-like symptoms that may occur during the hormone-free days.

Contraindications to the prescription of COCs

The International Planned Parenthood Federation recommends that women should not choose COCs if they have:

- A past or present history of venous or arterial thrombosis, ischaemic heart disease or severe hypertension
- Familial hyperlipidaemia
- Any condition favouring cerebral ischaemia, particularly severe focal migraine
- Acute liver disease and some forms of chronic liver disease
- Oestrogen-dependent cancer
- Undiagnosed vaginal bleeding.

Non-contraceptive benefits of COCs

As COCs are the most-used form of contraception in the world, it is important to note their non-contraceptive benefits:

- Most menstrual cycle disorders are reduced including menstrual blood loss, menorrhagia, dysmenorrhoea (by 80% or more) and the premenstrual syndrome. However, about 1% of COC users develop amenorrhoea.
- Pelvic infection (pelvic inflammatory disease) is reduced in women who have several sexual partners or whose partners have, or have had, several sexual partners.
- Benign breast disease and benign breast tumours are reduced by up to 50%.
- Breast carcinoma is not increased.
- Functional ovarian cysts are less common.
- Uterine myomata are less common, as is endometriosis.
- Endometrial and ovarian cancers are reduced.
- Rheumatoid arthritis appears to be reduced in COC users who have taken the medication for less than 5 years.

Clinical side-effects of COCs

The two main areas of concern are circulatory disease and certain cancers. Other clinical conditions may also occur.

Circulatory disease

Thromboembolism is slightly more common in COC users, although the risk is small (from 4–6 to 10–15 per 100000 women per year). The increase is due to an increase in fibrinogen concentration and of factors II, VII,

Table 31.2 Risk of developing DVT or pulmonary embolus

	RISK (PER 100 000 WOMEN)
Healthy women who neither smoke nor take sex hormones	4–6
Women taking low-dose COCs with 2nd generation progestogens	10–15
Women taking COCs containing 3rd generation progestogens	20–30
Pregnant and parturient women	50–60

IX, X and XII, and a decrease in antithrombin III. There is a concomitant increase in fibrinolysis, but it does not equal the coagulation changes. The risk is increased in smokers and in obese women. If these two variables are excluded the relative risk of developing thromboembolism in a woman taking low-dose COCs is small. (Table 31.2).

As major surgery adds to the risk of thromboembolism, women taking COCs should change to another form of contraception for 4 weeks before the surgery. Thrombotic stroke is increased sixfold (compared to women using no, or other, forms of contraception) but is very uncommon in this age group.

The use of COCs leads to a small increase in the systolic blood pressure, which is reversible. Hypertension of greater magnitude occurs in about 2% of women, particularly those who have a family history of hypertension, are overweight and over the age of 35. Women who have had pregnancy-induced hypertension are more likely to be affected. The cause is an increased sensitivity to the progestogen content of the pill, but oestrogen may be involved and so a low-oestrogen pill is to be preferred.

The use of low-dose COCs does not increase the risk of myocardial infarction unless the woman is a smoker, overweight and over 35, when there is a small increase in risk. Among these women, stroke (mainly haemorrhagic) is increased slightly (from 2 to 3 per 100000 per year).

Cancers

The use of COCs reduces the risk of developing ovarian cancer (by 40%) and endometrial cancer (by 50%). The prolonged use of COCs increases the risk of developing cervical cancer slightly, but this may be due to the sexual behaviour of the woman rather than to the use of COCs. The overall incidence of breast cancer does not increase except, perhaps, for a small subgroup of women presenting with breast cancer in their 30s who have taken the pill for at least 5 years before their first pregnancy.

Other clinical conditions occurring in women using COCs

Acne

The oestrogen content of the COCs tends to improve acne, whereas the progestogen tends to aggravate it. Monophasic COCs, especially those containing low-dose oestrogen and progestogen (20 μg ethinyl oestradiol), a second-generation progestogen (desogestrel), cyproterone or drospirenone should be chosen.

Breakthrough bleeding (BTB) and spotting

Many women starting to use hormonal contraception have episodes of breakthrough bleeding or spotting in the early months. In the first cycle 20% of women experience BTB; after 6 months less than 3% have the symptom. BTB is less likely if the woman takes the pill at the same time each day. BTB causes considerable concern to many women, and doctors should advise those starting to use the pill or 'switching' pills, that it may occur. The doctor should explain that in most cases it settles within a few months, and that it is not dangerous. If BTB continues for longer than 6 months, the woman should be prescribed a COC with a higher oestrogen content.

Chloasma

Hyperpigmentation of the skin may occur in susceptible women exposed to sunlight, but it is uncommon. The condition is thought to be due to oestrogen. Treatment consists of changing to a progesterone-only pill (POP) or using another form of contraception, avoiding direct sunlight, and if the woman is very concerned, applying 2% hydroquinone ointment. Even with these measures the chloasma takes up to 9 months to fade.

COCs and other drugs

Women who need to take antibiotics should take extra precautions during the time they take them, and for 7 days after, as absorption of the pill is reduced and pregnancy may occur. Women who are prescribed carbamazepine, griseofulvin, phenytoin or rifampicin should use a higher dose of COC preparation, as these antibiotics increase hepatic enzyme activity, which in turn increases the metabolism of contraceptive steroids and reduces their efficacy.

Eye problems

A few women who use contact lenses may experience discomfort owing to a change in the topography of the cornea.

Gallbladder disease

The development of gallbladder disease is accelerated in women taking a higher oestrogen dose COC (>50 μg).

Headaches and migraine

The prevalence of headaches among women taking COCs is variable and headaches may occur on days when no hormones are taken. If the headaches are severe and occur on days when the pill is not taken (or when a non-active pill is being taken in a 28-day pack), their frequency can be reduced by taking the pill continuously for 3 months. The woman will not have a withdrawal bleed until the end of the 3-month cycle, but will have fewer headaches each year.

A few women develop migraine when taking COCs. If the migraine is focal or persists severely for 3 days or more, the woman should change to another form of contraception.

Mood changes, including depression

Some women who have premenstrual mood changes find that the symptoms decrease when they take a monophasic COC, particularly if it contains a second-generation progestogen. Clinical depression is not increased in pill users.

Nausea and vomiting

These symptoms may occur in the first few months of taking COCs as the body adjusts to the hormonal milieu.

Sexual desire

A few women report a decrease in libido when taking COCs; others report an increase.

Vaginal discharges

An increased amount of vaginal secretions is usual, but candidiasis does not occur more frequently in women taking modern COCs.

Weight gain

This does not occur with the newer oral contraceptives. With the older-type pills a few women gained weight after a few months' use. Whether this is due to the progestogen content of the COC or to an increased appetite is unclear. The weight was usually lost when the COC was ceased.

Non-oestrogen hormonal contraceptives

Progesterone-only pill (POP) – the mini-pill

This oral contraceptive is a good choice for women who have contraindications for COCs, or who are breast-feeding. It is an alternative for some diabetic women, women who have risk factors for cardiovascular disease, women who have hypertension related to COCs or who need control by antihypertensives, and some migraine sufferers. The POP is associated with BTB and unpredictable menstruation in about one in four users. The failure rate (pregnancy rate) is shown in Table 31.1.

Long-acting injectable progestogens

This formulation contains medroxyprogesterone acetate (DMPA) 150 mg, injected 3-monthly, or norethisterone oenanthate (NET-OEN) 200 mg, injected every 2 months.

The advantage of the injectables is that they remove the need to take a pill every day. Their disadvantage is that during the first 4–6 months of use menstruation tends to be irregular. After this initial period amenorrhoea is usual and may lead to osteopenia.

Subdermal implants

The synthetic progestagen etonorgestrel (Implanon) is placed under the skin of the inner aspect of the non-dominant upper arm under local anaesthetic. The 68 mg implant is effective for 3 years and ovulation usually returns within 1 month of removal. It is a highly effective contraceptive agent with a Pearl Index of <0.07/100 woman years (Fig 31.5). As with other progestogen formulations such implants may provoke irregular episodes of uterine bleeding; oligomenorrhoea 26%, amenorrhoea 21%, frequent or prolonged bleeding 18% and normal menstrual cycle in 35%. Weight gain, breast tenderness and mood changes occur in 5–10% of women, and acne may be improved. If it is inserted in the first 5 days of the woman's cycle then it is effective immediately, otherwise it is important to make sure the woman is not already pregnant before insertion and then to use other contraception for 7 days.

Vaginal ring

This novel contraceptive, currently under study, has been developed in two forms:

- A ring containing an oestrogen and a progestogen, mimicking the COCs
- A ring containing levonorgestrel.

The ring fits in the upper vagina around the cervix. Its advantage is that it is the only long-acting method that is under the woman's control. The woman removes the ring

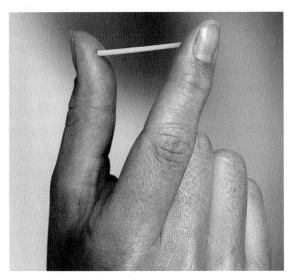

Fig. 31.5 Implanon.

at will but generally replaces it at once after it has been washed. The disadvantage is that the ring may be associated with irregular bleeding in the first months of use and may be expelled from the vagina.

Prescribing hormonal contraceptives

The history is taken and the woman is examined as described in Chapter 1. The choices of hormonal contraceptives available may be discussed with the woman, although often she has a good idea of the one she would prefer. She should be advised to read and to follow the instructions contained in the packet. Some doctors provide a pamphlet that reinforces these instructions.

The woman should be informed that these instructions include information on coping with forgotten pills to ensure maximum contraceptive effectiveness. If one OC pill is not taken at the regular time, it should be taken as soon as possible and the next pill taken at the regular time, even if this results in two tablets being taken on the same day. If two OC pills are missed, these two pills should be taken as soon as they are remembered, two pills should then be taken the following day, and then one pill each day until the pack is finished. Additional contraception, such as a condom, is needed for the next 7 days after two pills are missed.

Postcoital contraception

If a woman has unprotected sexual intercourse at ovulation time she has two choices. The first is to wait and see if she misses a menstrual period and then have an immunological pregnancy test. If this is positive, she can then choose to continue with the pregnancy or to have an induced abortion (see p. 105). The second choice is to use a form of postcoital contraception, provided she seeks help within 72 hours. Four methods are available:

- The method of choice is a single dose of 1.5 mg levonorgestrel repeated after 12 hours. This has fewer side-effects, particularly nausea and vomiting, than COC therapy.
- A commonly used alternative is a COC containing ethinyl oestradiol 50 μg and levonorgestrel 250 μg (the 'morning after' pill). (Yuzpe method). Two of these tablets are taken together with an antiemetic, because of the side-effects of nausea and vomiting. The dose is repeated after 12 hours.
- The woman is prescribed mifepristone (RU 486) in a dose of 600 mg, in countries where the drug is available. The advantage of mifepristone over the 'morning after' pill is that nausea and vomiting are less frequent.
- The woman may choose to have an IUCD inserted within 5 days of the unprotected intercourse. This method is inadvisable if the woman is nulliparous.

Pregnancy is prevented in 75% with Yuzpe, 88% with levonorgestrel and over 90% with an IUCD. It is important that the woman is given careful instructions to return a week after the time of her expected period for a pregnancy test if she fails to menstruate.

Intra-uterine device

Intra-uterine devices (IUCDs) were used in humans in the last years of the 19th century, but had so many adverse side-effects that their use was abandoned. The development of a polyethylene IUCD in 1950, which had a memory for its shape, revived interest.

A satisfactory IUCD should be easy to introduce, easy to remove, and have few side-effects and a high degree of efficiency in preventing pregnancy. In the 1980s, a series of legal actions against manufacturers led to the removal from the market of most IUCDs, and today only three types remain. Two of the devices have fine copper wire surrounding the stem, which permits a smaller device to be used and reduces some of the side-effects (Fig. 31.6). The third type contains levonorgestrel in its stem (Fig. 31.7). In the first 4 months of use some women have unpredictable episodes of spotting or bleeding, and may develop the unacceptable side-effects of negative mood change, acne and, sometimes, weight gain. After this time the levonorgestrel IUCD reduces the menstrual flow, controlling menorrhagia in women who have this menstrual disturbance; it may also cause amenorrhoea. This device may be chosen by women in their 40s who would otherwise consider tubal ligation.

Copper IUCDs prevent pregnancy by incapacitating the sperm, making them dysfunctional for fertilization. The progestogen IUCD releases 20 µg of levonorgestrel a day and acts in the same manner as the progesterone-only pill.

The 5-year cumulative pregnancy rate for the levonorgestrel IUCD is 0.5–1.0%, whereas that of the copper-containing IUCDs is between 2.0 and 5.5%.

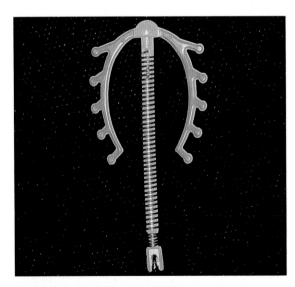

Fig. 31.6 Copper 375 multiload IUCD.

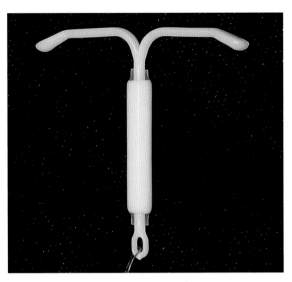

Fig. 31.7 The levonorgestrel IUCD.

Advantages of the IUCD

The IUCD requires only a single decision to have the device introduced into the uterus and, unless problems arise, will prevent pregnancy for 3–8 years (depending on the device). It is highly effective in preventing pregnancy (see Table 31.1).

Adverse effects of IUCDs

During insertion

Perforation of the uterine wall occurs in about 1 per 1000 insertions and is directly proportional to the skill of the individual performing the insertion. Perforation may cause bleeding and pain, but is often silent. If perforation is suspected, the location of the IUCD is determined using an ultrasound scan. If this indicates that the IUCD has perforated the uterus and is wholly or partly in the abdominal pelvic cavity, it should be removed because the copper may cause a tissue reaction leading to intra-peritoneal adhesions. The removal is effected by finding the IUCD using a laparoscope, or by performing a laparotomy.

Expulsion

The uterus tends to expel 'foreign bodies' and the IUCD is no exception: between 1 and 10 women in every 100 who have an IUCD inserted, expel the device. Expulsion may occur at any time after insertion, but usually occurs in the first 6–8 weeks, often during a menstrual period. Younger women and women who have never been pregnant are more likely to expel the device than other women.

Women using an IUCD should be encouraged to check once each month that they can feel the string; to aid their memory it is suggested this is done immediately after each menstrual period.

Cramping and bleeding

Over a 2-year period these complications have been shown to occur with a frequency varying from 4 to 10% of women in the case of the copper-containing IUCDs. The problem usually occurs in the first month after the insertion and diminishes as time passes. Half of the number of medical removals of an IUCD are for this reason.

Pelvic inflammatory disease

Pelvic inflammatory disease (PID), or pelvic infection, is discussed in detail in Chapter 33. The background incidence of PID in the community is 1 per 100 women aged 15–45 per year. It has been claimed that the IUCD increases the chance of developing PID. A recent meta-analysis has shown that this only applies if the infection occurs within the first month of insertion in women who have symptomless cervical infections due to *Chlamydia trachomatis*, *Neisseria gonorrhoeae* or, rarely, polymicrobial infection at the time of insertion.

These findings suggest that sexual activity rather than the IUCD is the cause of PID, and that the introduction of an IUCD through the infected cervix of a woman may increase slightly the chance that she will develop PID. It is good practice to take a high vaginal swab to screen for bacterial infections and an endocervical swab or first void urine sample for chlamydia PCR (polymerase chain reaction) before insertion.

Screening for actinomyces by taking an endocervical swab should be done before reinsertion. If detected the IUCD should be removed and penicillin treatment given. If actinomyces was found on a routine swab and had not caused PID then the IUCD can be reinserted after 3 months if swabs are then negative.

Tubal infertility

For a woman who has never been pregnant, the relative risk of developing tubal infertility (primary infertility) associated with the use of a copper IUCD is 1.6. Women who have only one sexual partner have no increased risk of primary infertility.

Pregnancy and the IUCD

Although the IUCD is highly effective (greater than 98%) in protecting against unwanted pregnancy, occasionally a pregnancy occurs with the IUCD in situ. The continued presence of the IUCD increases the risk of miscarriage to 25% (compared with a 10% risk in a woman who has no IUCD in situ), and thus, if the woman agrees, an attempt should be made to remove it from the uterine cavity. The procedure does not increase the miscarriage rate above that in the population. If the IUCD cannot be removed and the woman chooses to continue with the pregnancy, a miscarriage occurring in the second quarter of pregnancy may be

associated with infection (septic abortion), although the frequency of this complication is not known. Should infection occur, antibiotics should be given promptly and an attempt made to remove the IUCD, if feasible. These problems should be discussed with the woman. Given the information, she may choose to have an induced abortion.

Contraindications to the use of an IUCD

The IUCD should not be inserted into a woman:

- Who has, or has had, several sexual partners or whose partner has, or has had, several sexual partners
- With known or suspected pregnancy
- With current or previous PID which has been accurately diagnosed
- With a history of ectopic pregnancy
- With abnormal genital tract bleeding that needs to be investigated
- With congenital uterine abnormalities or myomata that distort the uterine cavity
- With valvular heart disease
- With Wilson's disease (copper-containing IUCD).

Insertion of the IUCD

An IUCD should only be inserted by a healthcare practitioner who has received training in the insertion technique. The most appropriate time to insert an IUCD is at midcycle, when the cervical canal is at its widest and the introduction of bacteria from the cervical canal is least likely.

PERMANENT METHODS OF BIRTH CONTROL

Vasectomy

The vasectomy operation is simple to perform, effective, and attended by little pain or inconvenience, particularly if the no-scalpel technique, developed in China, is used (Fig. 31.8). A few men develop scrotal swelling, bruising or a small haematoma, all of which settle quickly.

It is important that the medical practitioner discusses the procedure with the man and answers his questions. Many men equate vasectomy with castration; others are concerned that as sperm continues to be produced it will accumulate in the testes and swell them; others are anxious that after the vasectomy a man's desire and performance will diminish. None of these beliefs has any basis in fact. The man needs reassurance that vasectomy does not increase his risk of developing cardiovascular disease, prostatic disease, cancer, erectile failure or autoimmune disease.

He must be made aware that following vasectomy he is not immediately sterile, as the sperm in the epididymis proximal to the vasectomy are still potent. Until these have

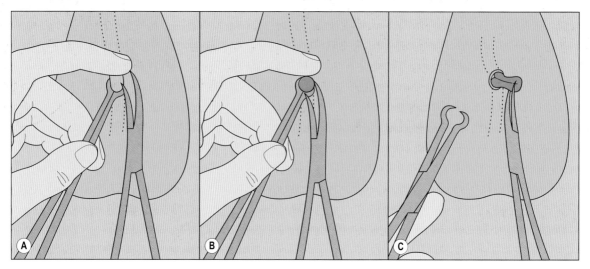

Fig. 31.8 In a no-scalpel vasectomy the vas (dotted line) is grasped by special ring forceps and the skin and the vas sheath are pierced by sharp-tipped dissecting forceps (A). The forceps then stretches an opening (B) and the vas is lifted out (C).

been ejaculated, which takes on average 12 ejaculations, contraception must continue. The man should also be made aware that vasectomy should be considered a permanent method of birth control. Although the operation can be reversed by microsurgery and patency obtained in 70% of cases, the pregnancy rate is less than 50%.

Tubal ligation

In most cases tubal ligation – or, more accurately, tubal occlusive clipping – is performed through a laparoscope. A few women have the operation via a small suprapubic incision (minilaparotomy).

Although a failure rate of 2 per 1000 procedures at 5 years is often quoted, a study in the USA of 10 700 women who had had a tubal ligation showed a failure rate of more than 7 per 1000. The highest rate was 36 per 1000 procedures following clip sterilization, and the lowest 7.5 per 1000 after unipolar procedures. The failure rate is three times lower if the operation is performed as an interval procedure, that is, not immediately postpartum or after an abortion. A woman should be made aware of this before she decides to have the operation.

In the discussion before recommending the operation, the alternative methods of permanent birth control, including vasectomy, should be mentioned. Also, the stability of the current relationship should be explored.

Provided the woman has made an informed decision that she wants the operation and is aware that tubal ligation should be considered a permanent method of birth control, adverse reactions are few. As in the case of vasectomy, tubal patency can be restored by microsurgery and about 60% of women treated will conceive. In general, tubal ligation should not be performed immediately after

childbirth, as 5% of women who have the operation at this time later regret their decision.

Hysteroscopically placed tubal occlusive device

The Selective Tubal Occlusive Device (Essure; Fig. 31.9) is a microcoil that is placed hysteroscopically directly into the tubal ostia under local anaesthesia. The localized inflammatory response causes tubal occlusion. The device appears to be well tolerated and clinical trials are reporting 85% successful placement and 99.8% efficacy.

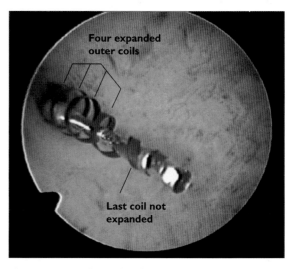

Fig. 31.9 Essure device placed hysteroscopically in the uterine ostium.

Chapter | 32 |

Infertility

A couple who have had regular unprotected intercourse for a period of 12 months without a pregnancy occurring is considered to be infertile and may seek help from a medical practitioner. Infertility affects 10–15% of couples. It is important to understand that humans like other primates are relatively subfertile.

During the first cycle 30% of couples will achieve pregnancy. During the second cycle a further 30% of couples will be successful and 80% will conceive in the first year. In the first three cycles, 30% of the conceptions will end in miscarriage, and almost half these miscarriages occur so early they are undetected except by a positive β-hCG pregnancy test

FACTORS IN INFERTILITY

The factors that may be involved in the couple's infertility vary depending on local conditions, the population investigated and the referral procedures. Analyses reported by several clinics of large numbers of patients in the past two decades are given in Table 32.1. In a quarter of cases, more than one of the factors is believed to be involved.

INVESTIGATION OF INFERTILITY

Of the many investigations suggested over the years, most have been found to be of little value, and today there is relative agreement about what tests should be made to reach a diagnosis.

In most cases the woman makes the first contact with a health professional. During this visit, the doctor should obtain information about the history of past illnesses and operations; the woman's menstrual history; and the couple's sexual behaviour, including frequency of sexual intercourse. Some women are concerned that they do not have an orgasm and that semen runs out of the vagina. The doctor should reassure the woman that neither of these affects her fertility.

A general physical examination, including a pelvic examination, is made to exclude any current disease. The pelvic examination is performed to detect any gross abnormalities of the genital tract, such as uterine myomata, ovarian tumours and endometriosis (see later). If a cervical smear (Pap smear) has not been taken in the previous year this should be done. Also, laboratory tests should be ordered and should include a full blood examination, including tests for syphilis, rubella and HIV infection, and a urine analysis. If the woman has attended during the luteal phase of her menstrual cycle, blood may be taken to measure the progesterone level to establish whether she is ovulating.

Having completed these initial investigations the medical practitioner should outline the investigations that will

Table 32.1 Factors in infertility

FACTOR	PERCENTAGE OF CASES
Male	
Defective sperm production, insemination difficulties	30–40
Female	
Ovulation factors	5–25
Tubal or uterine factors	15–25
Cervical/immunological factors	5–10
Unexplained after investigations	10–25

Box 32.1 **Normal seminal analysis**

Volume	>2 mL
Sperm concentration	>20 million per mL
Total sperm count	40 million
Motility 60 min after ejaculation	>50% with normal progression
Morphology	>30% with normal morphology

When the sperm count is less than 20 million per mL, abnormal morphology and motility is often found

be carried out, and their sequence. It is customary to start with a seminal analysis, as the man may have azoospermia or severe oligospermia. This finding would make further examinations of the woman unjustified initially.

Seminal analysis

Ideally, a man should accompany his partner at the first visit so that the investigation plan can be discussed with them both, a history can be obtained from the man, and the man can also be examined. However, it is unusual for a man to attend with his partner. Because of this, and intercourse, the first step is to arrange for a semen analysis, and only if this is abnormal need the man be seen.

The seminal specimen can be obtained in two ways. The man can either attend the laboratory and masturbate there and so provide a fresh seminal specimen, or he can masturbate at home (or have his partner masturbate him) and ejaculate into a clean, dry glass container. This is then taken to the laboratory within 1 hour, and the analysis made.

Standards for a normal seminal specimen have been developed by the World Health Organization (WHO) and are shown in Box 32.1. If the first seminal appraisal is abnormal, two further specimens should be evaluated before a prognosis is made. The most important predictors of male fertility are the percentage of motile sperm, the quality of the motility of the sperm, the motile sperm concentration, the total motile count and the sperm morphology. The absolute count is not a good predictor.

The semen analysis is traditionally graded as:

- Normal
- Oligospermia (a count of less than 20 million sperm per mL)
  - with normally motile sperm
  - with asthenospermia

- Severe oligospermia (less than 5 million sperm in total specimen)
- Azoospermia
- Asthenospermia with normal sperm count.

Abnormal results indicate that the man should be examined and a history taken. The history may show that he is exposed to high heat, certain chemicals, or is taking anticancer drugs. The examination of the man's genitals is important. The size of his testicles is evaluated and his scrotum is palpated, with the man standing, to detect if he has a varicocele. Treatment of the varicocele has been shown to be beneficial only if the man is oligospermic, as this will double the chance of pregnancy. If azoospermia or severe oligospermia is diagnosed, blood is drawn to measure the level of follicle-stimulating hormone (FSH). A raised level (three times the normal upper limit) indicates testicular failure. If severe oligospermia is diagnosed and the testicular volume and FSH levels are normal, a testicular biopsy is sometimes taken.

Absolute infertility is diagnosed if azoospermia and raised FSH levels are found. Severe infertility is diagnosed if severe oligospermia is found. Relative infertility is diagnosed if the sperm count is between 5 000 000 and 20 000 000/mL. Treatment may be offered to men with relative infertility, although it has to be said that none has proved more effective than placebo.

Investigating the woman

Factors that may delay or prevent fertility in women are:

- Anovulation or infrequent ovulation
- Tubal damage which prevents the passage of the sperm
- Uterine factors, such as intra-uterine adhesions (Asherman's syndrome)
- Cervical mucus 'hostility', which in most cases is an immunological defect.

These factors require to be investigated in the work-up of infertility.

Ovulation

The most effective way to determine whether the woman is ovulating is to measure the serum progesterone level in the midluteal phase of the menstrual cycle. The older methods of daily temperature charting and diagnostic curettage to determine whether endometrial luteinization had occurred are obsolete.

Anovulation is obvious if the woman is amenorrhoeic, and may occur in women who have normal menstrual periods. The investigation of anovulation is discussed in Chapter 28.

Time of ovulation

Knowledge of the time of ovulation is increasingly important in the treatment of some causes of infertility, because conception is most likely to occur on this day or on one of the 5 preceding days. The time of ovulation can be detected by measuring the plasma level of luteinizing hormone (LH) daily over this period. The peak of LH release coincides with ovulation.

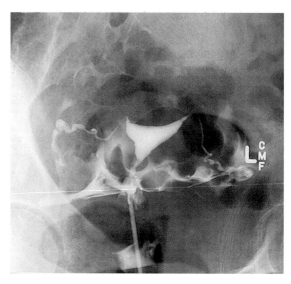

Fig. 32.1 Hysterosalpingogram showing a normal uterus and tubes.

Defective luteal phase

A number of infertility specialists believe that some cases of infertility are due to the poor development of the luteal phase endometrium, with the result that the fertilized egg is unable to implant. Other specialists deny that the condition exists. Many treatments have been tried to treat the condition, but none has been evaluated scientifically or proved to be of value.

Tubal factors

The patency of the Fallopian tubes can be evaluated in three ways:

- The first, hysterosalpingography, is performed by inserting a cannula, attached to a syringe, into the cervix and injecting a radio-opaque substance into the uterus under direct imaging. The passage of the dye is observed as it fills the uterine cavity and passes along the Fallopian tubes to spill into the peritoneal cavity. The advantages of hysterosalpingography are that it is a minor operation (the patient need not be admitted as a day-case) and that it will detect any intra-uterine abnormalities (Fig. 32.1).
- A more recent innovation is to use hysterosalpingo-contrast sonography. Under transvaginal ultrasound scanning, a galactose solution is injected into the uterus and passes along the Fallopian tubes, which delineates them more accurately than hysterosalpingography using a radio-opaque substance.
- The third method is to perform a laparoscopy and then to inject a water-soluble dye into the uterine cavity which is observed as it spills through the fimbrial ends of the Fallopian tubes. The advantage of laparoscopy is that, as well as ascertaining that the Fallopian tubes are patent, any peritubal adhesions and endometrial deposits can be detected. Endometriosis is the only abnormality found in about 10% of infertile women, and 40% of women who have endometriosis are involuntarily infertile, but the relationship between the two conditions is unclear. The topic is discussed further in Chapter 35.

Currently, the use of colour Doppler ultrasonography is being investigated, as is the use of tuboscopy.

Cervical hostility

Although this term is usually used to indicate that the sperm fail to penetrate the cervical mucus at the time of ovulation, it is more likely that the failure is due to defective sperm function, probably immunological.

Many gynaecologists continue to believe in cervical hostility, and test it by means of the postcoital test. This has been in use for over 100 years and was originally carried out to detect sperm in the cervix. Today, the test is performed as follows:

- The couple have intercourse on one of the two days before ovulation, or on the day of ovulation.
- After the man has ejaculated the woman lies on her back for 20 minutes, and attends the doctor 8–12 hours later so that a sample of cervical mucus can be removed (using a plastic tube attached to a syringe).
- The specimen is smeared on a slide and is examined to determine the degree of penetration of the mucus by actively moving sperm, and their numbers per field.

A positive test (more than 20 actively moving sperm per field) indicates that there is unlikely to be an immunological problem; a negative test provides no useful information. Because of this, more specific sperm–mucus tests have been developed. A second test is the mixed agglutinin reaction (MAR). Human red cells are sensitized with IgG and mixed with sperm. If the spermatozoa are coated with antibody, the mixed agglutinates will be visible. However, the value of these tests is unclear and the predictive value poor.

Unexplained infertility

After adequate investigation, up to 25% of infertile couples will still not have had a cause for their infertility found. Unexplained infertility is frustrating for both the couple and the health professionals.

TREATMENT OF INFERTILITY

Infertility in men

Azoospermia is an absolute barrier to conception, and it is unusual for a pregnancy to occur in a couple if the man has severe oligospermia. For these couples, donor insemination (DI) is a choice. Using DI monthly for 12 months, if necessary, will enable over 65% of women to become pregnant. If sperm can be recovered from the epididymis, a single spermatozoon can be microinjected into the space under the zona pellucida or into the ovum. The delivery rate per treatment cycle is 30%.

Improvement in the sperm count of men with non-severe oligospermia has been attempted using an oral form of testosterone (mesterolone), bromocriptine and antioestrogens, clomifene and tamoxifen, but none have been shown in controlled trials to have a significant effect on pregnancy rates.

An attractive alternative is to concentrate a seminal sample and fertilize several ova using the in vitro fertilization (IVF) technique.

Infertility in women

Anovulation (usually associated with amenorrhoea)

The treatment is as discussed in the treatment of amenorrhoea on page 223. Inducing superovulation with drugs can assist conception when the man has a low sperm count or the woman is experiencing oligomenorrhoea.

Tubal damage

Two choices are available, depending on the severity of the tubal damage and the wishes of the patient. The first approach is to attempt to make the Fallopian tubes patent, using microsurgery. If only the fimbrial ends of the tubes are blocked, a salpingostomy or fimbriolysis is carried out. This results in a 40% chance of the woman conceiving in the 2 years following the operation. Greater tubal damage necessitates a tubal anastomosis, with a success rate of no more than 20%, whereas reversal of a tubal ligation is followed by a pregnancy rate of 60%.

Given these relatively poor results (except in the case of reversal of a tubal ligation), the alternative approach – IVF – is recommended. The procedure is less invasive, the risk of ectopic gestation is lower and the chance of giving birth to a healthy baby is greater.

Cervical hostility (immunological infertility)

The oldest method of treatment is for the man to use condoms for 6 months in the hope that the antisperm antibodies will be eliminated. Other treatments are for the man to take low-dose corticosteroids (prednisone 20 mg twice daily for the first 10 days of the woman's menstrual cycle) for 3 months; to use washed sperm introduced into the uterine cavity; or to use IVF or gamete intrafallopian transfer (GIFT) techniques. None of these treatments has been properly evaluated, and it appears that as many pregnancies occur with treatment as when no treatment is given.

Unexplained infertility

Current opinion about the treatment of couples who have been diagnosed with unexplained infertility is confused. If no treatment beyond reassurance is given, over 40% of the women will become pregnant within 3 years. However, if the couple wish, or if the woman is over 35, IVF or GIFT may be used soon after diagnosis, rather than delaying for 3 years.

Assisted reproductive technologies

These technologies, that is, IVF and its variants (Table 32.2), have added a new dimension to the treatment of infertility. In the past decade considerable advances have been made in reducing the pain involved, the invasiveness of the procedure and the cost. The procedure is as follows:

1. The woman is given ovulatory drugs, FSH, gonadotrophin-releasing hormone agonists and human chorionic gonadotrophin, to produce superovulation.
2. The eggs are retrieved from the ovaries by the transvaginal route under ultrasonic guidance.
3. The eggs are prepared for fertilization and only good ova are selected.
4. Sperm are added to the selected eggs in vitro.

Table 32.2 Methods of assisted conception

TYPE	ASSISTED INSEMINATION WITH HUSBAND'S SPERM (AIH)	IN VITRO FERTILIZATION (IVF)	GAMETE INTRA-FALLOPIAN TRANSFER (GIFT)	INTRA-CYTOPLASMIC SPERM INJECTION (ICSI)	ZYGOTE INTRA-FALLOPIAN TRANSFER (ZIFT), TUBAL EMBRYO STAGE TRANSFER (TEST)
Indications					
Male	Impotence Retrograde ejaculation Severe hypospadias	Oligospermia Presence of sperm antibodies	Moderate oligospermia	Severe oligospermia or azoospermia Vasectomy	Severe oligospermia
Female	Localized cervical or uterine problem	Endometriosis Damaged or absent Fallopian tubes	Endometriosis		
Male and/or Female	Infrequent or absent sexual intercourse	Unexplained infertility		Failure of IVF	
Procedure	Sperm are transferred by catheter into uterus or Fallopian tube	Fertilized eggs are transferred into the uterus or Fallopian tube	Unfertilized eggs and sperm are transferred into one or both Fallopian tubes using laparoscopy or transvaginal ultrasound	Sperm is injected into the egg	Zygote or early embryo is transferred into the Fallopian tube using laparoscopy or transvaginal ultrasound the day after egg pickup
Pregnancy rate*	Up to 15% per cycle	10–25% per cycle; depends on maternal age	Up to 30–40% per cycle	More than 50% per cycle	Up to 30–40% per cycle

*'Take-home baby' rates are lower.

5. One or two (occasionally three) fertilized eggs are transferred into the uterus, or into the Fallopian tubes.

The GIFT technique involves similar procedures except that fertilization does not taken place before transfer of the ova and sperm into the Fallopian tubes.

Intracytoplasmic sperm injection involves the direct injection of the sperm into the nucleus of the ova and is the treatment of choice for male infertility due to oligospermia.

The calculation of the success rates of IVF procedures is complex because couples who have not been successful early in treatment cycles may not return for further treatment. The 'take-home baby' rates stratified by age are shown in Table 32.3.

Success rate of treatment

Four couples in every 10 treated for infertility will have a 'take-home baby', in most cases thanks to treatment, but about 20% of cases cannot be attributed to the treatment. The success rate for the treatment of various infertility factors is shown in Table 32.4.

PSYCHOSOCIAL PROBLEMS ASSOCIATED WITH INFERTILITY

The conception, and later the birth, of a healthy child is a significant life event. To most women, motherhood is the expression of their nurturing gender role and their

Table 32.3 Percentage cumulative live-birth rates after IVF according to maternal age (from Malitzia B et al. 2009 New Engl J Med 360: 236–243, with permission, © 2009 Massachusetts Medical Society. All rights reserved)

AGE (YEARS)	CYCLE					
	1	2	3	4	5	6
<35	33	49–52	59–67	63–76	65–82	65–86
35–37	28	44–47	51–58	55–67	56–74	57–78
38–39	21	32–35	40–47	43–55	45–62	46–67
≥40	9	15–16	19–24	21–32	22–37	23–42

Table 32.4 Pregnancy rates in infertility*

	PROPORTION OF ALL CASES OF INFERTILITY (%)	PREGNANCY RATE[†] (%)
Male:		
Azoospermia	7	65 (using DI)
Oligospermia	25	30
Female:		
Amenorrhoea	7	90
Other ovulatory	14	60
Tubal damage	16	20
Endometriosis (severe)	2	30
Uterine abnormalities	1	70
Male–female (immunological)	5	15
Unexplained	23	60

*'Take-home baby' rates are lower.
[†]Within 2 years of diagnosis with or without treatment.

femininity, and to most men the siring of a child is a visible demonstration of their masculinity and potency. For most couples, parenthood is an expression of their love for each other. However, society still regards infertility as an illness.

The psychological impact of infertility can be considerable and the necessary investigations psychologically disturbing, particularly to the woman, who has more tests performed than her partner. She may perceive these as invasive and intimate, involving a loss of control over her body.

If a bar to fertility is detected in either partner or, if after investigation and treatment a pregnancy does not occur, the couple may be subjected to considerable psychological strain and may develop psychosexual problems.

This possibility can be reduced in several ways, which involve the infertility specialist and the couple's general practitioner, who should have a key role as he knows the couple better. This implies that there must be good communication between specialist and doctor.

- As early as possible in the infertility work-up the medical practitioner should provide the couple with a clear detail of the investigations proposed, the reasons for them, and the sequence in which they will be performed. As the couple may be so anxious that they may listen to but not hear what is being said, it is helpful to suggest that they read a book about infertility or are provided with pamphlets.
- The investigations should be kept to a minimum, and only those that produce reliable information should be made. Once information is obtained, the couple should be told the results and be given the opportunity to ask questions.
- The attitude and behaviour of the doctor should be supportive, communicative and empathetic.
- If an absolute or severe barrier to conception is found, appropriate counselling should be offered. Inability to have a child represents a real loss, and mourning is an appropriate response. In counselling, the approach is to consider all the findings together as causing the couple's shared unhappiness, so that neither partner blames the other.

Couples who are in an IVF, GIFT or other assisted reproductive programme need special care, as in most cases these technologies are a 'last resort' in their attempt to have a child. The egg retrieval may be painful and the whole process psychologically traumatic, particularly if the woman perceives parenthood as a prerequisite for personal fulfilment. Most couples cope well, but one-third of women experience anxiety or depression and one in seven becomes severely distressed.

Infections of the genital tract

VULVOVAGINAL INFECTIONS

The skin of the vulva, in common with other parts of the skin that are liable to friction and chafing, may be infected by common skin pathogens. Boils may occur, particularly when the standard of hygiene is low. Multiple vulval ulcers occur occasionally, particularly in debilitated women, and are due to staphylococcal infection. The ulcers are shallow, with a grey, discharging base and surrounding oedema. The vulva is extremely tender. Treatment consists of antibiotics and 1% chlorhexidine cream if this can be applied without causing much pain.

Genital herpes

Herpetic infection of the genital tract is becoming increasingly common. The virus, herpes simplex virus (HSV), exists in two forms, HSV1 and HSV2. Type specific HSV1 usually causes oral cold sores, but in up to 40% of cases is the cause of genital herpes. In the remainder HSV2 causes genital herpes. Serological testing shows that between 10 and 40% of adults have been infected at some time, but the infection was symptomatic in less than a quarter.

The first clinical attack of genital herpes is usually worse than the recurrences. It follows sexual contact with an infected person who was either symptomatically or asymptomatically shedding the virus. The inner surfaces of the labia majora are most likely to be infected. After a short period of itching or burning, small crops of painful, reddish lumps appear which become blisters within 24 hours. The blisters ulcerate rapidly to form multiple shallow, painful ulcers (Fig. 33.1). The surrounding tissues become oedematous and secondary bacterial infection may occur, aggravating the oedema and pain. Micturition may be very painful. Over 5 days the ulcers crust over and heal slowly, the healing being complete in 7–12 days after the appearance of the blisters for a primary infection, and less for recurrences. During this time, and intermittently, the virus is shed from the infected area and in vaginal secretions. The virus also enters the sensory nerves supplying the affected area, and tracks to lie in the dorsal root ganglion. It may lie dormant for the rest of the person's life, or may be reactivated and track back along the nerves to cause a new attack of herpes. Second and subsequent attacks are less severe, but can cause considerable discomfort and affect relationships.

In 30% of infected women a single recurrence occurs, and between 2 and 5% have recurrent attacks, sometimes more than six times a year. As time passes the attacks (clinical and asymptomatic) become less frequent and may cease.

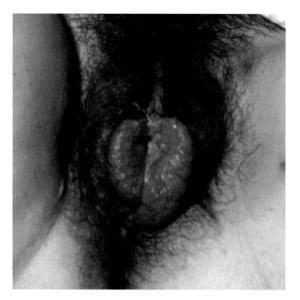

Fig. 33.1 Genital herpes – lesions are visible on the labia and the inner aspect of the left thigh.

In most cases the cause of the recurrence is not known, but recurrences are more common in the luteal phase of the menstrual cycle, if the woman has other sexually transmitted infections, or if she is emotionally stressed.

Intermittent asymptomatic shedding and atypical unrecognized lesions explain the unrecognized transmission to sexual partners. As HSV2 has a tropism for the genital area (HSV1 for the oral area) clinical recurrences are more frequent if the genital infection is HSV2 rather than HSV1.

Diagnosis

To make a definitive diagnosis of genital herpes, the blisters should be pricked to obtain vesicular fluid and the ulcers rubbed with a cotton tipped-bud to obtain virus-infected cells, and the swab sent in a virus transport medium for culture. Alternatively (particularly for older lesions) testing by polymerase chain reaction (PCR) is more sensitive. A full STI screen should be completed (Box 33.1).

Box 33.1 Screening for sexually transmitted infections (STIs)

Chlamydia
Gonorrhoea
Hepatitis B
HIV
Syphilis
Trichomonas
(check up-to-date with Pap smear)

Treatment

During an attack a woman should wash her hands after touching the infected area. If she is unable to pass urine because of pain or retention, a suprapubic catheter may need to be inserted. Local applications of ice or anaesthetic jelly provide some relief.

The antiviral drugs aciclovir, famciclovir and valaciclovir reduce the duration and severity of the initial and recurrent attacks, and shorten the time of viral shedding if given early in the attack. If a woman has five or more attacks each year, or the outbreaks are particularly severe, long-lasting or interfere with her psychosocial functioning, the drugs can be given daily as suppressive treatment for 6–12 months or longer.

Women who have recurrent genital herpes are often more concerned about the psychosocial sequelae of the disease, rather than the physical symptoms, and may need to be counselled.

Genital warts (condylomata acuminata)

Genital warts are caused by types 6 and 11 of the human papilloma virus (HPV), usually transmitted sexually. Vulval infections are the most common, although the virus may spread to infect the vagina, the perineum (Fig. 33.2) and occasionally the cervix.

Vulval warts usually present as cauliflower growths of varying sizes, but may be clinically undetectable. It has been estimated that 5–10% of sexually active adults are infected annually, and that 30% have evidence of previous infection with other HPV genotypes.

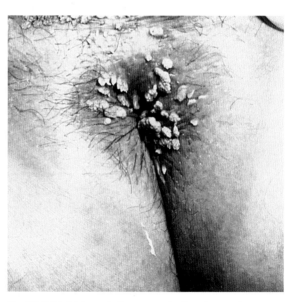

Fig. 33.2 Multiple genital warts on the introitus and surrounding the anus.

In most cases the warts are symptomless, but some women complain of vulval discomfort, including itching. If the warts involve the vaginal entrance or the vagina, the woman may complain of dyspareunia.

The importance of HPV infections is that they are surrogates for the exposure to and carriage of the oncogenic HPV types 16 and 18, which are the cause of cervical carcinoma. The risk of this occurring from vulval warts is small. This is discussed further in Chapter 37.

Treatment

Genital warts, if not too exuberant, may be treated with podophyllotoxin (twice daily for 3 days, repeated if needed after 4 days) applied by the woman herself, after trimming away any vulval hair around the wart; or the medical practitioner may apply 20% podophyllin in benzoin tincture to the wart without touching the surrounding skin, to avoid skin burns and ulceration. The mixture is allowed to dry and the woman washes it off 6 hours later. This is repeated once weekly, if necessary. This should not be used in pregnancy. Larger condylomata on the cervix may respond to the application of trichloroacetic acid. Imiquimod cream 5% can be applied before bedtime so that it is left on the skin for 6–10 hours, three times weekly.

Large warts, or warts that fail to respond to medical treatment, are treated by diathermy or by laser. The procedure is painful and anaesthesia is needed. Postoperatively, pain requires analgesics. A problem that has recently been reported is that neither diathermy nor laser may cure the woman, as the virus may have infected neighbouring normal cells and warts commonly recur. Because of the concern that HPV infection with types 16 and 18 may be involved with the development of cervical carcinoma, a woman who has vulval warts should have regular Pap smears.

Syphilitic vulval ulcer

Syphilis is caused by invasion of the tissues by *Treponema pallidum* and is sexually transmitted. The primary lesion, which is often unrecognized, is a small papule that appears at the site of inoculation, usually 14–28 days after the person is infected. In women, the usual site of infection is one of the labia majora, but the cervix may be infected instead. The papule rapidly enlarges to form an oval lesion of variable size, the centre of which becomes eroded and granulomatous. The edges of the eroded area are sharp, and outside this a thickened, indurated zone occurs, hence the name for the lesion – hard chancre. The chancre is painless and may be ignored by the woman or considered a small sore of no consequence, but as it is teeming with treponemas it is highly infectious. The primary lesion disappears in 21 days or so. Secondary lesions, which include mucous patches and condylomata lata (Fig. 33.3), appear 5–6 weeks later.

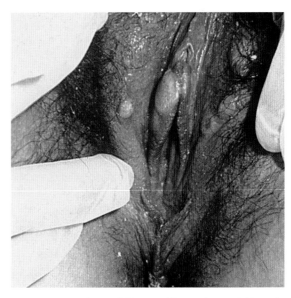

Fig. 33.3 Secondary syphilis – condylomata lata on labia and perianally.

Diagnosis

The diagnosis is confirmed by examining exudate expressed from the ulcer or mucous patches, through a microscope under dark-ground illumination. To obtain an accurate diagnosis the chancre is first cleaned with a swab, and then, if necessary, its edge and base are scarified with a scalpel so that exudate appears before the specimen is taken. The tests should be interpreted in conjunction with specialist sexual health physician or clinical microbiologist. A full STI screen should be ordered.

Treatment

Treatment consists of antibiotics, procaine benzylpenicillin 1 g daily for 10 days, a long-acting penicillin, benzathine penicillin, 1.8 g as a single dose or, for penicillin-sensitive individuals, doxycycline 100 mg twice daily for 14 days. Meticulous follow-up is essential.

Infection of Bartholin's gland (Bartholinitis)

The infection is usually due to *Escherichia coli* or staphylococci, but may follow *Neisseria gonorrhoeae* or *Clostridium trachomatis* infection. In the acute stage both the duct and the gland are involved. If it is not treated the infection may subside or a Bartholin's abscess may form. Occasionally the gland becomes chronically enlarged following an inflammatory conglutination of the duct epithelium, to form a Bartholin's cyst.

Diagnosis

In acute bartholinitis the woman complains of acute discomfort in the region of the gland, and a reddened, tender swelling appears beneath the posterior part of the labium majus.

Treatment

Treatment consists of excluding sexually transmitted infections (STIs) and prescribing analgesics and a broad-spectrum antibiotic. If an abscess has formed it should be marsupialized. An elliptical piece of the vagina and the abscess wall, just inside the hymen, is removed. The vaginal and abscess walls are sutured to maintain patency and a small drain is inserted.

Vaginal discharges and infections

The vagina of a woman in the reproductive years is lined by a layer of stratified epithelium, 10–30 cells thick. As is described on page 333, the superficial cells of the vagina are shed constantly into the vaginal cavity and release glycogen, which is acted on by Döderlein's bacilli (lactobacilli) to produce lactic acid and hydrogen peroxide (natural defences against vaginal infection) and to maintain the vaginal pH between 3.5 and 4.5.

The vagina harbours large numbers of bacteria, which constitute its normal flora (Table 33.1). However, a significant number of women harbour potential pathogens such as *E. coli*, anaerobes, *Candida* spp., and *Gardnerella vaginalis* (bacterial vaginosis). They produce symptoms in only a few women.

Table 33.1 Normal vaginal flora	
ORGANISM	**PERCENTAGE**
Lactobacilli	80–90
Staphylococci, micrococci	50–70
Ureaplasma	40–50
Anaerobes	20–50
Streptococci	20–30
Gardnerella	10–30
E. coli	5–15
Candida spp.	5–15
Bacteroides	5–10
Trichomonas	3–7

The vagina is normally kept moist by transudation of fluid through its walls, which mixes with the exfoliated vaginal cells, aliphatic acids and the microorganisms mentioned earlier. The quantity of vaginal secretions varies throughout the menstrual cycle, peaking at ovulation. The quantity is also increased by emotional stress. If an increased quantity of vaginal secretion is present it may form a white coagulum, which may cause concern to the woman when she notices a whitish discharge that may cause itching. The discharge is termed leucorrhoea, which is defined as a non-infective, non-bloodstained physiological vaginal discharge.

Leucorrhoea

When a woman presents with leucorrhoea, infection by pathogenic organisms must be excluded by obtaining an endocervical (for potential pathogens *Cl. trachomatis, N. gonorrhoeae*) or a vaginal smear (*Candida*, bacterial vaginosis, *Trichomonas*), which is examined or cultured.

Treatment

Treatment consists of reassuring the woman that the discharge is not pathogenic and exploring reasons for her concern. A few women have recurrent vaginal discharges that show no pathogens on repeated laboratory investigations. Some women have a dermatosis. Often these cases are difficult to treat. Some of these women have abnormal scores on psychometric tests, or have the somatizing syndrome, so the woman's lifestyle, including her sexuality, should be investigated rather than concentrating on the vaginal discharge. Some women repeatedly douche themselves for 'vaginal hygiene', a practice that may increase the chance of vaginal infection by reducing the number of vaginal lactobacilli.

If the woman wants medication, a vaginal acidifying jelly (Aci-Jel) may be prescribed. Antibiotics should be avoided as they may aggravate the discharge rather than relieve it.

Pathological vaginal discharges

The three common irritating pathological vulvovaginal discharges are caused by:

- Trichomoniasis
- Candidiasis
- Bacterial (amine) vaginosis.

In many cases they can be differentiated in the doctor's office or outpatient clinic by taking a sample of the discharge and looking at a 'wet preparation' under a microscope. Part of the swab is mixed with a drop of saline and part is mixed on a second slide with two drops of 10% potassium hydroxide (KOH). The saline preparation may reveal trichomonal flagellates, which can be observed moving and thrashing their tails (Fig. 33.4). Alternatively, the wet preparation may also show vaginal epithelial cells

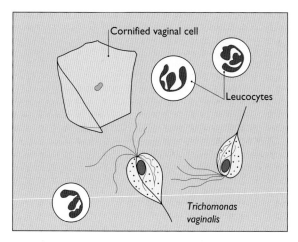

Fig. 33.4 *Trichomonas vaginalis.*

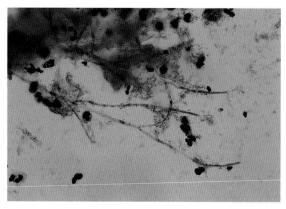

Fig. 33.6 *Candida albicans.*

with indistinct borders, 'clue cells' due to the 'hundreds and thousands' effect of the presence of large numbers of Gram-variable coccobacilli (Fig. 33.5), which suggest that the woman has bacterial vaginosis. Clue cells are more readily apparent on a Gram-stained slide. Bacterial vaginosis is also suggested by a strong fishy smell from the KOH preparation (the amine test). The KOH preparation is examined under a microscope, when hyphae of *Candida* species can be seen, if this is the cause of the discharge (Fig. 33.6).

The alternative is to take the vaginal swab and place it in a transport medium, and send it to a laboratory for microscopy and culture.

Trichomoniasis

The parasite *Trichomonas vaginalis* is a 20 mm long flagellate. It is a little larger than a leukocyte (see Fig. 33.4).

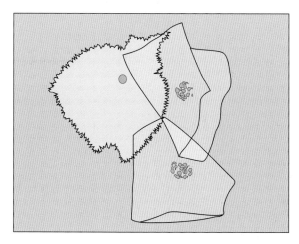

Fig. 33.5 'Clue cells', seen in bacterial vaginitis.

Once introduced into the vagina, it shelters at the bottom of the crypts of the velvet-like vaginal epithelium. It may be symptomless, or may cause vaginitis with discomfort and discharge. It is readily sexually transmitted and infects the man's urethra, where it is often symptomless.

Clinical aspects

The main complaint is a moderate to profuse vaginal discharge that produces itching and irritation inside the vagina and around the vaginal introitus. In longstanding cases the discharge is greenish and frothy. In pregnant women it is associated with prematurity. There is also an increased risk of HIV transmission.

Treatment

The patient is given a single oral dose of tinidazole 2 g or metronidazole 2 g. Alternatively, oral metronidazole is prescribed in a dose of 400 mg twice a day for 5 days. The woman's sexual partner should be invited to take the same treatment. These regimens cure 90% of infected women. A vaginal swab is taken 7 days after completing treatment, and if the flagellates are still present a second course of treatment is given. Side-effects of treatment are minimal: a few women feel nauseated and alcohol should be avoided while taking the tablets as it may lead to headaches and flushing.

Candidiasis (thrush)

Candida spp. infect the vaginal epithelial cells, particularly if in the fungal-germinating stage, when they develop spores and long threads (hyphae) (see Fig. 33.6). Inside the cells they may lie dormant until environmental conditions encourage germination. *Candida* spp. may also infect the vulval skin, the anogenital region, the mouth and the intestinal tract. For recurrent candidiasis underlying conditions such as diabetes, the recent use of broad-spectrum antibiotics or immunosuppressive therapy, e.g. corticosteroids, and HIV should be considered.

Clinical aspects

The woman complains of severe vulvovaginal irritation associated with a vaginal discharge. In some cases her sexual partner may complain of itching of his glans and foreskin.

Typically the discharge is thick, 'cheesy', and adheres to the vaginal wall in plaques, but often these findings are not present.

Diagnosis

A vaginal swab should be taken and processed as discussed earlier.

Treatment

One of the imidazole group of drugs (clotrimazole, econazole, isoconazole or miconazole) is prescribed as a vaginal tablet, either as a single dose or daily for 3 days. If vaginal treatment fails or oral treatment is preferred, a single dose of fluconazole or ketoconazole may be prescribed.

Alternatively, local treatment with an imidazole given every 2–4 weeks may control the infection. Vulval irritation may be intense and an imidazole cream may be applied at intervals. A course of treatment cures 85% of patients.

The woman should also be advised to wipe her vulva from the front to the rear to avoid possible faecal contamination.

Recurrent candidiasis

Between 5 and 15% of women with vaginal candidiasis have recurrent attacks, sometimes four times a year. Most are relapses of the initial infection, although the presence of a non-*albicans* candidal species with reduced susceptibility to azoles is possible. Recurrent attacks can cause a considerable disruption to the woman's personal and sexual life, and she may resort to alternative medicine.

Treatment

It is difficult to treat this condition. In women who have frequent recurrences, prophylactic ketoconazole 100 mg by mouth daily for 6 months, or fluconazole 150 mg weekly, may offer protection. Some women complain of nausea. In 1 in 15 000 users ketoconazole causes liver damage, and the woman should have liver function tests at the start of treatment and again after 3 months. The woman is usually told not to wear nylon pantyhose or tight jeans, but the value of this has not been established. Non-*albicans* candidiasis (*Candida glabiata*), which is resistant to conventional therapy, may respond to boric acid capsules.

Bacterial vaginosis

This vaginal infection is common, affecting 10–20% of women. In bacterial vaginosis the numbers of vaginal organisms are increased considerably, but only 6% of the lactobacilli produce hydrogen peroxidase, compared with the normal 60%. This leads to a rise in the vaginal pH and an increase in the growth of *Gardnerella vaginalis* and mixed vaginal anaerobes, *Mycoplasma hominis* and *Mobiluncus* spp. As mentioned on page 147, bacterial vaginosis may increase the chance of preterm birth.

Half of infections are symptomless; in others the woman complains of a thin, greyish discharge which has a strong fishy smell. The clinical diagnosis is difficult, but a vaginal smear that shows clue cells is diagnostic (see Fig. 33.5).

Treatment consists of metronidazole 2 g orally as a single dose. An alternative is clindamycin given orally, or as a vaginal cream, 5 g daily for 7 days. If these regimens do not clear the infection, metronidazole 400 mg three times a day for 7 days should be given. In pregnancy, metronidazole 400 mg twice daily for 2 days seems to clear the infection.

INFECTIONS OF THE INTERNAL GENITAL ORGANS

The fact that, apart from the lowest third, the genital tract derives from the Müllerian duct and has anastomosing systems of arteries, veins and lymphatics, means that infections of individual organs are less frequent than sequential ascending infection of the genital tract.

Ascending vaginal infection is controlled to some extent by the following mechanisms:

- First, the vaginal walls lie in apposition and the vaginal secretions are acidic, which inhibits bacterial growth.
- Second, the cervical mucus forms a meshwork, except at the time of ovulation, which limits upward spread.
- Third, the endometrium is shed each month during menstruation. However, if the cervix is infected directly, the above mechanisms are less effective.

Upper genital tract infections may be sexually acquired or result from ascending infection from endogenous vaginal flora, particularly after disruption of the normal cervical barrier following miscarriage, delivery or gynaecological surgery. Infections are usually not due to endogenous flora.

As it may be difficult, clinically, to determine which organ is infected, and as more than one organ is usually infected, the condition is generally diagnosed as acute pelvic infection or pelvic inflammatory disease (PID). Infection of the internal genital organs may also occur following an abortion or after childbirth. In these cases the infective agents (which are usually staphylococci, streptococci, *E. coli* or anaerobes) enter the tissues through cervical lacerations, or more frequently, through the placental bed. Infections following pregnancy or childbirth are discussed in Chapter 23.

Rarely pelvic infections occur either from haematogenous spread, as in tuberculosis, or from pelvic peritonitis.

STI-related pelvic inflammatory disease (PID)

The microorganisms invade the columnar cells lining the crypts of the cervical canal. They may be eliminated by the body's immune system, spread rapidly to cause an acute infection, or remain quiescent in the columnar cells, with the potential to spread to other pelvic organs. Spread occurs via the lymphatics, the veins or, possibly, by 'riding on the back of spermatozoa'. In a few instances the infection is carried into the uterus during the insertion of an intra-uterine device, and it is advisable to screen women for *Chlamydia* and *Neisseria gonorrhoeae* prior to insertion (see p. 248).

The endometrium is first infected, causing endometritis. From here the infection may spread to the myometrium, causing myometritis, or through the uterine cavity to the Fallopian tubes, causing acute or subacute salpingitis. In some cases the ovaries and the pelvic peritoneum may be involved (Fig. 33.7).

The two principal infecting agents are *Cl. trachomatis* and *Neisseria gonorrhoeae*. They require further discussion.

Chlamydial infection

Infection with *Cl. trachomatis* is commonly symptomless, but a few women (less than 20%) may complain of a mucopurulent discharge from the cervix, dysuria, or intermenstrual bleeding. Community studies have shown that between 15 and 30% of healthy women have circulating antichlamydial antibodies, indicating previous subclinical infection, and that between 4 and 12% have symptomless infection of their cervical cells (as have men who have symptomless infection of the urethral cells). Symptomatic infection affects between 1 and 3% of sexually active women aged 15–50 years (and rather more men) each year. With the availability of polymerase chain reaction (PCR) and ligase chain reaction testing on urine, greater diagnostic accuracy has been obtained. A higher incidence occurs in women under the age of 25, with multiple sexual partners, or whose sexual partners have had several partners.

Gonococcal genital infection

Gonococcal genital infection may be symptomless or may produce early symptoms of dysuria, urinary frequency and a purulent vaginal discharge. The discharge originates from infected endocervical cells and from Bartholin's gland, but not from the vaginal mucosa, as the gonococcus is unable to penetrate vaginal stratified epithelium. The severity of the initial infection varies, and in 50–80% of infected women the symptoms are so mild that they are ignored. Spread, if it occurs, is upwards to the endometrium and Fallopian tubes, or downwards to infect Bartholin's gland.

Clinical presentations of PID

Cervical infection has been discussed and endometritis is usually symptomless except when it follows a bacterial infection after abortion or childbirth.

Salpingitis may be symptomless or symptomatic. In acute symptomatic cases the growth of organisms in the cells lining the oviduct produces the acute phase of primary infection. A large amount of mucus is secreted, together with a fibrinous exudate which produces agglutination of the mucosal folds of the endosalpinx. The Fallopian tubes become inflamed and oedematous, producing recognizable signs and symptoms. These are:

- Severe bilateral lower abdominal tenderness and pain
- Abdominal muscle spasm (guarding)
- Pelvic tenderness and pain on moving the cervix (cervical excitation)
- Fever (>38°C), often with rigors
- Leukocytosis, raised ESR and C-reactive protein (CRP).

On examination the lower abdomen is tender, and on pelvic examination bimanual palpation of the lateral vaginal fornices is excruciatingly painful.

In particularly virulent infections pus may collect in the Fallopian tube, producing a pyosalpinx, or the infection may spread to the ovaries.

Low-grade infections will either be symptomless or associated with non-specific lower abdominal pain.

Diagnosis

The diagnosis may be established clinically, but confirmation by laparoscopy is required in most cases as the

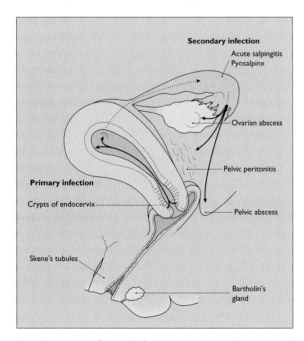

Fig. 33.7 Route of spread of non-gonococcal and gonococcal infection.

symptoms are non-specific and may occur in tubal pregnancy, accompany a complication of an ovarian cyst, or have a psychosomatic basis. Ideally a definitive diagnosis can be made from an endometrial sample (using a protected triple-lumen sampler) sent to a laboratory to detect plasma cells. Transvaginal pelvic ultrasound scanning is as accurate as laparoscopy and less invasive. The transvaginal ultrasound looks for:

- Multiple ovarian cysts
- Thickened fluid-filled Fallopian tubes
- Free fluid in the pelvis.

Laboratory tests should be made: urethral and endocervical swabs should be taken and sent in appropriate transport media for microscopy and culture for N. gonorrhoeae and potentially pathogenic endogenous flora. Screening for chlamydia is largely by PCR from first-void urine (FVU), endocervical swab or self-collected genital swab.

Treatment

In most cases treatment should be started before the exact infective agent has been identified. In severely ill patients antibiotics should be started intravenously. In less severe cases intramuscular or oral antibiotics should be given. Because of the frequent association of chlamydia and gonococcal infection, and the increasing prevalence of penicillin-resistant N. gonorrhoeae, the Center for Disease Control in the USA and the Therapeutic Guidelines in Australia recommend that the current treatment of doxycycline and metronidazole should be replaced with a single dose of probenecid 1 g and ceftriaxone 250 mg intramuscularly (one dose), followed by doxycycline 100 mg orally twice daily for 14–21 days. Alternative regimens include clindamycin 450 mg four times a day for 10 days, or gentamicin 4–6 mg/kg IV daily.

In severe infections, including tubo-ovarian abscess, intravenous treatment should be started with cefoxitin 2 g four times daily plus doxycycline 100 mg twice daily. This regimen is continued for 4 days and is followed by doxycycline 100 mg twice daily for a further 10 days. Such cases may require either surgical or radiologically guided drainage.

Oral azithromycin 1 g stat has a major role in combating bacterial sexually transmitted diseases, particularly chlamydia infections, and may be superior to other treatments. As the recommended antibiotic treatment is constantly changing it is important for the doctor to keep up to date and adopt the latest recommendations.

Surgery is indicated if the drug treatment fails in the presence of obvious abscesses that do not respond to antibiotics. The surgery should be as conservative as possible, drainage being preferred. 'Total clearance' of the genital organs is rarely indicated.

Prevention

Both chlamydia and gonorrhoea are sexually transmitted. Prevention is therefore best obtained if people are prepared to use 'safer sex', that is, limiting the number of sexual partners and insisting on the use of a condom, particularly if either partner cannot be relied on to disclose their previous sexual behaviour. This advice is idealistic and usually ignored. An alternative is to suggest that a person who has had several sexual partners, or whose partner has had several sexual partners, is screened for chlamydia and gonorrhoea every 6 months or so.

Long-term effects of PID

A first chlamydial genital infection, unless treated, causes damage to the Fallopian tubes in 10% of cases. If a second infection occurs the proportion of women who develop tubal damage increases to 25% and, after a third infection, to over 50%. Gonococcal infection, unless treated, is associated with an even higher chance of tubal damage. As many infections, particularly with chlamydia, are symptomless, it is not surprising that evidence of previous tubal infection is often first detected during investigations for infertility. If a previously infected woman who has had tubal damage does succeed in becoming pregnant, she has five to seven times the risk of having an ectopic pregnancy compared with a woman who has not had PID.

Subacute salpingitis

This is often symptomless, but the woman may feel unwell. A vaginal examination may show a tubal mass. This is found in half the number of women infected with gonorrhoea, but in only a quarter of those infected with chlamydia.

Chronic genital infection (chronic PID)

Chronic genital infection is a long-term sequela of acute or subacute infection and may follow post-abortion or puerperal infection. It may present as a pyosalpinx, a hydrosalpinx or a chronic tubo-ovarian abscess (Fig. 33.8). In other cases the infection involves the connective tissues of the pelvis, causing chronic pelvic cellulitis.

Pyosalpinx

Pyosalpinx, or 'chronic pus tube', forms as a result of blockage of the lumen of the oviduct at the fimbrial end and at one or more points along the Fallopian tube. This occurs in the acute phase of the infection, and exudate accumulates, distending the oviduct to a greater or lesser degree (Fig. 33.9). The distension of the oviduct flattens the endosalpinx and the wall of the oviduct is thickened by the inflammatory process. Because the inflammatory process extends through the wall of the oviduct, adhesions to surrounding structures are common. The ovary may be involved to form a chronic tubo-ovarian abscess.

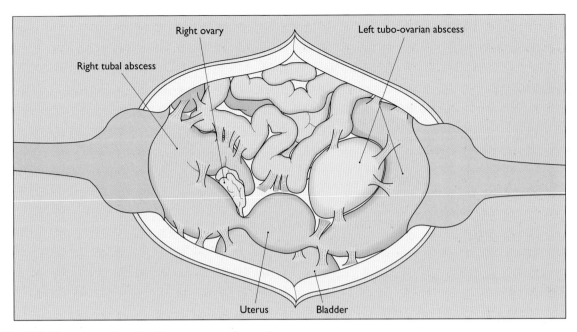

Fig. 33.8 Bilateral pyosalpingitis – the appearance at operation.

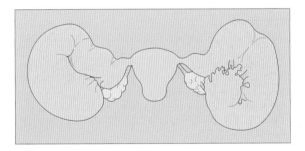

Fig. 33.9 Bilateral chronic salpingitis.

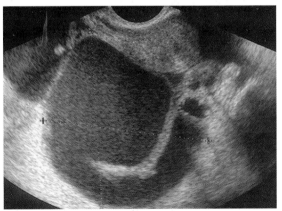

Fig. 33.10 Vaginal ultrasound showing a 7 cm diameter fluid-filled hydrosalpinx.

There may be no symptoms, or vague pelvic pain may occur which is intermittent or constant. It is often worse in the premenstrual phase of the menstrual cycle, and some women complain of deep dyspareunia. These symptoms are not specific for chronic pelvic infection and may be due to psychosomatic conditions. The symptoms may vary in severity, possibly because of an exacerbation of the infective process. This may occur months or years after the first infection. Laparoscopy may be needed to establish the diagnosis. In some cases the woman becomes acutely ill.

Treatment of chronic pyosalpinx which is causing symptoms is surgical. The extent of the surgery depends on the severity of the condition and, in general, requires bilateral salpingectomy and often oophorectomy, although some ovarian tissue may be saved. Hysterectomy is also usually performed in case residual infection is present.

Hydrosalpinx

Hydrosalpinx (Fig. 33.10) is the end result of burnt-out pyogenic salpingitis, which was of low virulence but highly irritating, producing large quantities of clear exudate within the closed portion of the oviduct. The distended oviduct has a thin wall, which is translucent and usually retort-shaped (Fig. 33.11). Adhesions to contiguous structures may be present.

Hydrosalpinx may be symptomless, but if symptoms are present they are many and variable. They include general ill-health, lassitude, disturbances of menstruation

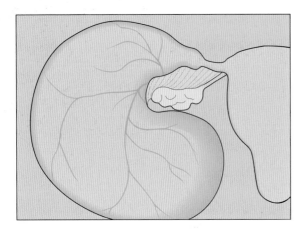

Fig. 33.11 Hydrosalpinx. Note the retort-shaped distension of the oviduct.

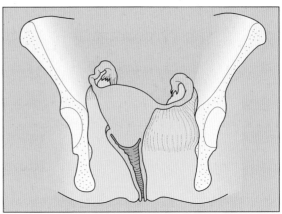

Fig. 33.12 Chronic pelvic cellulitis.

and chronic aching in the lower abdomen, which is worse premenstrually. Abdominal examination often shows no abnormality. Vaginal examination may reveal generalized tenderness or a smooth cystic enlargement. Because of these non-specific complaints, laparoscopy is often required to make a diagnosis. Treatment is surgical. The extent of the surgery is determined by the condition of the other Fallopian tube and the woman's desire to have children.

Chronic pelvic cellulitis

Chronic pelvic cellulitis is less common today but still occurs. It is usually the sequela of acute pelvic cellulitis and results in thickening and fibrosis of the connective tissues of the parametrium, with the result that the position of the uterus is distorted and it is relatively or absolutely immobilized (Fig. 33.12). The symptoms of chronic pelvic cellulitis are variable. The most common complaint is a chronic deep pelvic ache, often localized to one side, and backache. Deep dyspareunia is frequent, and may be so severe as to prevent sexual intercourse. Vaginal examination shows a tender uterus drawn to one side and relatively fixed in position.

Treatment is unsatisfactory; some patients respond to pelvic short-wave diathermy, and hysterectomy is another option. Unfortunately, in spite of treatment, in many women the pain persists.

Tuberculous infection of the genital tract

In the developed countries genital tract tuberculosis is very uncommon, accounting for less than 0.5% of all pelvic infections. In regions where *Mycobacterium tuberculosis* is endemic the incidence is much higher. The disease is spread in the postprimary haematogenous phase of tuberculosis. If this happens to coincide with puberty, when increased growth both of the internal genital organs and of the supply of blood thereto occurs, infection may also occur. The disease may be limited to the oviducts, but spread to the endometrium is common. Symptoms are minimal, and the condition is detected when investigations for infertility are made. Treatment is that for pulmonary tuberculosis, surgery only being used when there are large adnexal masses and after medical treatment has been tried.

Chapter | 34 |

Atrophic and dystrophic conditions

In the years after the menopause the internal genital organs become smaller and atrophic. These changes occur because the amount of circulating oestrogen falls to a very low level.

ATROPHIC CHANGES OF THE INTERNAL GENITAL ORGANS

Vulval atrophy in older women

By the time a woman reaches the age of 75 the uterus, the Fallopian tubes and the ovaries have shrunk considerably (Fig. 34.1). In the uterus, the endometrium has become atrophic and the muscle fibres of the myometrium have been progressively replaced by fibrous tissue. The cervix has atrophied and the cervical canal may become obliterated. If the woman develops uterine infection the pus might not escape, leading to a pyometra. This may also occur if the woman develops an endometrial or cervical carcinoma. The woman may complain of lower abdominal pain, and an examination shows that the uterus is larger than expected for her age. The diagnosis is confirmed by ultrasound scanning, which shows that the uterine cavity is enlarged and filled with fluid. If carcinoma is detected it is treated appropriately; if it is not present, the cervix is dilated and a drain inserted for a few days.

The vagina

The changes in the vagina depend on levels of oestrogen, which continues to be synthesized in peripheral tissues, but in most women the vaginal epithelium becomes atrophic. The superficial cells diminish in number, and intermediate and parabasal cells predominate. These changes show clinically as vaginal discomfort and burning, and painful intercourse.

The pelvic floor

Deprived of oestrogen, the blood supply to the muscles of the pelvic floor diminishes. The pelvic floor muscles lose their tone and the connective tissue loses its elasticity, with the result that pelvic floor tissues damaged during childbirth are likely to relax, with varying degrees of prolapse (see Ch. 38).

The vulva

As a woman's age increases, the labia majora lose their fat and elastic tissue content and become smaller, and the vaginal introitus is exposed. In very old women, only a narrow cleft indicates the presence of the vaginal introitus.

The vulval epithelium becomes thin, with loss of elastic and collagen fibres. These changes may lead to vulval irritation, although this may occur at earlier ages.

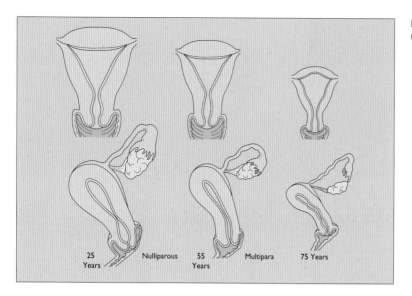

Fig. 34.1 Reduction in the size of the uterus in old age.

Vulval atrophy in younger women

Vulval atrophy may occur in a few younger women. It can cause considerable distress, not only because it is uncomfortable but because it prevents sexual intercourse, or makes it painful. The woman should be investigated for the presence of impaired glucose tolerance, and allergic conditions sought. Treatment is not very effective. The woman should be advised not to wear pantyhose, as these garments prevent ventilation and increase vulval moisture. Most medications are ineffective.

PRURITUS VULVAE (ITCHY VULVA)

One woman in 10 who attends a medical practitioner for genital tract disorders will say, among other complaints, that she has an itchy vulva. The reason may be infection, general skin or medical disease, or emotional problems. Emotional problems are thought to cause vulval itch in some women because both the skin covering the vulva, and its underlying capillaries, are unstable. Thus sexual or marital problems, anxiety and depression may manifest somatically as vulval itch.

Whatever the cause, the itch, mediated by a release of histamines, leads to scratching, which aggravates the itch. Over a period of months, the itch–scratch cycle may initiate a variety of histological changes in the vulval skin – non-neoplastic epithelial disorders of the skin and mucosa.

There have been a number of attempts to classify the disorders of the vulval epithelium. The most recent is shown in Box 34.1.

The most common vulval problem is lichen sclerosis, which presents with chronic pruritus, pain and

> **Box 34.1 Non-neoplastic vulval epithelial disorders: classification recommended by the International Society for the Study of Vulvar Disease (ISSVD)**
>
> **Non-neoplastic epithelial disorders of skin and mucosa**
> Lichen sclerosus
> Squamous hyperplasia
> Other dermatoses
>
> **Mixed non-neoplastic and neoplastic epithelial disorders**
>
> **Intraepithelial neoplasia**
> Squamous intraepithelial neoplasia
> VIN 1
> VIN 2
> VIN 3
> Non-squamous intraepithelial neoplasia
> Paget's disease
> Tumours of melanocytes, non-invasive

dyspareunia if there is ulceration and fissures. The skin may be reddish or normal in colour, and atrophic shiny white plaques are seen. A skin biopsy shows that the horny layer is unchanged or hyperkeratinized, with thinning of the epidermis and the disappearance of the rete pegs. The dermis is oedematous, with some degree of hyalinization, and collections of round cells are seen (Fig. 34.2).

Biopsy of the affected areas is indicated if there is any doubt about the diagnosis and/or malignancy or premalignancy

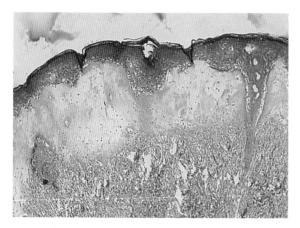

Fig. 34.2 Lichen sclerosis (atrophic pattern).

is suspected. Treatment is with topical corticosteroids, the most effective being clobetasol propionate applied nightly for 4 weeks, alternate nights required. The woman should be encouraged to use a soap substitute. Topical testosterone has been shown to be no more effective than emollients.

Squamous hyperplasia

The skin is usually reddened with exaggerated folds. In certain areas lichenified white patches may be seen. A biopsy specimen will show a thickened epithelium, with elongated papillae which retain their normal shape. The dermis is oedematous and contains numbers of plasma cells (Fig. 34.3).

Vulval intraepithelial neoplasia (VIN) is discussed in Chapter 37.

Aetiology

Studies of women who have pruritus show that this disease has a varied aetiology.

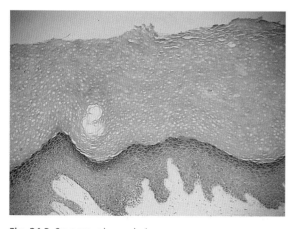

Fig. 34.3 Squamous hyperplasia.

General skin diseases

The conditions listed in Table 34.1 are the usual skin diseases that may manifest as pruritus vulvae. Fungal infections may also cause vulval itch, although the itch is generally intercrural.

General diseases

The most common general disease causing pruritus vulvae is diabetes mellitus. In diabetes, as well as being itchy, the vulva is swollen and dark red.

Allergic dermatitis

Sensitivity to soap (usually perfumed), some detergents used to wash pantyhose, and other contact allergens may cause vulval itch.

Vaginal infections

The most common causes of vulval itch, particularly in younger women, are vaginal infections, particularly candidiasis and trichomoniasis. As candidal infection of the vulval skin is common, vulval skin scrapings should be taken in cases where general diseases and allergic causes have been eliminated. It may also be helpful to inspect the vulval skin through a magnifying glass or a colposcope.

Human papilloma virus (HPV) infection is no longer thought to be a cause of pruritus vulvae but may be found on biopsy.

Psychosocial causes

Pruritus vulvae is of organic aetiology in more than two-thirds of women with the disease. It is thought that psychosocial causes account for the remainder.

Table 34.1 The itchy vulva: aetiology

	PERCENTAGE OF CASES
General skin diseases (psoriasis, leucoderma, lichen planus, intertrigo, scabies)	5
General diseases (diabetes, ? deficiency diseases)	5
Allergic dermatitis	5
Vaginal discharges Trichomoniasis Candidiasis	50
Psychosomatic conditions	35

Investigation of pruritus vulvae

Because psychosocial factors are involved in many cases, the history of the condition is crucial and questions should be asked about the period before the itching became distressing. The patient's general health should be assessed and questions asked about her general and sexual relationships (including, when appropriate, sexual abuse in childhood). Any concerns raised should be explored. The history will determine whether the main area of itch is vulval, anal or intercrural. If it is one of the last two, the cause is probably threadworms, tinea or intertrigo. The woman should be asked about any allergic conditions, including contact dermatitis and drug sensitivity. The duration of the pruritus should be determined. If it is longer than 12 months, multiple skin biopsies using a dermatome should be considered, irrespective of the age of the woman or the appearance of the vulva.

General skin condition should be assessed by examining the patient in a good light and inspecting all body surfaces, including the interdigital folds of the feet and hands.

General medical causes should be considered, particularly glycosuria. The urine should also be checked for protein. In elderly women, a 2-hour postprandial or fasting blood sugar test should be ordered.

The vagina should be inspected and swabs taken, on more than one occasion, to exclude candidiasis and trichomoniasis. A skin scraping for vulval candida infection should be taken if the pruritus has persisted for more than 6 months.

Candidal infection of the vulval skin may cause cyclic, episodic itching or burning and, occasionally, postcoital vulvovaginal irritation. The syndrome is termed cyclical vulvovestibulitis.

Treatment

Any aetiological factor detected should be treated. Medical treatment is the appropriate course in cases of lichen sclerosis and squamous cell hyperplasia, unless a skin biopsy shows VIN3, when surgical or laser treatment is indicated. Surgery by simple vulvectomy has been largely abandoned because pruritus recurs in more than 50% of cases. The patient must be made aware that to obtain a cure, medical treatment must be continued over a long period. During this time, attempts should be made to discover any psychological upsets that might have precipitated the pruritus.

Perfumed sprays, creams or lotions should not be applied to the vulva: in fact, it is preferable to apply nothing but water. Douching, if used, should cease and close-fitting pants and pantyhose should be avoided.

Topical corticosteroids are prescribed. Initially, a high-potency topical steroid cream, such as diprosone OV or clobetasone (Dermovate), is applied twice daily for 2–3 weeks, and then daily for 1 month. After this, a less potent topical corticosteroid, such as hydrocortisone or Trimovate, is prescribed.

If the itch is severe, a sedative should be prescribed to help the woman sleep at night. Elderly women may obtain relief if hormone replacement treatment (see p. 325) is tried. The patient requires a good deal of support and reassurance over the period of treatment, but should be made aware that, in time, the itch ceases in about 90% of patients.

VULVODYNIA (CHRONIC VULVAL BURNING OR PAIN)

Vulvodynia is a disorder with a prevalence of 9–12%. The woman experiences chronic burning, stinging, irritation, rawness and, sometimes, pain in the vulvo-vestibular area. In a subset of vulvodynia the woman complains of severe vulval pain after sexual intercourse, during penile entry, or when one or more areas of the vulva is touched with a cottonwool swab. The area of tenderness may be reddened. The aetiology of the condition has not been resolved but it is considered to be multifactorial with both organic and functional elements. There is evidence of proinflammatory markers and increased intraepithelial innervation in biopsies taken from the affected sites. There is also increased central sensitization so that the woman may experience abnormal sensory and motor pain elsewhere in her body. A diagnosis of vulvodynia is made by exclusion, and the symptoms may last for months or years. Vulvodynia can have profound effects on a woman's life, leading to depression, low self-esteem, the avoidance of sexual intercourse and relationship problems. A good psychosocial and sexual history is necessary. Vaginismus may precede or follow the vulval symptoms. A previous and current history of stressful events, psychological and psychiatric problems may help plan management.

Treatment by a multidisciplinary team is recommended, and may include topical xylocaine 5% ointment, an antidepressant (SSRI (selective serotonin reuptake inhibitor)), cognitive behavioural and pain management therapy, and psychotherapy. Dilatation of the vaginal introitus and Kegel exercises will help pelvic floor and vulval tension and help patients overcome anxiety and their fear of vulval pain. In carefully selected cases vestibulectomy gives good long-term relief of symptoms.

Endometriosis and adenomyosis

ENDOMETRIOSIS

Endometriosis denotes presence of functioning endometrial tissue in an abnormal location, in other words, outside the uterus (Box 35.1). The locations and the approximate chance of the lesion affecting the organ or structure are shown in Figure 35.1.

The incidence of endometriosis is difficult to determine, as in many instances it is only discovered at laparoscopy when the patient presents with infertility or abdominal pain. A probable estimate is that between 5 and 10% of women in their reproductive years have endometriosis. Endometriosis is found more commonly in women who have more spontaneous menstrual cycles, for example when menarche is early or childbearing delayed. The incidence is lower when women are taking oral contraception and have a history of smoking. There is emerging evidence of a genetic component to the development of endometriosis as the incidence is up to seven times greater in the relatives of affected women compared with those without a family history. It appears to be linked to chromosomes 7 and 10.

Aetiology

How the endometrium reaches the ectopic locations is not entirely understood. The explanation to account for most of the endometrial lesions is retrograde passage of endometrial tissue along the Fallopian tubes during menstruation. This is supported by the observation that endometriosis only occurs in primates that menstruate and that explains the majority of sites where it is found: on the ovaries, the uterosacral ligament, or in the cul-de-sac (pouch of Douglas). It is believed that retrograde menstruation occurs in most women, but the development of other than temporary endometrial nodules (blisters) only occurs in some women. To explain the rare deposits of endometriosis in distant sites, for example the umbilicus, the lung and eye, lymphatic or haematogenous spread has been suggested. Metaplasia of mesothelial coelomic cells into endometrial cells has also been suggested.

Once viable endometriotic tissue has reached and adhered to the ectopic location, it still has to be explained why it survives and grows, instead of being eliminated by macrophages. A current theory is that there may be a defect in cell-mediated immunity which permits the endometrial tissue to survive. In order to grow in these ectopic sites, the endometrial tissue has to respond to cyclical oestrogen and, to a lesser extent, progesterone. If a constant oestrogen milieu occurs, as in pregnancy, the lesions tend to be attacked by macrophages and become fibrotic.

Box 35.1 **Endometriosis**

What is it?	Functioning endometrial tissue which is outside the uterus, most commonly found on the uterosacral ligament and ovary
Aetiology	Not understood, as retrograde menstruation (along the fallopian tubes) occurs in most women
	Why the endometrial lesions fail to be attacked by macrophages in some women is not understood
Prevalence	Probably occurs in 5–10% of women and can regress, remain unchanged or progress
	More common among women with more spontaneous menstrual cycles
Diagnosis	Can only be diagnosed at laparoscopy and confirmed by biopsy
Symptoms	Frequently symptomless, the main reasons for investigation being menstrual irregularities, premenstrual 'dysmenorrhoea' pain, non-cyclical pelvic pain, dyspareunia and infertility
Management	Depends on the woman's age, her desire for pregnancy, the severity of the symptoms and the extent of the lesions
	Hormonal – to prevent the cyclical ovarian production of oestrogen, and to a lesser extent progesterone
	Surgical – laser or diathermy ablation of the lesions, ovarian cystectomy, conservative surgery or hysterectomy with bilateral oophorectomy
Outcome	All treatments are beneficial in the short term
	Five years after either hormonal or surgical treatment has ceased endometriosis recurs in 20–40% of women
	Cystectomy is superior to drainage for endometriomata
	Surgery is superior to hormonal treatment for pain symptoms if bilateral oophorectomy is performed

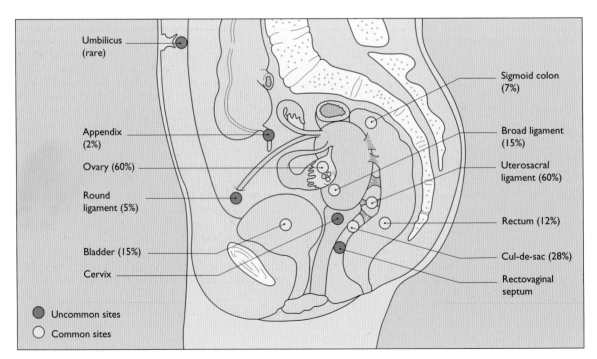

Fig. 35.1 Common and uncommon sites of extra-uterine endometriosis. The figures given in parentheses indicate the approximate chance of the lesion affecting the organ or structure.

Why endometriosis spontaneously regresses or fails to progress in half of the cases is also not fully understood.

Pathology

Whatever the location, the ectopic endometrium, surrounded by stroma, implants and forms a miniature cyst, which responds to the cyclic secretion of oestrogen and progesterone, just as the uterine endometrium does. During menstruation, bleeding occurs in the cyst, and the blood, endometrial tissue and tissue fluid are trapped. Over the next cycle, the tissue fluid and the blood plasma are absorbed, leaving dark, thickened blood. The cycle recurs each month and slowly the cyst enlarges, containing increased amounts of tarry, chocolate-coloured inspissated blood. The maximal size of the cyst depends on its location. Small cysts may remain small, or be attacked by macrophages and become small fibrotic lesions. Ovarian cysts (endometriomata) tend to be larger than other cysts, but do not usually become larger than a medium-sized orange. As the cyst grows, internal pressure may destroy the active endometrial lining, making the cyst non-functional.

Rupture or leakage of material from even small cysts is not uncommon. The released inspissated blood is very irritating, with the result that multiple adhesions surround the cysts. The ectopic endometrium and stromal cells also tend to infiltrate adjacent tissues, leading to more pelvic adhesions and fixation (Fig. 35.2). If an ovarian cyst is found which looks like an endometrioma, but there are no adhesions, the diagnosis is unlikely to be endometriosis.

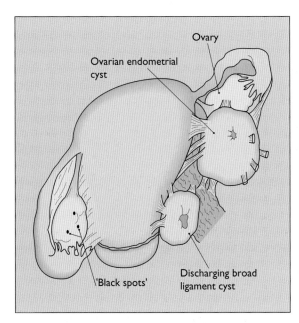

Fig. 35.2 Extra-uterine endometriosis.

Endometriotic tissue, compared with endometrium, has increased levels of oestrogen, prostaglandins and acute inflammatory cytokines such as interleukin-1β, interleukin-6 and tumour necrosis factor. These inflammatory cytokines in company with increased proteolytic metalloproteins may promote implantation of the endometrial fragments. The prostaglandin release is enhanced by increased cyclooxygenase (COX) expression and is mediated by increased oestradiol, including endometriotic oestradiol, and vascular endothelial growth factor (VEGF) levels. The increased prostaglandin production directly induces pain (PGE_2), vasoconstriction and uterine contractions ($PGF_{2\alpha}$) and inflammatory and immune responses. Progesterone does not appear to have a major role in the pathogenesis and endometriotic tissue has very low levels of progesterone receptors.

As mentioned, the ovary is most often involved, and ovarian endometriosis may present as small superficial implants (red or black spots) or a larger endometrial cyst. Lesions on the surface of the broad ligament occur either directly from implanting endometrial tissue or as a secondary spread from the ovarian deposit. In these locations the endometrial deposits cause puckering of the peritoneum and adhesions to the posterior surface of the uterus, often fixing it in retroversion. Lesions in the cul-de-sac are of interest, as they may not be palpable or visualized by a laparoscope unless the laparoscopy is made during menstruation.

Clinical features

The clinical features of endometriosis are often non-specific. In at least a quarter of women who have the disease it is symptomless. The symptoms may be bizarre because of the varying locations of the disease and, in many cases, the lack of correlation with the extent of the lesions. They include pain, menstrual irregularities, dyspareunia and infertility.

Pain

Typically, lower abdominal crampy pain starts premenstrually, reaches its peak in the last few days of menstruation and then slowly subsides. This symptom is often referred to as acquired dysmenorrhoea. If the endometrial cysts are large and adhesions are present, or if lesions involve the peritoneum over the bowel, the woman may complain of constant lower abdominal or pelvic pain which varies in intensity, and she may have pain on defecation.

Menstrual disturbances

In 60% of women menstrual irregularities occur. The woman may complain of premenstrual staining or spotting, heavy menstrual periods (menorrhagia), or more frequent periods, which may be heavy.

Dyspareunia

If the endometriotic lesions involve the cul-de-sac, particularly if the uterus is retroverted and fixed by adhesions, the woman may complain of dyspareunia on deep penile penetration.

Infertility

Although endometriosis is associated with infertility, whether it is a cause of infertility is disputed, unless the lesions are severe and distort the anatomy. Usually endometriosis is not suspected until a laparoscopy, made during the course of infertility investigations, reveals the disease.

Clinical examination

Abdominal and pelvic examination may show no abnormality if the lesions are small. It has been suggested that the pelvic examination should be made during menstruation, or soon after, to detect lesions in the pouch of Douglas that may not be apparent at other times of the menstrual cycle. Larger cysts cause fixed, tender nodular swellings and may be easily palpable.

Diagnosis

It is often difficult clinically to distinguish endometriosis from pelvic inflammatory disease or an ovarian cyst. Because of this, it is necessary to visualize the lesions through a laparoscope and to biopsy them to confirm the diagnosis. At laparoscopy the extent of the disease should be determined, as this will influence the treatment (Table 35.1).

Management of endometriosis

The management of endometriosis depends on the extent of the disease (see Table 35.1), on the severity of the symptoms, and on the desire of the woman to retain her fecundity. In primary care the combined oral contraceptive and non-steroidal anti-inflammatory drugs should be included. Figure 35.3 is an algorithm showing the management of this disease, details of which will now be discussed.

Table 35.1 The management of endometriosis

STAGE	CHARACTERISTICS	DIAGNOSIS	TREATMENT
I, II	**Minimal, Mild**		
	Small surface nodules with no scarring or peritubal adhesions	Only by laparoscopy in investigation of infertility	At most, electrocautery or CO_2 laser to lesions Do not give hormones
III	**Moderate**		
	Small scattered surface lesions with scarring; ovarian endometriomata, <2.5 cm, few periovarian or peritubal adhesions; nodules in the cul-de-sac or uterosacral ligaments	Often symptoms but confirmation by laparoscopy needed	Electrocautery or CO_2 laser to lesions Hormones Conservative surgery if hormones fail to relieve symptoms
IV	**Severe**		
	Ovarian endometriomata >2.5 cm; marked adhesions of ovary or tubes, cul-de-sac obliteration	Symptoms and signs Laparotomy confirms	Conservative surgery Hormones Hysterectomy and salpingo-oophorectomy
V	**Very severe**		
	Stage III plus involvement of bowel, bladder, ureter, etc.	Laparotomy Barium enema Intravenous pyelogram	Surgery Hormones, if surgery incomplete

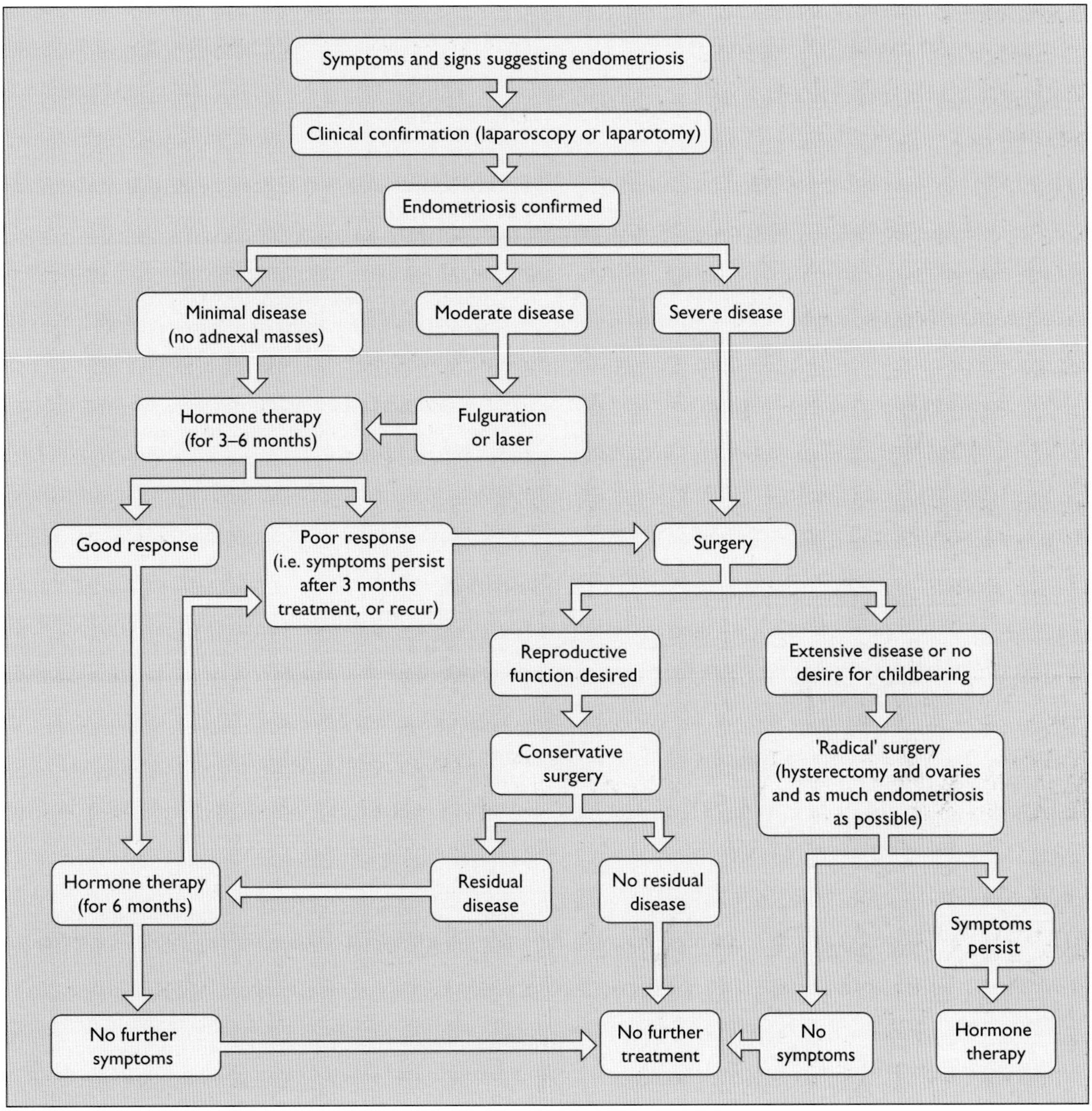

Fig. 35.3 Management of endometriosis.

Hormonal treatment

Oral contraception may be useful for symptomatic relief. Four additional regimens of hormonal treatment have been used. These treatments suppress or reduce oestrogen synthesis and release. In consequence, menstruation ceases and this inhibits further growth of the lesions, permits the body defences to absorb the contents of the lesions, and leads to their fibrosis. The hormonal treatments are danazol, gonadotrophin-releasing hormone (GnRH) agonists, gestrinone and medroxyprogesterone acetate.

Danazol

Danazol, an isoxazole derivative of 17α-ethinyl testosterone, reduces the number of GnRH receptors in the pituitary gland and causes a reduction in the level of sex hormone-binding globulin (SHBG). The fall in SHBG causes an increase in free testosterone and a fall in unbound oestradiol. Danazol may also act directly on the ovary to reduce steroid synthesis.

Danazol is given for 3–6 months, depending on the extent of the lesions and on the response. The symptoms are usually relieved in 2–6 weeks in three-quarters of women treated. The effect of danazol on the endometriotic lesions is discussed later. Adverse effects include:

- Amenorrhoea in 60% of women and oligomenorrhoea in the remainder
- An increase in weight, often more than 3 kg
- Oily skin or acne in 20% of women
- Deepening voice in 10% of women (irreversible).

GnRH agonists

GnRH agonists render the pituitary gonadotrophs insensitive to stimulation by endogenous GnRH, with resulting suppression of ovarian steroid secretion. The drug is given intranasally or as a long-acting injection for 3–6 months. The effect on the endometriosis is similar to that of danazol. Adverse effects include:

- Nearly all women experience hot flushes, which may be severe.
- Amenorrhoea develops in 70% of women.
- Reversible bone loss of 2–4% over a 6-month period occurs in 3% of women. However, fewer patients complain of side-effects than with danazol.

Gestrinone

Gestrinone is a progestogen with mixed agonist and antagonist effects and has actions similar to those of other androgen analogues, including danazol.

Medroxyprogesterone acetate

This progestogen has been used for the past 30 years. Side-effects of nausea, weight gain, oily hair, acne and mood disturbances are common.

Levonorgestrel intrauterine systems (Mirena)

LNG-IUS effectively reduce the pain associated with endometriosis and this is maintained over the life of the IUS.

Complementary treatments

There is a paucity of good evidence on the effectiveness of such treatments as acupuncture, homeopathy, reflexology, traditional Chinese medicine, herbal treatments, vitamin B_1 and magnesium. Some women do report that they find them beneficial as part of a holistic approach to their care.

Longer-term adverse effects of the medications

The first four regimens of treatment, if continued for more than 6 months, lead to bone loss, which is increased if GnRH agonists are used. Some women develop severe hot flushes and other symptoms of oestrogen deficiency. These women, and those who require a longer course of GnRH agonists, can be treated with hormone replacement therapy (HRT) (see p. 325), the so-called 'add-back' treatment.

Outcome

The effect of each of these hormonal treatments is similar in terms of relief of pain and reduction in the severity of the endometriosis, as judged by a second-look laparoscopy after treatment has ceased and the woman has had at least one menstrual period. Danazol and GnRH agonists have been shown to reduce the pain for longer than placebo after treatment is ceased, but have no effect on infertility. The results are:

- In 30% of the women complete regression of the disease will have occurred.
- In 60% partial regression will have occurred.
- In 10% the extent of the disease is unchanged, although the symptoms have been relieved or cured. The findings suggest that further courses of treatment may be needed. Once hormonal treatment ceases, the mean duration for pain to recur is 5–6 months.

It should be noted that the more extensive the disease the greater the chance of recurrence.

Surgery

Small lesions detected with laparoscopy can be treated by diathermy or laser ablation under laparoscopic vision. Laser ablation results in an improvement in symptoms in over 60% of women. Larger lesions, particularly those involving the ovaries, require more extensive surgery. The procedure depends on the patient's age, her desire for children and the difficulty of the operation. If the woman desires a pregnancy (provided there are no other bars to conception), the aim should be to conserve as much ovarian tissue as possible by dissecting out or marsupializing the endometrial cysts. Cystectomy is more effective than simple drainage. A multicentre RCT has shown that laparoscopic ablation increases conception rates and reduces dysmenorrhoea and dyspareunia, although there is a significant rate of recurrence after 6 months. In women who have no desire for a further pregnancy total hysterectomy and bilateral oophorectomy may be appropriate, provided that they are informed about the procedure and have had the opportunity to think about it and discuss it with the surgeon. In some cases hysterectomy will not relieve the symptoms as the endometrial nodules are extra-uterine and often deep in the pouch of Douglas. These deposits are difficult to access.

Psychological aspects of endometriosis

The knowledge that she has endometriosis can cause considerable distress to a woman. In part, this is because of the poor correlation between the size and number of the lesions and the symptomatology, and in part it is due to the publicity that endometriosis receives in the popular press.

The doctor should explain what endometriosis is and what it is not. The differentiation between endometriosis and the premenstrual syndrome needs to be discussed because some symptoms are similar. The relationship between endometriosis and infertility needs to be discussed and treatment strategies outlined. The woman should be made aware of the choices of hormonal treatment and surgery (or a combination of the two), and of their relative merits in her case. The fact that endometriosis may recur following either treatment needs to be brought to her attention. However, the doctor should offer qualified optimism about the outcome, and should stress the importance of adequate follow-up.

ADENOMYOSIS

Adenomyosis is the presence of functioning endometrial tissue which has penetrated the myometrium by direct spread from the uterine lining (Box 35.2).

Pathology

The cells that infiltrate the muscle derive mainly from the basal layer of the endometrium. As this layer is relatively insensitive to hormonal stimulation the adenomyotic nodules tend to be small, containing little blood, but they provoke a marked stromal reaction. The lesion also appears to stimulate myometrial proliferation, causing the tumour to enlarge slowly (Fig. 35.4). Clinically, adenomyosis may be indistinguishable from a myoma, and both may coexist. As the growth of the clinical adenomyoma takes time, clinical adenomyosis tends to occur later in the reproductive years, often in parous women after a long period of secondary infertility.

Clinical features

One-third of patients are asymptomatic. In the remainder the main symptoms are:

- Progressively increasing pain, usually associated with menstruation. In this case the pain increases throughout menstruation, reaching its peak towards the latter stages.
- Menstrual irregularities, such as premenstrual staining and spotting, increased flow, or more frequent periods.

Management of adenomyosis

At pelvic examination the uterus is found to be enlarged and tender, and there may be discrete adenomyomata which are indistinguishable from myomata. If the woman has no symptoms and the adenomyoma is not large, no treatment is needed. If the woman has symptoms, hysterectomy is the preferred treatment as adenomyosis does not respond well to hormone treatment.

Box 35.2 **Adenomyosis**	
What is it?	Infiltration of basal endometrial cells into the uterine muscle
Aetiology	Unknown
Prevalence	Greater in women who are of later reproductive age
Diagnosis	Pelvic examination, uterus large and tender
Symptoms	Symptomless in a third of women, menstrual irregularities, pain of increasing severity, frequently occurring during menstruation
Management	Depends on size and severity of symptoms, no treatment or hysterectomy

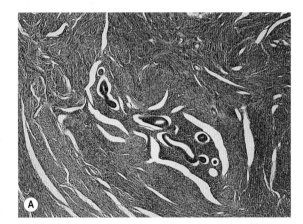

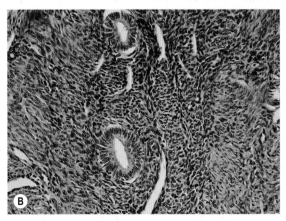

Fig. 35.4 The microscopic appearance of adenomyosis. (A) The adenomyotic nodule is lying deep in the myometrium, and both glands and stroma are present. (B) Another specimen at higher magnification showing the glands and the stroma, which is quite dense.

Chapter 36

Benign tumours, cysts and malformations of the genital tract

Benign tumours or cysts may form in any part of the genital tract. Benign tumours occur most often in the uterus and most benign cysts occur in the ovaries. Malformations tend to involve the uterus and the vagina.

MALFORMATIONS OF THE GENITAL TRACT

In a female fetus the Müllerian ducts develop from the paramesonephric ducts, growing caudally on each side. By the 35th day after fertilization the lower part of the ducts change direction and grow towards the midline, where they meet and fuse with each other and then grow caudally once again. By the 65th day they have completed the fusion and their medial walls have gradually disappeared to form a single hollow tube (Fig. 36.1). The most caudal portion, which will become the vagina, becomes solid and fuses with an ingrowth of endodermal cells from the cloaca. By the 20th gestational week, the solid growth has recanalized and the external genitalia have formed (Fig. 36.2).

Malformations of the genital tract occur when the process described above does not occur. The error may be one of failure of the recanalization process, or may be a failure of the two Müllerian ducts to fuse.

Failure of recanalization

The most common defect is an imperforate hymen or transverse septum, which should be detectable during the examination of the neonate. If it is not detected until after puberty, menstrual discharge may collect in the vagina and, in long-term cases, may distend the uterus and tubes (Fig. 36.3). Treatment is to make a cruciate incision in the hymen septum and permit the inspissated fluid to escape slowly. Less common defects produce complete or partial vaginal atresia.

Failure of the ducts to form or to fuse

One or other duct may fail to form, and only one Fallopian tube and a distorted unicornate uterus may be found. If both ducts fail to form the woman will be amenorrhoeic.

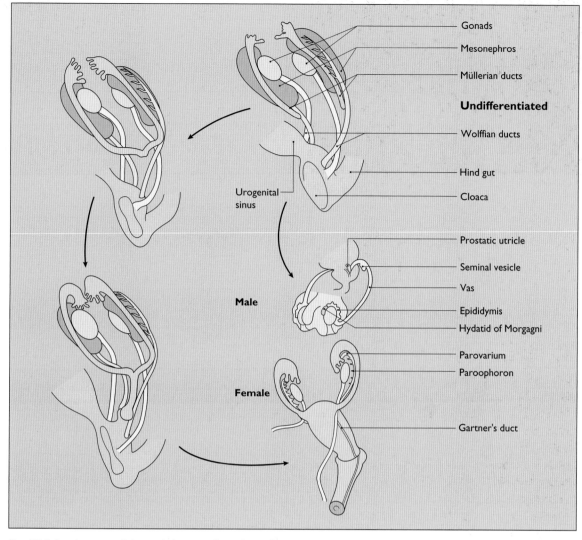

Fig. 36.1 Development of the genital organs, from the Müllerian duct in the female and the Wolffian duct in the male.

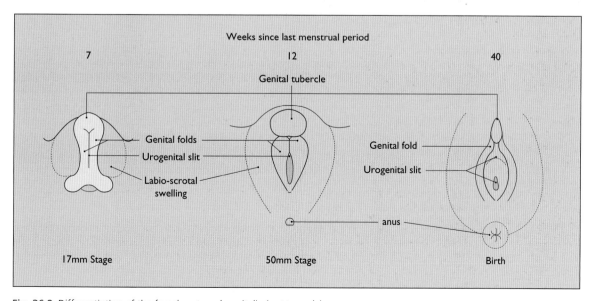

Fig. 36.2 Differentiation of the female external genitalia (not to scale).

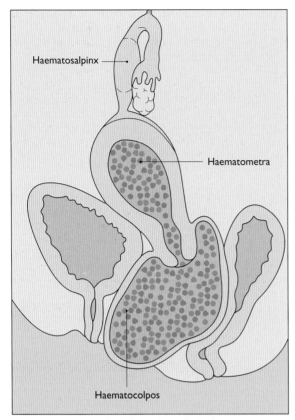

Fig. 36.3 Haematocolpos due to imperforate hymen septum.

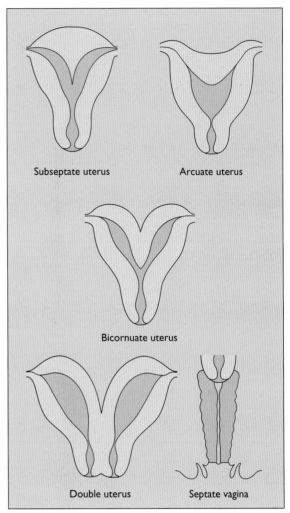

Fig. 36.4 Common genital tract malformations.

Failure of the two Müllerian ducts to fuse leads to one of several malformations (Fig. 36.4). Most of these malformations do not reduce the woman's fertility, but should pregnancy occur there is an increased risk of late miscarriage and premature labour. A subseptate uterus may lead to recurrent abortion, and can be treated by excising the septum by surgery or laser. If the woman has a bicornuate uterus and becomes pregnant, the fetus may present as a transverse lie in late pregnancy.

VULVAL TUMOURS

Because the tissues of the vulva are covered by skin, tumours arising in them are similar to those occurring in any part of the integument. A few women develop vulval varicosities, which may cause discomfort and are more marked in pregnancy.

VAGINAL TUMOURS

Vaginal cysts are uncommon, but occasionally one develops in the lateral wall of the upper vagina. It is a cyst of a remnant of the degenerate Wolffian duct and is referred to as a Gartner's duct cyst. A cystic swelling may occur in the anterior wall of the vagina, directly below the urethra: this is a urethral diverticulum. If it becomes infected, the woman complains of dysuria and frequency of urination. Occasionally, a myoma may develop beneath the vaginal epithelium.

CERVICAL TUMOURS

The most common cervical tumour is a cervical polyp, which occurs as the result of localized hyperplasia of the epithelium and stroma covering a ridge between two clefts in the cervical canal. The columnar epithelium covering the polyp may undergo squamous metaplasia, or ulcerate. The main symptoms are intermittent or postcoital bleeding, although many cervical polyps are symptomless. The diagnosis is made on inspection of the cervix. The polyp can be removed by twisting the pedicle, and the tissue should be sent for histopathology. Other tumours that may be detected occasionally are genital papillomata and fibroids.

UTERINE TUMOURS

Endometrial polyps

Endometrial polyps may occur in association with endometrial hyperplasia and may be a cause of abnormal uterine bleeding. They are detected by curettage, provided a polyp forceps is also introduced into the uterus (Fig. 36.5), or by hysteroscopy.

Uterine fibroids (leiomyomata, fibromyomas)

These are the most common tumours of the genital tract. A uterine fibroid is composed of smooth muscle bundles interspersed with strands of connective tissue, surrounded by a thin capsule (Box 36.1). The tumour may arise in any part of the Müllerian duct, but occurs most often in the myometrium, where several may develop simultaneously. The tumour may vary from the size of a pea to that of a football.

Fibroids occur in about 5% of women during the reproductive years. They grow slowly and may only be detectable clinically in the fourth decade of life, when the incidence increases to about 20%. They are more common in nulliparous women or women who have had only one child.

Their aetiology is unclear. They may arise from normal muscle cells, from immature muscle cells in the myometrium, or from embryonal cells in the walls of uterine blood vessels. Whatever their origin, the tumours begin as tiny multiple seedlings which are scattered through the myometrium. The seedlings grow very slowly but progressively (over years rather than months), under the influence of circulating oestrogens, and, unless detected and treated, as most are today, may form a tumour weighing 10 kg or more. At first the tumour is intramural, but as it grows it may develop in several directions. This is shown in Figure 36.6. After the menopause, as oestrogen is no longer secreted in any great quantity, fibroids tend to atrophy.

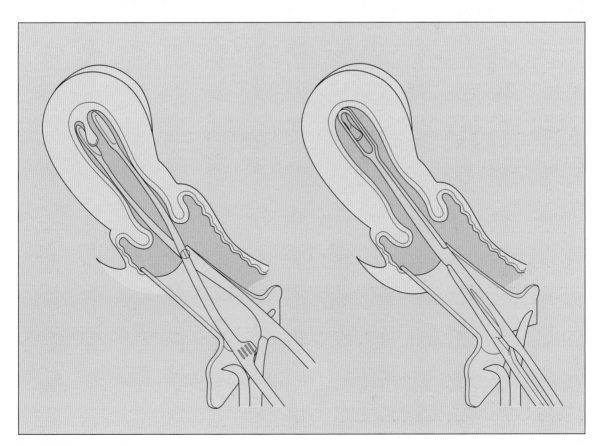

Fig. 36.5 The use of polyp forceps to secure and remove endometrial polyps.

Box 36.1 **Fibroids**

What are they?	Encapsulated smooth muscle fibres interspersed with strands of connective tissue usually developing in the myometrium. They may remain intramural or grow outwards or into the uterine cavity. Dependent on an intact blood supply
Aetiology	Unclear
Prevalence	Increases from 5% to 20% of women during their reproductive years. More common in nulliparous women and those of low parity. Very slow growing in response to oestrogen. Regress after menopause
Diagnosis	Examination and confirmatory ultrasound
Symptoms	Depend on size and position and are frequently symptomless. Two most common symptoms are abnormal vaginal bleeding, usually heavy and/or prolonged, and pelvic discomfort, crampy or pressure
Management	Depends on rate of growth, size, symptoms and desire for pregnancy • Relief from bleeding, anaemia • Wait and see • Myomectomy to preserve fertility, possibly in conjunction with a GnRh analogue to shrink the tumour temporarily • Hysterectomy
Outcome	Hysterectomy is the treatment of choice for women comfortable with its psychological and physical sequelae Myomectomy is associated with a 40% chance of successful conception and a 5% recurrence of the fibroid or menorrhagia GnRH analogue is not suitable for long-term treatment
Pregnancy complications	Early pregnancy bleeding, premature rupture of membranes, obstructed labour and postpartum haemorrhage

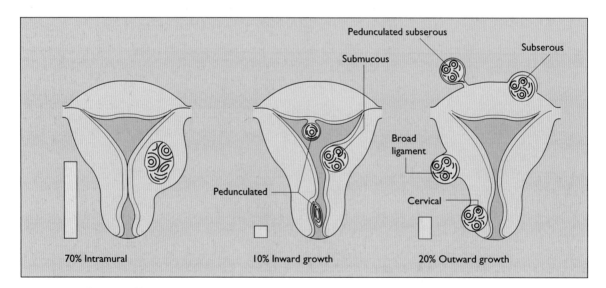

Fig. 36.6 Development of fibroids.

Pathology

If the tumour is cut, it pouts above the surrounding myometrium as its capsule contracts. Whitish-grey in colour, it is composed of whorled intertwining bundles of muscles in a matrix of connective tissue (Fig. 36.7). At its periphery the muscle fibres are arranged in concentric layers, and the normal muscle fibres surrounding the tumour are similarly oriented. Between the tumour and the normal myometrium a thin layer of areolar tissue forms a pseudocapsule, through which the blood vessels enter the fibroid.

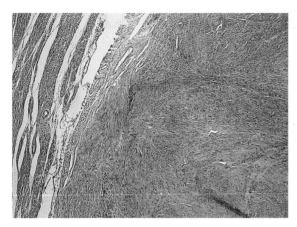

Fig. 36.7 Gross appearance of a fibroid.

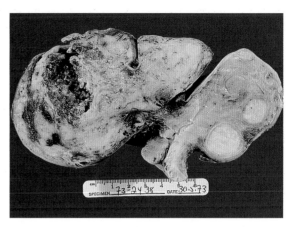

Fig. 36.9 Transvaginal ultrasound of a submucous fibroid 1 cm in diameter. Image enhanced by infusion of saline through transcervical catheter seen in upper-left on scan.

On microscopy, groups of spindle-shaped muscle cells, with elongated nuclei, are separated into bundles by connective tissue (Fig. 36.8). As the entire blood supply of the fibroid is derived from the few vessels entering from the pseudocapsule, the growth of the tumour means that it often outstrips its blood supply. This leads to degeneration, particularly in the central portion of the fibroid. Initially, hyaline degeneration occurs, which may become cystic, or calcification may occur over time – the 'womb stones' of 19th-century gynaecologists. In pregnancy, a rare complication (red degeneration) may occur. This follows extravasation of blood through the tumour, giving it a raw beef appearance. In less than 0.1% of tumours sarcomatous change occurs.

Symptomatology

The symptoms depend on the size and the position of the fibroid. Most small fibroids, and some larger ones, are symptomless and are only detected during a routine examination. If the fibroid is submucous, it may be associated with menorrhagia (Fig. 36.9). This may result from an increase of the endometrial surface, increasing uterine vascularity and blood flow, and changes in the ability of the uterus to contract.

If the heavy bleeding persists the woman may become anaemic and, as the uterus contracts, it may cause crampy pains. Submucous fibroids which become pedunculated may cause a persistent bloody discharge from the uterus.

Irrespective of their position in the uterus, large fibroids may cause pressure symptoms in the pelvis, dysuria and frequency, and constipation or backache if the enlarged uterus presses on the rectum. A cervical fibroid may cause pelvic pain and make sexual intercourse impossible.

Diagnosis

Abdominal and vaginal examination may show a 'knobbly' uterus, or a smooth enlargement of the uterus. When the cervix is moved the whole firm mass moves. In some cases the diagnosis is obvious, in others the smooth enlargement may be due to a pregnancy or to an ovarian mass. A pelvic ultrasound examination will establish the diagnosis.

Management

Four choices exist:

- To continue to observe the fibroid
- To perform a myomectomy
- To perform a hysterectomy
- To offer the woman gonadotrophin-releasing hormone analogue (GnRHa).

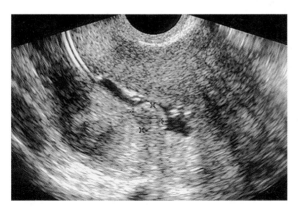

Fig. 36.8 The microscopic appearance of a fibroid. The bundles of spindle-shaped muscle cells run in several directions and tend to form a whorl-like pattern.

Observation

Symptomless fibroids smaller than a 14-week pregnancy may be observed. Other types of fibroids:

- Distort the uterine cavity and are considered a factor in the couple's infertility
- Are situated in the lower part of the uterus or the cervix, which would complicate childbirth
- Grow rapidly, which might suggest sarcomatous change.

If the fibroid is associated with menstrual disturbances a hysteroscopy is advisable to exclude intrauterine pathology.

Myomectomy

If the woman wishes to preserve her reproductive function, myomectomy may be chosen. Depending on the size and position, and the experience of the surgeon either a laparoscopic or an open abdominal approach will be selected. The operation removes all detected fibroids and reconstitutes the uterus. The woman must accept that, if problems arise during myomectomy, the surgeon may have to proceed to hysterectomy. Following myomectomy, 40% of women who have the opportunity to conceive will do so. If the surgeon did not have to open the uterine cavity then the woman can consider a vaginal delivery. In 5% of women the fibroids recur, and a similar number of women continue to have menorrhagia, which necessitates the use of medication (see p. 227), hysteroscopic resection or hysterectomy.

Hysterectomy

Total hysterectomy is the treatment of choice in older women, women who have no wish for a further pregnancy, and those who have menorrhagia or marked pressure symptoms. A patient should not be rushed into making a decision to have a hysterectomy. She should be given time to think and to ask questions about the procedure. The gynaecologist should also make sure that misconceptions about the operation are addressed. This is discussed on page 227.

GnRH analogue

Given by injection at intervals, the drug will suppress oestrogen secretion and consequently the fibroids will atrophy. The greatest effect is in the first month when, on average, there is a 27% reduction in size. After 3 months little further reduction in the size of the tumour is apparent. In 10% of cases the treatment is ineffective, and after cessation of treatment the fibroids will grow again. GnRH analogue has a small role in the treatment of selected cases of symptomatic fibroids prior to myomectomy. However, this drug produces a hypo-oestrogenic state, and bone loss may increase and predispose the woman to osteoporosis.

Fibroids and pregnancy

The prevalence of fibroids complicating pregnancy is 1 in 200, but the majority of fibroids are small and cause no problems. The complications that may occur depend on the number, the size and the position of the fibroid in the uterus.

Effect of pregnancy on the fibroids

The increased vascularity of the uterus, together with the increased circulating levels of oestrogen, often leads to an increase in the size and a softening of the fibroid. If the fibroid grows too fast it may outstrip its blood supply, causing degenerative changes in the tumour. The most serious outcome is necrobiosis (red degeneration). The patient may complain of pain and low-grade fever, usually in the second quarter of pregnancy. Palpation reveals that the fibroid is very tender and treatment entails giving analgesics. The pain resolves within a few days and the pregnancy continues.

Effect of the fibroid on the pregnancy

This depends on the size and position of the tumour. If it distorts the uterine cavity, the risk of spontaneous miscarriage is doubled and there is an increased chance that labour will start prematurely. Large tumours in the myometrium may also distort the uterine cavity, causing malposition or malpresentation of the fetus. Tumours in the lower part of the uterus may obstruct the birth canal, preventing vaginal delivery. Large tumours may cause pressure symptoms on the bladder or the rectum. Post-delivery they can interfere with uterine muscle contraction, leading to postpartum haemorrhage.

Diagnosis

If the patient presents early in pregnancy the fibroid may be felt on vaginal examination. A single fundal fibroid may cause diagnostic difficulty, but this can be resolved by an ultrasound examination.

Management

In most cases no treatment is needed during pregnancy. Myomectomy is inadvisable as the operation is attended by marked bleeding, and haemostasis can be difficult. In late pregnancy the position of the myoma in relation to the fetal presenting part and the pelvic cavity will affect the decision regarding the method of delivery. The patient and her partner should be involved in the discussion and the reason for the final decision explained.

As the tumour is usually in the upper segment of the uterus, vaginal delivery is possible for most patients. A few women with low-lying fibroids that obstruct the birth canal require caesarean section. Myomectomy should not be performed during this operation because of the dangers of haemorrhage and infection.

FALLOPIAN TUBE TUMOURS

Benign tumours and cysts of the Fallopian tubes and the broad ligament are rare. Occasionally, cysts are found in remnants of the Wolffian duct at surgery (hydatid of Morgagni). Parovarian cysts are often large and may be thought to be ovarian until exposed at surgery.

BENIGN OVARIAN CYSTS AND TUMOURS

The ovary consists of:

- Coelomic epithelium
- Oocytes, derived from primitive germ cells
- Mesenchymal elements which form the medulla.

These tissues are particularly dynamic, being affected by hormonal stimuli from puberty to the menopause. This may be the reason why so many benign cysts and tumours arise in the ovary.

Classification of benign ovarian cysts and tumours

There is no entirely satisfactory classification of ovarian cysts and tumours. This is because of the complexity of ovarian new growths and because the distinction between some of them can only be made after histological examination. Table 36.1 presents a classification and shows the proportions of benign cysts and tumours encountered.

Functional cysts

A follicular cyst is an enlargement of an unruptured Graafian follicle that has continued to secrete fluid. The cyst is usually unilateral and less than 5 cm in diameter (Fig. 36.10). The cells may secrete oestrogen or be relatively

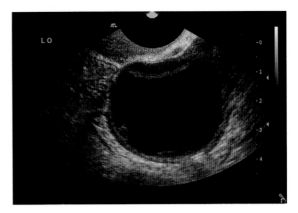

Fig 36.10 Transvaginal ultrasound scan showing a simple 4 cm diameter ovarian cyst.

quiescent, and because of this the symptoms vary. The woman's menstrual cycle may be lengthened and menorrhagia may occur, or it may be of normal length or shorter.

Multiple follicle cysts may occur following the use of clomiphene or gonadotrophins for inducing ovulation.

Corpus luteum cysts occur when, instead of degenerating when the embryo fails to implant, the corpus luteum survives and grows. Theca lutein cysts occur in gestational trophoblastic disease (see p. 143).

If the clinical findings are insufficient to reach a diagnosis, a transvaginal ultrasound examination will help to diagnose an ovarian cyst. However, small cystic enlargements should not be reported as ovarian cysts without qualification. For example, just before ovulation follicles may measure 20 mm (±10 mm). A simple cyst measuring less than 30 mm on ultrasound scanning is better described as a follicle, to avoid unnecessary investigations and, perhaps, surgery.

Treatment

The cyst should be observed for 2–3 months, during which time it will probably disappear. Should it still persist and be unilocular, showing no solid areas on ultrasound, it may be

Table 36.1 A classification of benign ovarian cysts and tumours			
TUMOUR (BENIGN)	**CELL ORIGIN**	**TYPE**	**PROPORTIONAL INCIDENCE %**
Functional cysts (follicle, corpus luteum)	Normal follicle	Cystic	24
Serous cystadenoma	Coelomic epithelium	Cystic	20
Mucinous cystadenoma	Coelomic epithelium	Cystic	20
Teratoma (dermoid cyst)	Oogonia	Cystic	15
Endometrioma	Ectopic endometrium	Cystic	10
Fibroma (incl. Brenner's tumour)	Mesenchyme	Solid	5

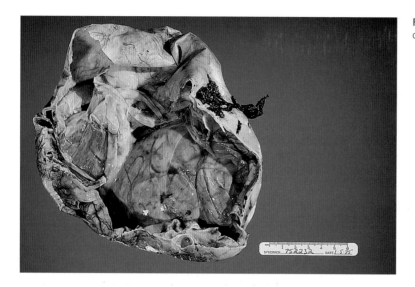

Fig. 36.11 Benign mucinous cystadenoma.

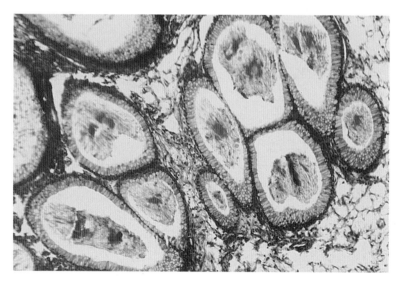

Fig. 36.12 Microscopic appearance of mucinous cystadenoma – note that the cells lining the tumour resemble those of the endocervix.

aspirated under ultrasonic or laparoscopic guidance. If needle aspiration shows bloodstained fluid a laparotomy is needed. Multilocular persistent cysts require surgical removal.

Benign ovarian neoplasms

Mucinous cystadenoma and serous cystadenoma account for 40% of benign ovarian cysts and tumours. Both derive from the multipotential coelomic epithelium, which forms the Müllerian duct and can imitate tubal, uterine or cervical epithelium.

Mucinous cystadenoma

These cysts occur most frequently between the ages of 35 and 55. They can grow to a considerable size and are multilocular

(Fig. 36.11). They are usually unilateral and rarely become malignant. The cyst is lined with tall columnar cells, each of which has a basal nucleus and cytoplasmic mucin (Fig. 36.12). Mucin is constantly secreted into the cyst, with the result that its wall becomes tense. Often a portion of the wall bulges outwards and a depression may form at the neck of the bulge, which may become occluded, forming a daughter cyst (Fig. 36.13). Occasionally the cyst may rupture, releasing mucinous cells, which may become attached to the peritoneum and omentum, leading to an intraperitoneal accumulation of mucin (pseudomyxoma peritonei).

Serous cystadenoma

These cysts are also more frequently detected in women aged 35–55. They are lined with cuboidal epithelium, resembling that of the oviduct (Fig. 36.14). The cells secrete thin,

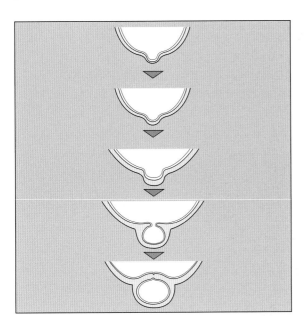

Fig. 36.13 Formation of daughter cysts in the wall of a mucinous cystadenoma.

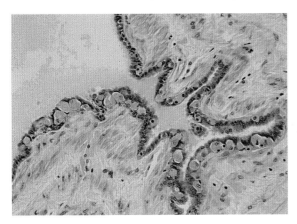

Fig. 36.14 Microscopic appearance of a serous cystadenoma. Note that the cells lining the tumour resemble those of the endosalpinx (×256).

watery fluid, but the quantity secreted is not great. In consequence, the tension inside the cyst is low and the epithelial cells proliferate to form intracystic papillomata. In some cases the cells penetrate the cyst wall to form external papillary projections. Serous cystadenoma are uni- or multilocular and in 30% of cases are bilateral (Fig. 36.15). They only grow to a moderate size, with malignant changes occurring in one-third of cases, usually when the woman is in her 50s.

Endometriomata

These ovarian tumours (chocolate cysts) are usually associated with other evidence of endometriosis. They

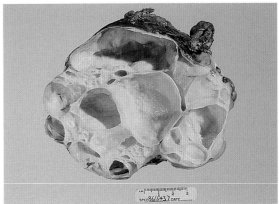

Fig. 36.15 Gross appearance of a serous cystadenoma.

rarely become malignant. Endometriosis is discussed in Chapter 35.

Benign teratoma (dermoid cyst)

Deriving from germ cells, benign teratomata are relatively common. The cyst contains epithelial, mesodermal and endothelial elements. Thus the dermoid may contain hair, teeth and pultaceous material from sebaceous glands. In 10% of cases the tumour is bilateral. It may occur at any age, but mostly is detected when the woman is aged between 20 and 40. The nature of the tumour is confirmed by ultrasound examination or radiology (Fig. 36.16).

Connective tissue neoplasms

Fibromata constitute 5% of benign ovarian neoplasms. The tumour may consist entirely of connective tissue or may be found in association with serous cystadenoma, or with the rare Brenner tumour. Fibromata are usually small, and in 10% of cases are bilateral. Rarely, the fibroma is associated with hydrothorax and ascites (Meigs' syndrome).

Diagnosis of ovarian tumours

Benign ovarian cysts and tumours grow silently and are often undetected for years. They do not cause pain, but if large may cause discomfort. They rarely affect menstrual function. Periodic abdominal and vaginal examinations will detect benign tumours. A painless cystic or solid mass in the cul-de-sac, or in the position of an ovary, or distending the abdomen, which is cystic to firm on palpation, suggests an ovarian tumour. The diagnosis can be confirmed by an abdominal or transvaginal ultrasound scan, which differentiates the tumour from pregnancy, obesity, pseudocyesis, a full bladder or cystic degeneration of a fibroid (Figs 36.10, 36.16).

287

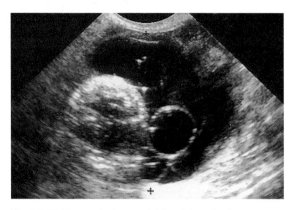

Fig. 36.16 Transvaginal scan of 4.8 × 4.0 cm benign teratoma ovarian cyst.

Management of benign ovarian tumours

The treatment of mucinous cystadenoma is surgical, the extent of the operation depending on the age of the patient. In younger women ovarian cystectomy is possible; the ovary being reconstructed after the tumour has been shelled out. A similar approach can be used in cases of serous cystadenoma, but in women over the age of 40 bilateral salpingo-oophorectomy and total hysterectomy is preferred, because of the possibility of malignant change. Endometriomata, benign teratomata and fibromata can often be shelled out of the normal ovarian tissue and the ovary reconstructed.

Ovarian tumours and pregnancy

One pregnancy in 1500 is complicated by a clinically detectable ovarian tumour measuring more than 50 mm in diameter. If an ultrasound examination of the pelvis is made routinely, ovarian tumours are detected in 1 in 200 pregnancies. Most of them are cysts, usually an enlarged corpus luteum which resolves spontaneously. Neoplastic tumours are less common in pregnancy. Most are serous cystadenomas, a few are mucinous cystadenomas, and these two account for 65% of all neoplasias complicating pregnancy. Teratomata account for 25% and the remaining 10% is made up of a wide variety of ovarian tumours. Pregnancy can also cause lutein cells to hypertrophy (luteoma). Conditions producing high levels of hCG, hydatidiform mole, choriocarcinoma, multiple pregnancy or hyperstimulation during ovulation induction, can cause massive ovarian enlargement.

Effect of the pregnancy of the tumour

The size of the tumour may not change during the pregnancy, but the growing uterus may displace it so that it becomes more obvious. Rarely, torsion of the ovary containing the tumour may occur and, even more rarely, the tumour may rupture.

Effect of the tumour on the pregnancy

The only problem is that the tumour may become incarcerated in the cul-de-sac and obstruct the birth canal (Fig. 36.17).

Diagnosis

In early pregnancy a vaginal examination may reveal two masses, the pregnant uterus and the ovarian tumour. If there is any doubt a pelvic ultrasound examination will clarify the diagnosis.

Treatment

Treatment depends on the size and consistency of the tumour and its ultrasound appearance. Ovarian tumours less than 80 mm in diameter and echo-free can be observed, repeat scans being made to see if the tumour increases in size. If treatment is decided upon, the cyst may be aspirated or a cystectomy performed. A multilocular cyst or a tumour greater than 80 mm in size which is thick-walled or semisolid, requires surgical removal after the 12th gestational week. A tumour detected after the 30th gestational week may be difficult to remove surgically and premature labour may follow. The decision to operate can only be made after careful consideration and involvement of the patient and her partner. If the tumour obstructs the birth canal and cannot be moved digitally, the patient should be delivered by caesarean section and cystectomy performed.

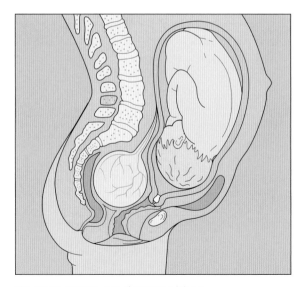

Fig. 36.17 Ovarian cyst obstructing labour.

Chapter | 37 |

Premalignant and malignant conditions of the female genital tract

Only four cancers can be either prevented or diagnosed at a stage when treatment is curative in most cases:

- Skin cancer can be prevented by avoiding excessive exposure to the sun.
- Lung cancer can largely be prevented by avoiding smoking tobacco.
- Cancer of the uterine cervix by cervical smear screening to detect precancerous changes and vaccination against HPV strains 16 and 18.
- Breast cancer by mammography screening to detected tumours at a stage when treatment is curative.

CERVICAL PRECANCER AND CANCER

The cervical epithelium undergoes changes throughout the menstrual cycle and is readily accessible for examination. The epithelium covering the ectocervix is stratified and identical to that of the vagina (Fig. 37.1). It is separated from the underlying stroma by an apparent basement membrane. Superior to this is a layer of basal cells from which the other cell layers differentiate. Above the basal layer are five or six layers of parabasal cells. Above these are intermediate and superficial cell layers. The intermediate cell layer consists of large cells, each with reticulated nuclei and vacuoles of glycogen in the cytoplasm. The superficial cell layer varies in thickness, depending on the oestradiol : progesterone ratio.

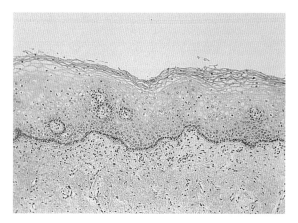

Fig. 37.1 Normal squamous epithelium covering the vaginal portion of the cervix.

The superficial cells are flattened and have small nuclei, the cytoplasm containing glycogen (Fig. 37.2). A small amount of keratin is produced in some of the cells, which becomes 'cornified'. During the reproductive years the superficial cells are constantly shed or exfoliated into the vagina, and differentiation of cells from the basal layer also proceeds constantly.

The characteristics of the superficial cells can be studied by taking a smear from the cervix and staining it with Papanicolaou's stain. In some women the nuclei become abnormally shaped or dyskaryotic, which may indicate a precancerous change; this can be detected by cervical smears.

Epidemiology of cervical cancer

Cervical cancer occurs almost exclusively in women who are or have been sexually active. There is strong molecular biological and epidemiological evidence that the predominant cause of cervical cancer is sexually transmitted human papilloma virus (HPV). There are four HPV types that are considered to be high risk (16, 18, 45 and 56), a further 11 types that are intermediate risk (31, 33, 35, 39, 51, 52, 55, 58, 59, 66 and 68) and eight that are low risk (6, 11, 26, 42, 44, 54, 70 and 73) By the age of 35, 60% of sexually active women have acquired HPV infection of the genital tract (including the vulva). This proportion is higher if the woman or her partner has had several sexual partners. In most cases the infection is symptomless and disappears within a few months (see p. 258).

Possible cofactors in cervical carcinogenesis include cigarette smoking, immunosuppression, hormonal factors and vitamin deficiencies. Prophylactic vaccination is now available either as a bivalent against the high risk HPV 16 and 18 or as the quadravalent HPV 16, 18, and the lower risk 6 and 11. A number of countries offer the vaccination from age 12–13 up to 27 years; consideration is also being given to offering the vaccine to young men before they become sexually active.

Cervical exfoliative cytology

The development of cervical carcinoma is preceded by the appearance of abnormal (dyskaryotic) cervical cells. These can be detected by microscopically examining an exfoliative cervical smear, stained using the Papanicolaou stain (the Pap test). As this is a screening test false negatives may occur, estimated at 5–15%. The proportion of false-negative smears will be reduced if strict criteria are adopted for taking and for examining the smear.

A further refinement is liquid-based cytology that involves taking cervical cells with a Cervex sampler brush and rinsing the brush into a vial of fixative. The cells are not obscured by blood or mucus and are all fixed properly. In the laboratory, a monolayer of cells is made which is easier to interpret. If the result is inconclusive, the remaining cells in the vial can be used to make a hybrid capture test, which will detect the presence of oncogenic HPV. This methodology reduces the unsatisfactory/inconclusive smear rate by 80% and has been shown to be cost-effective. A further advantage of this test is that it is likely to reduce the number of colposcopies that gynaecologists make when an inconclusive Pap smear abnormality is found. The technique has the potential to be used for the detection of other sexually transmitted diseases, such as chlamydia and gonorrhoea.

The recommended smear regimen is summarised in Box 37.1. In women aged 30 and over, the doctor or nurse taking the smear should also examine the woman's breasts, teach her breast self-examination, and after the age of 40 measure her blood pressure.

Technique for taking a cervical smear

A tray is provided on which a bivalve vaginal speculum, some slides, a spray-on fixative plastic, a modified Ayre

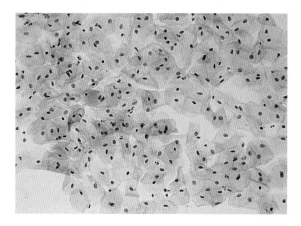

Fig. 37.2 Normal exfoliated cervical cells.

spatula and an endocervical brush are placed. Before performing a vaginal examination, the warmed speculum is inserted to expose the cervix. The cytobrush is inserted into the cervical canal and rotated. The sample is smeared on to the slide. The ectocervix is sampled with the Ayre spatula or Cervex brush by rotating it twice through 360° and the sample is smeared on to a slide (Fig. 37.3). If liquid-based cytology is being used the brush is placed in the liquid medium.

The smears are sent to a reliable, quality assured cytological laboratory for examination.

REPORTING ON SMEARS

Cytologists have agreed that nuclear abnormalities should form the basis of a cytological diagnosis. They have agreed to report smears as follows:

- **Unsatisfactory**. A diagnosis cannot be made because there are too few cells, there are no endocervical cells, or the slide has been processed incorrectly. The smear should be repeated 4 weeks later.
- **Inflammatory or inconclusive**. The nuclei are distorted by the effects of vaginal infections, such as trichomoniasis and gardnerella. The referring doctor is asked to treat the infection appropriately and then to repeat the smear.
- **Normal**. Repeat the smear in 1–2 years.
- **Mild dyskaryosis** (predictive of CIN 1). The slide may show HPV infection with no dyskaryosis, HPV infection and dyskaryosis, or dyskaryosis without HPV infection.
- **Moderate dyskaryosis** (predictive of CIN 2).
- **Severe dyskaryosis** (predictive of CIN 3) (Fig. 37.4).

The Bethesda Classification

An alternative classification is used in the USA (the Bethesda Classification). Smears showing abnormal cells are categorized as:

Squamous cell

- Atypical squamous cells of uncertain significance
- Low-grade squamous intraepithelial lesions, which includes HPV infection as shown by koilicytosis (a halo around the nucleus of some cells) and mild dyskaryosis (CIN 1)
- High-grade squamous intraepithelial lesions, which includes moderate dyskaryosis (predictive of CIN 2) and severe dyskaryosis (predictive of CIN 3)
- Squamous cell carcinoma.

Glandular cell

- Endometrial cells cytologically benign in a postmenopausal woman

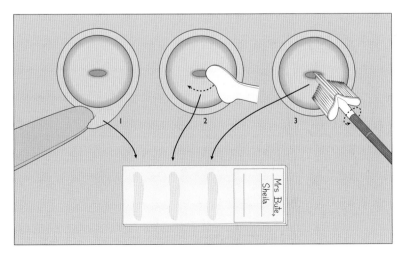

Fig. 37.3 Methods of obtaining cells from the cervix for cytological examination, using (1) a special wooden spatula, (2) an Ayre spatula, and (3) a Cervex sampler.

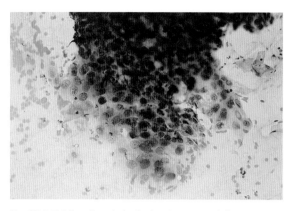

Fig. 37.4 Exfoliated cervical cells showing severe dyskaryosis.

- Atypical glandular cells of undetermined significance
- Adenocarcinoma
  - Endocervical
  - Endometrial
  - Extra-uterine
  - Not otherwise specified.

New cervical screening techniques

Meta-analysis of conventional screening found a sensitivity of 58%, a specificity of 69% and a false-negative rate of 20%. This has led to the exploration of other technologies to improve diagnostic accuracy. In the ThinPrep method, the sample is placed into a 20 mL vial of buffered alcohol, which is then prepared for automated image analysis. A study by Duke University and the American Association of Obstetrics and Gynaecology reported that this technique was cost-effective and would reduce cancer cases, deaths and serious interventions, including hysterectomy, by 57% if screening was performed every 2 years.

Detection of HPV in women:

- With negative smears carries an increased risk of developing CIN

- With low-grade abnormalities carries an increased risk of progression to a high-grade abnormality.

HPV-negative women should have repeat cervical cytology at recommended intervals. HPV-positive women should be offered colposcopic evaluation.

Telling the patient

The result of the smear should be reported to the woman by phone or by letter. This applies to all smears, not just abnormal ones. If an abnormal smear is reported, the need to counsel and explain is imperative.

To many women, the finding of a dyskaryotic smear suggests the presence of cancer. If HPV is found, many women question their own and their partner's previous sexual behaviour. Either finding can lead to guilt, misery and anxiety. Doctors should be aware of this and should talk with the woman, explaining the meaning of the result and that HPV is not always sexually transmitted. The woman should also be told, in clear non-jargon language, what procedures may be needed. In one reported study, the term 'precancer' was perceived as threatening and the authors suggested that a better term would be 'early warning cells'.

Management of abnormal cervical smears

Approaches to the management of abnormal cervical smears are summarized in Table 37.1.

HPV infection with no evidence of dyskaryosis

Smears should be taken at 6-monthly intervals until they are negative for HPV, then annually for 2 years. If there is no evidence of HPV at this time, the patient should return to having a smear every 2 years. If dyskaryosis appears in any smear, treat as recommended below.

Table 37.1 Management of an abnormal Pap smear

LESION	LOW-GRADE SQUAMOUS INTRA-EPITHELIAL		HIGH-GRADE SQUAMOUS INTRA-EPITHELIAL	
Normal	HPV infection	Mild dyskaryosis	Moderate dyskaryosis	Severe dyskaryosis
If first Pap smear repeat within 1 year: otherwise every 2 years	Repeat Pap smear every 6 months, 3 times. If HPV persists, refer for colposcopy	Either repeat Pap smear 3 times every 6 months and if persists refer, or refer at once for colposcopy	Refer for colposcopy and biopsy	Refer for colposcopy and biopsy

Mild dyskaryosis (predictive of CIN 1) with or without HPV

There are three potential management options:

1. Repeat the cervical smear in 12 months: if the abnormality persists refer for colposcopy, if this smear is reported as normal repeat in 12 months.
2. Refer for immediate colposcopy. There is, however, no evidence from randomized controlled trials that this early intervention conveys any benefit over option 1.
3. HPV testing and then instituting further investigation if a high risk HPV strain is identified. Again there is currently insufficient evidence to support this option.

Consequently the National Health and Medical research Council of Australia recommends option 1.

Moderate and severe dyskaryosis (predictive of CIN 1 or CIN 2)

These degrees of dyskaryosis require referral for colposcopy and cervical biopsy.

Colposcopy

Dyskaryosis is a cytological diagnosis and observer error is not uncommon. For this reason, a colposcope is often used to verify abnormal findings. A colposcope is a system of lenses that magnifies the cervix 5–20 times and enables a trained observer to translate changes in colour tone, opacity, surface configuration, vascular pattern and intercapillary distance into a diagnosis (Figs 37.5–37.8).

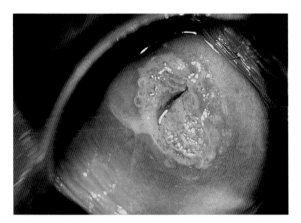

Fig. 37.5 Normal cervix. Opening the bivalve speculum exposes the endocervical canal, allowing examination of the full transformation zone.

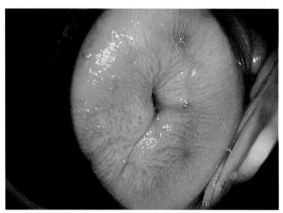

Fig. 37.7 The appearance of the cervix following diathermic ablation of the dysplastic epithelium. The abnormal transformation zone has been replaced by mature squamous epithelium.

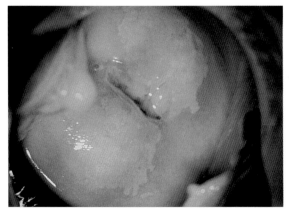

Fig. 37.6 CIN 1. The abnormal epithelium is visible on both the anterior and posterior margins of the cervix, having turned white after the application of acetic acid.

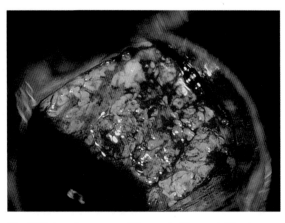

Fig. 37.8 Invasive cancer of the cervix. The cervix bleeds readily on contact.

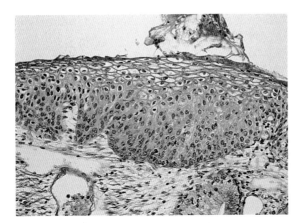

Fig. 37.9 Dysplasia (moderate) (CIN 2).

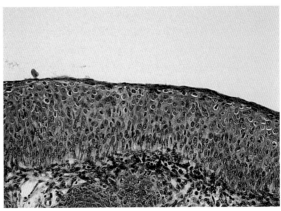

Fig. 37.10 Dysplasia (severe) (CIN 3).

Abnormal epithelium is white after the application of aqueous acetic acid solution (acido-white epithelium), white keratotic patches may be seen (Fig. 37.6), and the blood vessels may appear as punctate dots or as a mosaic arrangement. Bizarre branching vessels usually denote invasive cancer. A trained observer can differentiate between the minor and major cervical precancer lesions and carcinoma with a reasonable degree of accuracy. The predicted diagnosis is confirmed by punch biopsies, which are examined histologically.

Histology

Mild dysplasia is characterized by nuclear abnormalities in the basal third of the epithelium; the upper layers are not affected. In moderate dysplasia some dyskaryotic nuclei are found in the upper layers of the epithelium, and abnormal nuclei are more common (Fig. 37.9). In severe dysplasia the abnormal nuclei occupy all the epithelial layers and there is a high nuclear : cytoplasmic ratio (Fig. 37.10). Severe dysplasia may be difficult to differentiate from carcinoma *in situ*. In carcinoma *in situ* there is no differentiation as the surface layers are reached; the nuclei vary in size and stain deeply, the cells are crowded and the cytoplasm is scanty (Fig. 37.11).

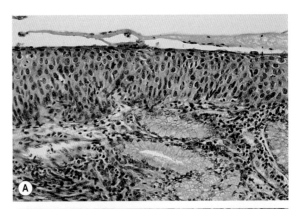

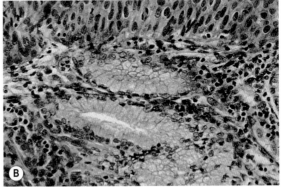

Fig. 37.11 Cervical biopsy from the patient whose cervical smear is shown in Fig. 37.4. Carcinoma *in situ* was found. (A) (× 40). There appears to be invasion of the tissues, but in reality the cells have only crept into endocervical crypts. (B) (× 160). The lack of stratification and pleomorphism of the cells is seen at higher magnification.

CERVICAL INTRAEPITHELIAL NEOPLASIA (CIN)

In some cases there is uncertainty about the exact histological diagnosis and whether the identified lesion will regress, persist or progress. This has led to a classification that includes all grades of dysplasia, the CIN classification (Table 37.2).

Natural history of CIN

The current belief about the natural history of CIN is shown in Figure 37.12.

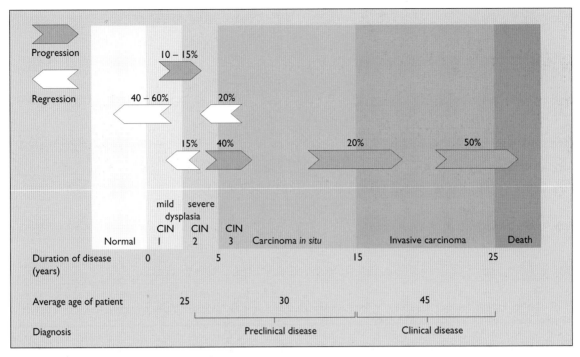

Fig. 37.12 The 'lifecycle' of unstable cervical epithelium.

Table 37.2 CIN classification	
GRADE	**DESCRIPTION**
Grade 1	Mild dysplasia
Grade 2	Moderate dysplasia
Grade 3	Severe dysplasia/Carcinoma *in situ*

Management of CIN

The management of CIN depends on the age of the woman, her desire to reproduce, and on the location and extent of the lesion. Current recommendations for treatment are described below.

CIN grade 1

There is a lack of agreement about management if colposcopically controlled biopsy shows mild dysplasia (CIN 1). Some gynaecologists recommend careful observation, as the majority of lesions will resolve spontaneously, but increasingly specialists are recommending that the lesion be obliterated using one of the methods outlined in the management of CIN 2 and 3.

CIN grades 2 and 3

These major-grade lesions require either local destructive treatment or excision of the suspect area. Local destructive treatment includes laser, cryosurgery and electrocoagulation diathermy. The selection of patients is important, the whole lesion must be visible and invasive cancer must have been excluded. All treatments can be given under local anaesthesia or general anaesthesia depending on the patient's and the gynaecologist's preference. Following ablation the smear and colposcopy returns to normal in over 90% of women.

Each of these treatments may be followed by a blood-stained or clear discharge for 1–3 weeks. About 5% of women have vaginal bleeding, and the patient may complain of pain or severe discomfort. Sexual intercourse and the use of tampons should be avoided for 4 weeks to allow complete healing. The treatments do not affect the woman's fertility or alter the course of a subsequent pregnancy.

An alternative method of treatment is large loop excision of the transformation zone (LLETZ), with ball cautery to the exposed area of the cervix if needed to achieve haemostasis. The advantage is that the tissue can be examined histologically to exclude invasive cancer, particularly if the suspect areas extend up the cervical canal and their upper limit cannot be identified by colposcopic inspection. The whole transformation zone and some of the cervical canal area is excised. If the procedure is performed by an experienced gynaecologist there appears to be no adverse effect on the duration of a subsequent pregnancy.

If the upper limit of abnormality cannot be adequately visualized then a cone biopsy is indicated. Knife conization, usually with suturing to repair the cervix, is associated with a 10% chance of postoperative haemorrhage. If the woman becomes pregnant, there is an increased risk of miscarriage in the second quarter of pregnancy and she may give birth to a preterm baby, as a result of an incompetent cervix. The risk increases with the size of the cone excised. Ultrasound surveillance of the cervical length during the second trimester will help identify those at risk of premature delivery. Conversely, scarring can cause stenosis of the cervical canal, which can result in cryptomenorrhoea or can prevent the cervix dilating during labour, necessitating delivery by caesarean section.

Depending on age, the presence of other gynaecological conditions (for example, fibroids or menorrhagia) and personal preferences, some women with CIN 3 may choose hysterectomy.

As mentioned, follow-up is essential. The woman should be reviewed 6 and 12 months after treatment, when a cervical smear is taken and a colposcopic examination performed. If the cytology is negative and the colposcopy normal, annual smears are made from then on. Following hysterectomy for CIN, 6-monthly smears should be made for the first year and every 2 years thereafter, as abnormal cells may be found in the upper vagina, signifying vaginal CIN.

Psychological effects of CIN on women

Many women diagnosed as having CIN become depressed and upset, particularly if a health professional implies that they have been sexually promiscuous.

The woman may be concerned that her partner has been or is continuing to be unfaithful. Her attitude to sexual intercourse may change, and she may want to avoid sex.

The anxieties and uncertainty should be resolved, as far as possible, by giving the woman a full explanation of CIN and giving her the opportunity to ask questions. She may also need continued psychological support.

CERVICAL CARCINOMA

Carcinoma of the uterine cervix is the second most common gynaecological cancer (after breast cancer). The annual risk for women over the age of 35 is 16 per 100 000, but is much greater in developing countries. The peak incidence is between the ages of 45 and 55, the mean age being 51.4 years, with a recent trend towards a younger age. Cervical cancer usually grows outwards, becoming a fungating mass; occasionally it grows inwards, enlarging the cervix. More

than 85% of cervical cancers are squamous cell carcinomas; the remainder are adenocarcinomas, which arise from the cells lining the cervical canal or its clefts. With time, the cancer spreads either by direct extension upwards to involve the uterine cavity, downwards to involve the vagina, or via the lymphatic drainage to the external iliac lymph nodes (47% of cases); the obturator lymph node (20%); the hypogastric nodes (7%); or the paracervical nodes (2%).

Clinical staging is not able to detect spread to the liver and lymph nodes. Ultrasound, computed tomography (CT) and magnetic resonance imaging (MRI) are used. CT can detect lymph node metastases, plus liver, urinary tract and bone involvement. MRI has a role in detecting parametrial spread and is particularly useful in evaluating pregnant women, as it avoids exposing the fetus to radiation. The place of positron emission tomography (PET) is still being assessed but it has the potential to accurately determine the extent of spread from the cervix and lymph node involvement.

Accurate staging of the disease is critical to determine the optimal mode of treatment, and the International Federation of Obstetrics and Gynaecology (FIGO) classification is summarized in Table 37.3. The higher the stage on the initial examination, the greater the chance of lymph node involvement and the poorer the prognosis (Table 37.4). In early-stage disease (stages 1B and 2A, see later) lymph node metastases are present in 25–30% of cases.

Table 37.3 International Federation of Obstetrics and Gynaecology (FIGO) classification for staging of carcinoma of uterine cervix

STAGE	DESCRIPTION
Stage 0	Cervical intraepithelial neoplasia 3 (CIN 3), Carcinoma *in situ*
Stage 1	The carcinoma is confined to the cervix 1A Invasion can only be diagnosed by microscopy with maximum depth ≤5.0 mm and horizontal spread of ≤7.0 mm 1B Clinically visible
Stage 2	The carcinoma invades beyond the uterus but does not reach pelvic wall or lower third of the vagina 2A No obvious parametrial involvement 2B Obvious parametrial involvement
Stage 3	The carcinoma has reached the wall of the pelvis and/or the lower third of the vagina 3A Reached lower third of the vagina 3B Extension to pelvic wall or hydronephrosis or non-functioning kidney
Stage 4	The carcinoma has spread beyond the true pelvis or has invaded the bladder or rectum 4A Spread to adjacent organs 4B Spread to distant organs

Table 37.4 Lymph node involvement and 5-year survival rates of cervical carcinoma related to stage of the disease

STAGE	LYMPH NODE INVOLVEMENT	5-YEAR SURVIVAL (%)
0	0	100
1A	0.5	95
1B	15	80
2A	25	66
2B	35	64
3	55	35
4	>65	14

Diagnosis

In its earliest stage an abnormal smear is the only way to detect cervical cancer, as symptoms tend to occur only with established invasive disease. Irregular bleeding per vaginam, particularly after sexual intercourse, or a pink vaginal discharge after urination, demands investigation by vaginal examination using a speculum and a cervical smear. Diagnosis is confirmed by a cervical biopsy, if necessary under colposcopic direction or, if gross evidence of cervical cancer is detected, by biopsy and endocervical curettage.

Treatment

The best results of treatment for cervical cancer are obtained in oncological units staffed by gynaecological and radiological oncologists. The treatment of microinvasive (stage lA) cancer depends on whether or not the woman wants to retain her uterus. In this circumstance a cone biopsy with clear margins is adequate treatment. Otherwise it can be treated by simple total hysterectomy.

Stage 1B and early 2A cancer is usually treated by radical hysterectomy followed by radiotherapy. Radical hysterectomy includes removal of the parametrium and pelvic lymphadenectomy, and radiotherapy includes a combination of external beam and intracavity radiation. In younger women the ovaries can be preserved and relocated out of the potential radiotherapy field. More advanced cervical carcinoma is treated by radiotherapy, although in some centres chemotherapy is being tried.

Bladder dysfunction, lymphoedema and sexual dysfunction are complications of treatment, especially of radiotherapy.

Chemotherapy has been used in both early stage (1B) and advanced disease. This improves the 2-year survival rate from 79 to 89% and 63 to 75%, respectively.

ENDOMETRIAL CARCINOMA

Endometrial carcinoma is a disease of women in their middle years, the peak incidence occurring in the 55–65-year age group. Women whose menopause is delayed beyond the age of 55, who are relatively infertile, and overweight or hypertensive are more likely than other women to develop endometrial cancer. This profile suggests that unopposed oestrogen may play a role in the development of the cancer. As discussed on page 297, unopposed oestrogen may lead to endometrial hyperplasia (Fig. 37.13). Endometrial hyperplasia has several pathological appearances, and if the pathology shows complex hyperplasia with atypia 17–43% of women will develop endometrial cancer, unless they are treated.

The tumour may originate in any part of the endometrium, and grows slowly, tending to spread over a part of the endometrium before invading the myometrium. If the growth starts in the lower part of the uterus, the fungating mass may block the cervix and fluid or pus may collect in the uterus (pyometra). Various histological patterns of adenocarcinoma are found on the histological examination of an endometrial biopsy or curettage. The more undifferentiated the endometrial cells, the worse the prognosis. The cancer is staged using the FIGO classification (Table 37.5).

Clinical features

The usual symptoms of endometrial carcinoma are a bloody vaginal discharge or irregular bleeding, which is slight in amount and recurrent. Some women have a watery vaginal discharge, but this is uncommon. Examination usually shows a normally sized uterus, unless there are associated myomata or a pyometra. Any

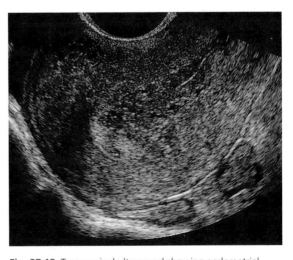

Fig. 37.13 Transvaginal ultrasound showing endometrial hyperplasia.

Table 37.5 Surgical–pathological staging of endometrial carcinoma (FIGO, 1989)

STAGE	DESCRIPTION
IA	Tumour limited to endometrium
IB	Invasion to <1/2 myometrium
IC	Invasion to >1/2 myometrium
IIA	Endocervical glandular involvement only
IIB	Cervical stromal invasion
IIIA	Tumour invades serosa and/or adnexae and/or positive peritoneal cytology
IIIB	Vaginal metastases
IIIC	Metastases to pelvic and/or para-aortic lymph nodes
IVA	Tumour invades bladder and/or bowel mucosa
IVB	Distant metastases including intra-abdominal and/or inguinal lymph node

peri- or postmenopausal woman who has symptoms of irregular bleeding per vaginam or a bloody vaginal discharge must be examined and endometrial and endocervical canal tissue sampled. Using a hysteroscope, the uterine cavity can be inspected and a biopsy taken under direct vision. An alternative is to measure the thickness of the endometrium by transvaginal ultrasonography. If the endometrium is less than 5 mm thick, endometrial cancer can be excluded. Confirmation is by hysteroscopy and biopsy or by curettage, either using a biopsy curette (this can be done as an outpatient procedure) or a formal curettage under general anaesthesia. Two biopsy curettes are commonly used (Gynescan and Pipelle). They are introduced through the cervix and rotated in the uterine cavity. The procedures are said to be relatively painless, but 60% of women experience discomfort or pain. A negative biopsy in a symptomatic woman should be followed by a formal hysteroscopy and biopsy/curettage under anaesthesia, as there is a 10% false-negative rate.

Screening for endometrial cancer

Mass screening for endometrial cancer is neither practical nor justifiable with currently available techniques. Papanicolaou smears will detect 50% of cases but is too unreliable to be used for screening asymptomatic women. Three groups are at high risk: postmenopausal women taking unopposed oestrogen therapy, women with a familial history of non-polyposis colorectal cancer, and premeno-

pausal women with anovulatory cycles. These women should be offered regular surveillance, including transvaginal ultrasound examination. Women taking tamoxifen are only at risk if they have abnormal vaginal bleeding.

Treatment

Over 75% of cases are diagnosed when the cancer is at an early stage. Total hysterectomy and bilateral oophorectomy is the treatment of choice in these cases. As lymphatic spread is a later development, pelvic lymphadenectomy is performed only with grade 3 disease (>50% non-squamous or non-morular growth pattern), grade 2 (6–50% non-squamous or non-morular growth pattern) tumours >2 cm in diameter, adenosquamous, clear cell or papillary serous carcinomas, >50% myometrial invasion, or in those with cervical extension. The excised uterus is examined histologically, and if the myometrium has been invaded to more than half its thickness, either whole pelvis irradiation (50 Gy over 5 weeks) or hormone treatment is given. Some gynaecological surgeons arrange for intravaginal irradiation 3–4 weeks after the hysterectomy, giving 40 Gy. The objective is to prevent recurrence in the vaginal vault. Problems with this approach are that the vaginal vault may become stenosed, making intercourse uncomfortable, and that bladder or rectal symptoms may occur as a result of radiation damage.

If the patient is unfit for surgery or if the cancer is advanced, hormone treatment such as medroxyprogesterone acetate 200–400 mg orally daily may be used as an alternative.

Prognosis

The prognosis depends on the stage of the disease, the histological grade of the tumour and the age and health of the woman (Table 37.6).

Women who have received treatment for low-stage endometrial carcinoma and who have severe menopausal symptoms may be prescribed hormone replacement therapy with no increased development of any residual cancer.

Follow-up is recommended at 4-monthly intervals for the first 3 years, and annually thereafter. The woman is examined abdominally and vaginally, checked to detect any enlarged lymph nodes, and a chest X-ray is taken.

VULVAL DISEASE

Vulval intraepithelial neoplasia (VIN)

This condition is being increasingly diagnosed during the colposcopic investigation of women presenting with pruritus vulvae or vulval warts. The best treatment is unknown. The options are watchful expectancy or local excision of the area in high-grade VIN 3. Follow-up is important, as one-third of patients have recurrent disease.

Between 4 and 8% of women with Paget's disease have an underlying adenocarcinoma. Treatment is by wide excision,

Table 37.6 The recommended treatment and 5-year survival rate of endometrial cancer related to the stage of the disease

STAGE	RECOMMENDED TREATMENT	5-YEAR SURVIVAL RATE (%)
IA	Hysterectomy	90
IB	Hysterectomy	88
IC	Hysterectomy followed by vaginal vault and pelvic irradiation	80
IIA	As for carcinoma of cervix	77
II B	As for carcinoma of cervix	67
III	Hysterectomy and bilateral salpingo-oophorectomy if feasible plus radiation therapy	40
IV	Palliative surgery, radiation therapy and progestogenic therapy	10

including the underlying dermis. Because of the high rate of recurrence these women need long-term surveillance.

Carcinoma of the vulva

Vulval carcinoma accounts for 3% of genital tract cancers and affects elderly women. The growth usually starts as a lump or an ulcer on one labium majus (50% of cases) or on a labium minus (25% of cases). In some cases several areas are affected. In recent years a number of younger women have been presenting with malignant change in a vulval condyloma.

The affected woman may have complained of vulval itching for months or years, or may have had few symptoms and has only noticed the lump or the ulcer recently.

Clinical

The lesion presents as a hard nodule or an ulcer with a sloughing base and raised edges, which may be small or large depending on the duration of the disease (Fig. 37.14). If the cancer is large, lymph node involvement will have occurred in more than 50% of cases.

Treatment is either simple vulvectomy with dissection of the inguinofemoral lymph nodes for stage 1 disease

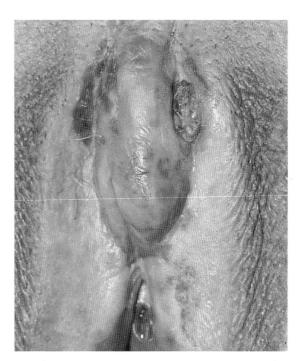

Fig. 37.14 Vulval carcinoma in the anterior part of the vulva.

(tumour = 2 cm), or radical vulvectomy for stage 2 (confined to the vulva and >2 cm in diameter) with inguinal, femoral and pelvic lymphadenectomy. Wound necrosis is a troublesome complication after radical vulvectomy, and persistent leg oedema occurs in 20% of women. For women with advanced disease the treatment needs to be individualized and depends on the degree of spread, the age of the woman and her general state of health. The modalities employed include surgical excision, radiotherapy and chemotherapy.

The overall 5-year survival is 70%; for stage I 90%, stage II 75%, stage III 50%, and stage IV 15%.

CANCER OF THE OVARY FOLLOWED BY ULTRASOUND (FIG. 37.15)

Malignant ovarian tumours are rarely diagnosed early and, in consequence, carry a high mortality. About 6% of ovarian tumours are found to be malignant at surgery, the proportion increasing as a woman grows older.

The tumour may arise in several ways, as shown in Table 37.7.

Primary ovarian carcinoma accounts for about 20% of all gynaecological cancers. In more than 70% of cases the growth has spread beyond the ovaries when first detected. By this time the prospect of 5-year survival is less than 25%.

Up to 10% of ovarian epithelial cancers have a genetic origin, with several family members being affected. The strongest

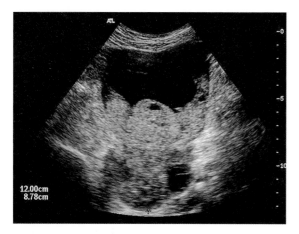

Fig. 37.15 Transvaginal scan showing 12 × 9 cm malignant ovarian tumour. Note the irregularity and the solid and cystic areas.

association is with the *BRCA1* gene, located on chromosome 17, and a smaller number with the chromosome 13 *BRCA2* gene. About 40% of current female family members with a *BRCA1* mutation will develop ovarian cancer, and up to 87% with *BRCA1* or *BRCA2* mutations will develop breast cancer. Some authorities suggest a prophylactic bilateral oophorectomy when the woman has completed her family.

Clinical features

The woman, who is usually aged 50 or more, may notice that her abdomen is becoming larger (from the mass, or from ascites), or she may complain of pressure symptoms on her bladder or rectum. Abdominal discomfort and gastrointestinal symptoms may be present. She may have lost weight and have a poor appetite. In most cases the symptoms are few if any and the tumour is detected during a routine examination Germ cell malignancies can affect women under the age of 30, the most common being dysgerminoma. The FIGO staging of ovarian cancer is shown in Table 37.8.

Management

Ovarian malignancies should be treated in oncological units, not by a general gynaecologist or a surgeon. The initial management is surgical, as much malignant tissue being removed (including the omentum) as is surgically possible without causing severe damage. Following surgery, chemotherapy is initiated, including cisplatin (or carboplatin) and paclitaxel (Taxol) taken every 21 days. Some pelvic surgeons make a 'second-look' laparotomy after six courses of treatment to assess the response, and possibly to debulk persisting or recurrent disease.

Combination chemotherapy is toxic: 60–80% of patients have severe nausea and vomiting during treatment; severe hair loss occurs in 50–60%; peripheral neuropathy

Table 37.7 A classification of the commoner malignant ovarian tumours			
TUMOUR	**PEAK AGE INCIDENCE (%)**	**PROPORTIONAL THAT ARE BILATERAL (%)**	**PROPORTIONAL INCIDENCE OF ALL OVARIAN TUMOURS (%)**
Surface epithelial tumours			
Serous of low malignant potential	40–60	25–30	10
Serous carcinoma	50–70	60	40–50
Mucinous of low malignant potential	30–45	7–35	7
Mucinous carcinoma	50–60	10	10
Endometrioid	>55	33	25 (20% concomitant endometrial cancer)
Clear cell carcinoma	45–65	40	10
Sex cord-stromal tumours			
Granulosal cell	50–55	<10	1–2 (10% concomitant endometrial cancer)
Sertoli–stromal	20–40	0	1
Germ cell tumours	20–30	10	1–2
Dysgerminoma			
Metastatic			
From endometrium, gastrointestinal tract and breast		Most	5

Table 37.8 FIGO staging and 5-year survival of ovarian cancer

STAGE		5-YEAR SURVIVAL (%)
I	Growth limited to ovaries	85
II	Growth involving 1 or both ovaries with pelvic extension	60
III	Peritoneal implants outside the pelvis	30
IV	Distant metastases	10

in 5–30%; and renal toxicity in 15–60%. Because of the high death rate following a diagnosed ovarian cancer, studies are being carried out to determine whether a cancer can be detected at an early stage in a postmenopausal woman. Trials of transvaginal ultrasound, the measurement of CA125 antigen and Doppler colour flow mapping (to detect the early angiogenesis that occurs in a malignant tumour) have been conducted. The high false-positive rates have meant that they are not suitable for routine screening except in women with a strong family history of ovarian cancer.

VAGINAL CANCER

Primary vaginal cancer is rare, comprising between 1 and 2% of female genital tract malignancies; 85% of vaginal cancers are secondary cancers from cervix, endometrium, colon and rectum, ovary and vulva.

There is a strong association between primary vaginal cancer and previously treated CIN 3 and invasive cervical cancer (in up to 30%). This suggests that HPV infection may play an aetiological role.

Squamous cell carcinoma of the vagina is diagnosed at a mean age of 60 years. Most cases present with abnormal bleeding.

Upper vaginal tumours are treated as for cervical carcinoma and lower tumours by radiotherapy.

The 5-year survival is poorer than for cervical and vulval carcinoma, being around 45%.

FALLOPIAN TUBE CARCINOMA

This is very uncommon, contributing only 0.3% to all female genital tract malignancies. Its behaviour and management are similar to those of ovarian cancer. The mean age is 55–60 years and the 5-year survival is 55%.

TELLING THE PATIENT SHE HAS GYNAECOLOGICAL CANCER

The fear of cancer is widespread in the population, many people believing that it is a death sentence. If cancer is diagnosed the woman and her family may be devastated. The doctor should understand the patient's fears, and anticipate her possible reaction to the news (anger, distress with crying, silence, etc.).

Before talking with the woman and, if she wishes, her partner or a near relative, the doctor should have the case records, including test results, available. The discussion should take place in a quiet, private room. The information (including providing an honest appraisal of the prognosis) should be given in non-jargon language, and time should be allowed for the information to 'sink in'. The patient's understanding of her condition should be checked in a supportive, empathetic manner, and time given for her to react. If the reaction is anger, the doctor should respond by being sympathetic. If the patient responds by showing shock, or distress or crying, the doctor should let her recover and not try to stop her releasing her emotions. Time should be given for her or her relative to ask questions. Most importantly, the patient should be offered the opportunity for a further talk with the doctor, as she may be so upset by the news that she is unable to ask questions that concern her. She may not remember very much of the information given to her on the first occasion.

PSYCHOLOGICAL IMPLICATIONS OF GYNAECOLOGICAL CANCER

During and after treatment for gynaecological cancer many women become depressed, which may adversely affect their relationship with their partner. Surgery of the genital tract, especially if it involves the vagina or vulva, threatens the woman's identity. Her vagina may be shortened, her vulva mutilated, she may no longer lubricate when sexually stimulated, and she may perceive sexual activity as inappropriate. Her husband may be concerned that sexual intercourse may damage her or lead to his developing cancer. He may find difficulty in accepting his 'mutilated' wife as a sexual partner. Women who have cervical cancer may be concerned that the disease is a result of her or her partner's past sexual behaviour (see pp. 292, 295). These feelings are commonly associated with reduced or absent sexual desire.

Strategies to reduce these psychosexual concerns include preoperative explanations of the effects of surgery or radiotherapy, sexual counselling, and the use of oestrogen vaginal creams, tablets or ovoids when the surgery involves the vagina, or the ovaries are extirpated or irradiated. Sexual explanation and counselling should include discussion about ways other than sexual intercourse they enjoy or could enjoy to obtain sexual pleasure. The counselling session should include both partners and be conducted in a non-threatening environment, with ample time for discussion.

Chapter | 38 |

Uterovaginal displacements, damage and prolapse

UTERINE DISPLACEMENTS

The uterus is an organ that normally pivots about an axis formed by the cardinal ligaments at the level of the internal cervical os. In 90% of women the uterus is anteflexed and anteverted, lying on the urinary bladder and moving backwards as the bladder fills. In 10% of women the uterus is retroflexed and may be retroverted (Fig. 38.1). This is a developmental occurrence. The uterus is mobile and can be moved by inserting a finger in the posterior vaginal fornix. In spite of anecdotal statements, a mobile retroverted uterus is not a cause of infertility, abortion or backache.

Acquired uterine retroversion may occur, but is less common. It is associated with endometriosis of the uterosacral ligaments or the cul-de-sac; with adhesions resulting from pelvic inflammatory disease; or caused by a tumour in front of the uterus pushing it backwards.

Symptoms

Developmental retroversion is symptomless; only when the retroverted uterus is 'fixed' may symptoms occur. These include the symptoms associated with the underlying cause. In addition, the woman may complain of dyspareunia on deep penetration, pelvic pain and low backache. A few women who have chronic pelvic pain and are told by their doctor that their uterus is retroverted, will obtain some relief if the uterus is manipulated to become anteverted. They often remain pain free when the uterus becomes retroverted again, as it usually does.

Diagnosis

A clinical finding that the uterus is retroverted and is accompanied by symptoms should alert the medical practitioner to determine whether the retroversion can be corrected by manipulation (Fig. 38.2). If it can, it is not the cause of the symptoms. If it cannot be manipulated it may be the cause of the symptoms.

Treatment

In most cases the woman needs reassurance that the retroverted uterus is not the cause of any symptoms she may have, and does not require treatment. If the uterus is 'fixed' and the woman has symptoms of deep dyspareunia

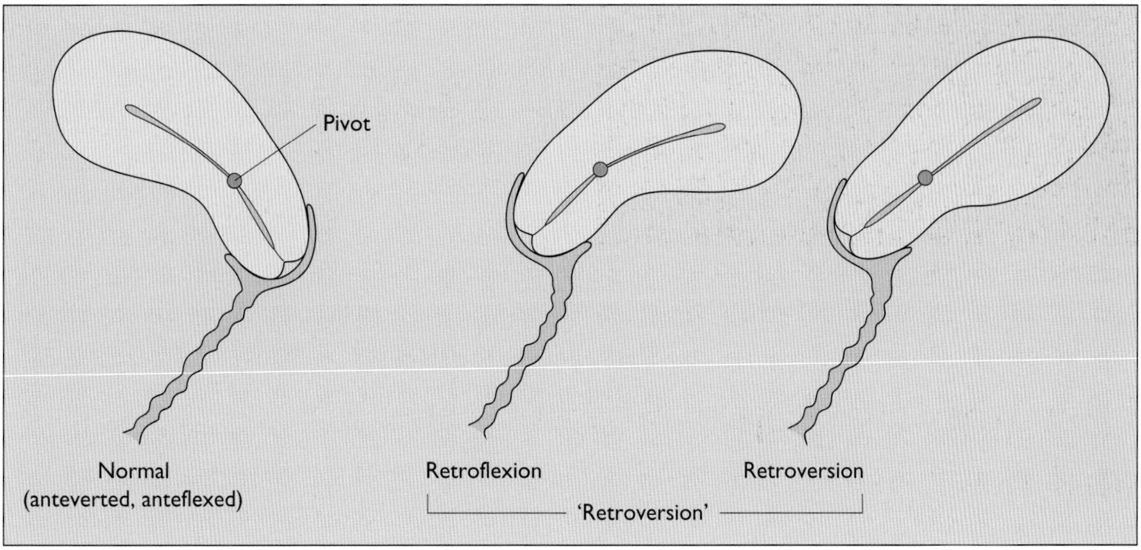

Fig. 38.1 Retroversion and retroflexion of the uterus.

or chronic pelvic pain, surgery may be suggested, but the patient should be told that, although it may correct the position of the uterus, the symptoms may not be relieved permanently. The procedure is aimed at shortening the round ligaments by plication and treating any pelvic pathology at the same time.

UTEROVAGINAL DAMAGE AND INJURIES

Injury to the vulvovaginal area may occur, for example if a girl or woman falls astride some object or is kicked. The vagina may be damaged or a haematoma may form in the vulva (Fig. 38.3). Injury may also occur if a young girl or a postmenopausal woman is sexually assaulted.

During the first sexual intercourse, the hymen is stretched and torn and a small amount of bleeding results; very occasionally more severe bleeding occurs if a large blood vessel is damaged.

Injury resulting from childbirth is discussed on page 81. Occasionally a vaginal tear is not sutured immediately, and the woman attends a medical practitioner some time later. On inspection the vaginal entrance is seen to gape and the perineal muscles are separated (Fig. 38.4). The woman may complain that water enters her vagina when she bathes, or that vaginal flatus occurs.

Vaginal burns may occur following a very hot vaginal douche, or the deliberate insertion of a caustic agent, such as rock salt, to procure an abortion or, in a few cultures, following tightening of the vagina after childbirth to make sexual intercourse more satisfying to the man.

Cervical damage may occur during rough cervical dilatation. The laceration is usually small, but may extend from one or other lateral angle of the external cervical os. This may cause marked bleeding. Cervical damage may also occur during childbirth and is discussed on pages 81, 82.

GENITAL TRACT FISTULAE

Genital tract fistulae occasionally follow childbirth, but in developed countries they usually result from a complication of surgery or following radiotherapy. Fistulae are very uncommon in the developed countries. They may develop between the vagina and uterus and any adjacent organ. The most frequently encountered fistulae lie between the vagina and the bladder (vesicovaginal fistula) or between the vagina and rectum (rectovaginal fistula).

Obstetrical and surgical fistulae occur immediately after the procedure or 5–14 days after the operation, when the traumatized ischaemic tissue sloughs. The woman complains of continuous leakage of urine in cases of a vesicovaginal fistula, or faeces in the case of a rectovaginal fistula. If the fistula is large it can be seen on vaginal inspection with a Sims speculum, the woman lying in the left lateral position. Small fistulae may require tests to pinpoint the damaged area. One such test is shown in Figure 38.5. Small vesicovaginal fistulae may close spontaneously if the bladder is drained continuously for 14 days, but rectovaginal fistulae and larger fistulae require surgery.

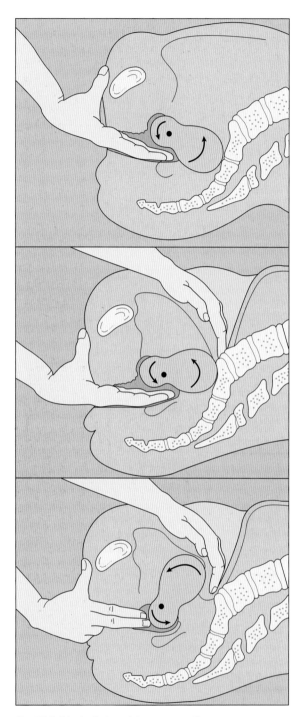

Fig. 38.2 Manipulation of the retroverted uterus.

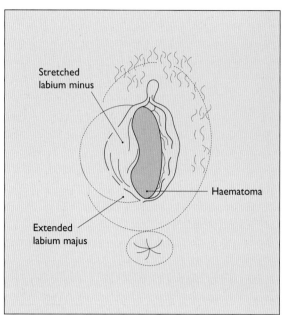

Fig. 38.3 A large vulval haematoma.

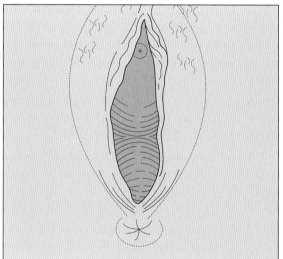

Fig. 38.4 Marked perineal deficiency.

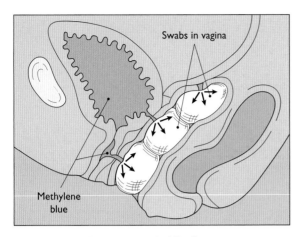

Fig. 38.5 Detecting a vesicovaginal fistula.

UTEROVAGINAL PROLAPSE

Uterovaginal prolapse is defined as a descent of the uterus or vagina. A vaginal prolapse may occur independently of any uterine descent, but a prolapsed uterus always carries some part of the upper vagina with it.

To understand how uterovaginal prolapse occurs some knowledge about the supports of the uterus is required. The uterus is supported in the midpelvis by three structures. These are:

- The vagina, the walls of which lie in apposition and are muscular.
- The transcervical (cardinal) ligaments, which stretch from each pelvic wall and attach to the uterus at the level of the supravaginal cervix. They are not ligaments in the true sense as they are composed of a felted mass of collagenous connective tissue through which blood vessels pass to supply the uterus and bladder (Fig. 38.6). The cardinal ligaments act as the middle support of the uterus and their function can be explained in terms of chicken wire. If the strain is not too great the ligaments have considerable tensile strength, but if the strain is increased or the ligaments are damaged, they stretch (Fig. 38.7). Posteriorly, on each side, condensations of the tissue form the uterosacral ligament.
- The upper supports of the uterus, i.e. the relatively weak round ligaments, which operate mostly by maintaining the uterus in an anteverted position so that the increase in intra-abdominal pressure on straining forces the uterus on to the bladder, rather than directly down towards the vulva.

Acting in conjunction, these supports prevent uterine prolapse (Fig. 38.8). However, this state of affairs may be altered if the supports are stretched during childbirth. This may occur if the woman tries to expel the fetus before

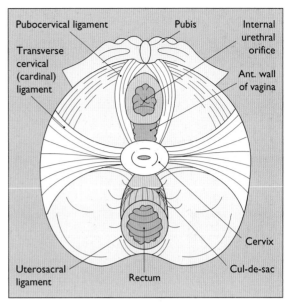

Fig. 38.6 The transverse cervical ligament.

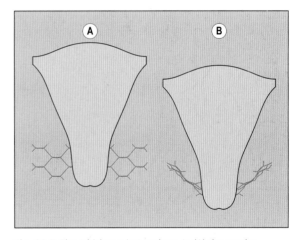

Fig. 38.7 The 'chicken wire' analogy. In (A) the areolar tissue is not stretched; in (B), because of the uterine descent, condensation of the tissue occurs, with the appearance of a ligament.

the cervix is fully dilated, strains for a long time in the second stage of labour, or if undue force is used to expel the placenta. In these circumstances the cardinal ligament may be stretched, making a uterine prolapse more likely. In consequence, prolapse is more common in women who have had several children and are obese.

Uterovaginal prolapse is more common in the later reproductive years and after the menopause. In most cases it is due to damage to the supporting tissues and pudendal nerve damage occurring during childbirth, but is not

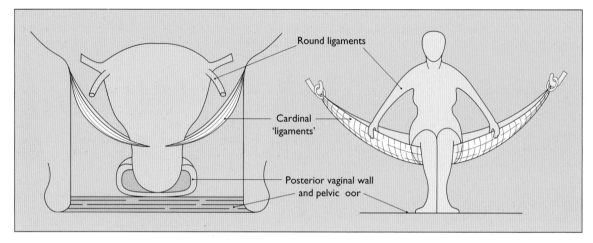

Fig. 38.8 Mechanism of prolapse: if the 'holding apparatus', or the 'supporting apparatus' is stretched, some descent of the uterus, or of the vagina, will occur, particularly if the intra-abdominal pressure is increased.

apparent until the tissues atrophy in middle age when, deprived of oestrogen, the collagen tissue of the ligaments diminishes and the vaginal muscle becomes weaker, permitting the prolapse to occur. An additional cause may be chronic constipation leading to straining.

A further way in which prolapse occurs in a very few nulliparous women is through the supporting tissues failing to develop properly.

Degrees of uterine prolapse

For descriptive purposes uterovaginal prolapse is divided into three degrees of increasing severity (Fig. 38.9). In each of these the cervix elongates and may become congested or oedematous. When the cervix protrudes from the vagina, as in the third degree of prolapse, the cervical epithelium becomes dry and its superficial layers are keratinized.

With better obstetric care the frequency of uterovaginal prolapse is diminishing and severe cases are not so often seen.

Prolapse of the anterior vaginal wall (cystocele)

This occurs during childbirth, when the fibres of the levator ani muscle, which supports the vagina, are stretched. The weakened anterior vaginal wall bulges into the vagina, bringing the adjacent bladder with it (Fig. 38.10).

Prolapse of the posterior vaginal wall (rectocele)

In this situation the supporting tissues of the distal posterior wall, including the perineal muscles, are stretched or damaged during the delivery of the baby.

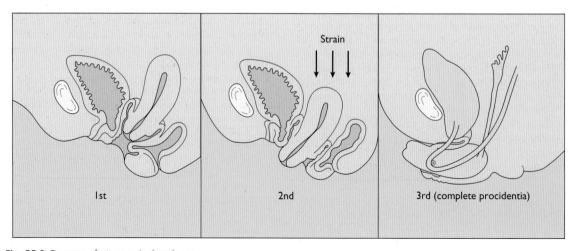

Fig. 38.9 Degrees of uterovaginal prolapse.

With diminished support, the posterior vaginal wall, together with the anterior rectal wall, bulges into the vagina (Fig. 38.11).

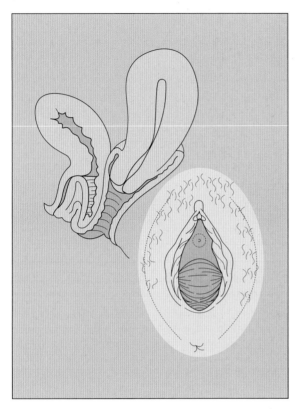

Fig. 38.10 Cystocele.

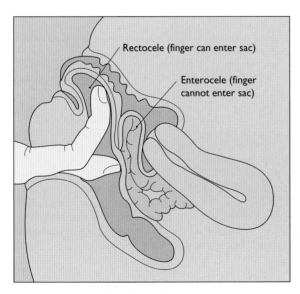

Fig. 38.11 Enterocele and rectocele.

Rectocele (finger can enter sac)

Enterocele (finger cannot enter sac)

If the supports of the proximal vaginal wall are weakened (for example after hysterectomy) it may bulge into the vagina, often containing bowel. This is termed an enterocele.

Symptoms and diagnosis

Many women have no symptoms but are concerned that 'something is bulging in my vagina'. Some women feel dragging pains in the lower pelvis, and have difficulty or discomfort when they try to micturate or defecate. Other women are mildly incontinent.

The type and degree of uterovaginal prolapse can be diagnosed by looking at the woman's vulvovaginal area when she coughs or strains. A vaginal examination using a Sims speculum will confirm the prolapse. A rectal examination may be needed to differentiate a rectocele from an enterocele.

Treatment

Treatment depends on the age of the woman, her desire to have further children, and the degree of the prolapse. Younger women with mild degrees of symptomless prolapse can delay treatment until the prolapse worsens or the menopause is reached. They should be taught pelvic floor exercises (see p. 311), which alone may control the symptoms. It is preferable not to treat a prolapse surgically if the woman wishes to have a further child, as the delivery must then be by caesarean section to avoid damage to the repair. If the woman has a cystocele, a midstream urine sample should be taken to exclude bacteriuria. If the urine is sterile, surgery is not required unless the woman desires it. She should be checked periodically.

If the prolapse is marked and is causing symptoms, surgery can be recommended. There are two choices, which should be discussed with the woman. The first is vaginal hysterectomy and vaginal repair. The second is the Manchester operation, which involves shortening the cervix and the cardinal ligaments and plicating them in front of the shortened cervix (to keep the uterus anteverted), and then performing a vaginal repair. If urinary incontinence is present it should be treated.

Elderly women should be given oestrogen for 4–6 weeks before the operation to improve the quality of the vaginal tissues. Old frail women, or women who decline an operation, may choose to have a polythene ring pessary introduced into the vagina. The size chosen should prevent descent of the vaginal walls or the uterus and be comfortable. The woman should have the pessary removed at intervals for cleaning and then replaced.

The treatment of a cystocele or a rectocele consists of repairing the vagina by excising a triangular piece of the anterior or posterior vaginal wall, depending on whether a cystocele or a rectocele is present, pushing the bladder or rectum proximally, and suturing the supporting muscles beneath it and then rejoining the cut edges of the vagina.

Chapter | **39** |

The urinary tract and its relationship to gynaecology

The close connection of the bladder to the vagina and the short urethra give rise to more problems in a woman's urinary tract than in a man's. The anatomy of the urinary tract is described on page 343. The function of the urinary tract is to permit waste products of metabolism to be removed from the body in the urinary flow. For this reason the mechanics of micturition will be discussed first.

MECHANICS OF VOLUNTARY MICTURITION

The bladder fills as urine trickles down the ureters. To accommodate the urine the bladder distends, and it can accommodate 300–400 mL of urine without any increase in the resting intravesical pressure, which remains below 10 cmH$_2$O. In the resting state the urethrovesical junction is flat and there is an angle of about 90° between the bladder and the urethra (the urethrovesical angle) (Fig. 39.1A).

Continence is maintained because of the inherent tone of the urethra and by the muscles that envelop the urethrovesical junction and the proximal urethra, which keep the intraurethral pressure 7–10 cmH$_2$O higher than the pressure within the bladder.

When more than 350 mL of urine distends the bladder, cholinergic muscarinic stretch receptors in the bladder wall are stimulated. This causes the detrusor muscle to contract and the intravesical pressure rises. Paradoxically, the extension of the detrusor muscle, which surrounds the proximal urethra in a spiral fashion, relaxes, with the result that the intraurethral pressure falls below the intravesical pressure. By the age of 5 most children have learned to inhibit the detrusor contractions and to keep the urethra closed, so that micturition can be delayed until an appropriate time. In some women, this higher centre control cannot be maintained and micturition occurs inappropriately. A second line of defence against involuntary micturition is provided by the muscles forming the external urethral sphincter and the fibres of the pubococcygeal muscle that surround and support the distal urethra.

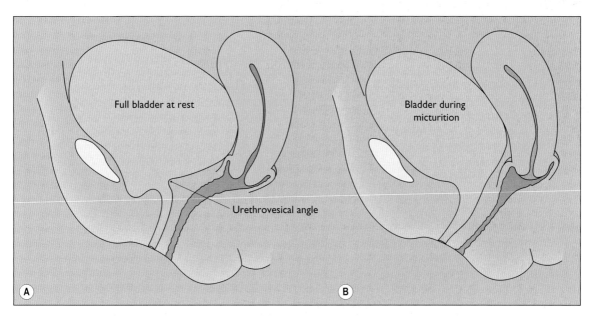

Fig. 39.1 Tracing from radiographs of the bladder and urethra. (A) At rest; (B) during micturition.

When the person is ready to pass urine the detrusor muscle is permitted to contract strongly, which raises the intravesical pressure above the intraurethral pressure. The detrusor contractions also cause funnelling of the bladder base and obliterate the urethrovesical angle (Fig. 39.1B).

At the same time, the person contracts the abdominal muscles, which raises the intravesical pressure further. These changes and the relaxation of the proximal urethral muscle permit urine to pass into the urethra. The person now relaxes the muscles surrounding the distal urethra, and urine is voided until the bladder is empty. When this occurs the detrusor ceases to be stimulated and relaxes, and the urethrovesical angle is restored. The proximal urethra contracts from its distal end to the urethrovesical junction, 'milking' back a few drops of urine into the bladder. Finally, the external sphincter closes.

URINARY INCONTINENCE (INVOLUNTARY MICTURITION)

As women grow older the incidence of urinary incontinence increases, often causing social isolation or psychological problems. In the 35–50-year age group 5% of women are incontinent at least once each week. By the age of 60, 15–20% of women complain of urinary incontinence, and by the age of 80 one woman in four is incontinent.

In women two main and two subsidiary forms of urinary incontinence occur. The two main forms are:

- Urge incontinence
- Urethral sphincter incontinence (genuine stress incontinence).

The two subsidiary forms are:

- Reflex incontinence
- Overflow incontinence.

Of the subsidiary forms, reflex incontinence is an involuntary loss of urine due to abnormal reflex activity in the spinal cord in the absence of a desire to pass urine. Overflow incontinence (urinary retention with overflow) occurs in:

- Motor neurone disease
- Urethral obstruction, which is rare in women
- Cases of chronic bladder distension.

The proportion of women complaining of the two main forms of incontinence is not known. The best estimates are shown in Table 39.1.

Urge incontinence (overactive bladder syndrome)

In this disorder the detrusor muscle contracts involuntarily. There are two categories of urge incontinence. In the first, sensory incontinence, the woman passes urine, not because of involuntary detrusor activity but because it hurts if she does not empty her bladder. The woman has to micturate frequently, often several times at night as well as

Table 39.1 Percentage prevalence of the types of urinary incontinence

TYPE OF INCONTINENCE	AGE (YEARS)	
	<70	>70
Urethral sphincter	50	26
Urge incontinence	20	33
Mixed	30	41

during the day, and may have dysuria. In some cases there is obvious urinary tract infection. In others no evidence of this is found.

In the second category, motor urgency (detrusor instability), the urge to micturate before the bladder is full occurs at variable intervals and variable amounts of urine are voided. This may be accompanied by urinary frequency and incontinence if the woman is unable to reach a toilet. At night she may wet the bed. Pain on micturition is not a feature.

Urethral sphincter incontinence

In urethral sphincter incontinence, involuntary loss of urine occurs when the intravesical pressure exceeds the intraurethral pressure in the absence of detrusor activity. Two defects are thought to be present. The first is that the proximal urethra has been displaced downwards through the urogenital diaphragm. When the abdominal pressure rises, as occurs when a woman sneezes, coughs or is jolted, the pressure is not transmitted to the urethra, with the result that the intravesicular pressure rises although the intraurethral pressure does not. The second mechanism is that, either because of defective development of the urethral supporting muscles or damage to the bladder neck supports during childbirth, when the bladder is at rest its base is funnelled, not flat. This impairs the normal closure mechanism at the urethrovesical junction.

The combined effect of these mechanisms is to increase the intravesical pressure above the intraurethral pressure in the absence of a voluntary pressure increase. This results in a leak of urine into the urethra when only a small increase in intra-abdominal pressure occurs.

Clinical findings

The mechanisms explain the clinical findings, which are that the woman complains that a small amount of urine leaks if she laughs, coughs or jumps. The leak can be confirmed if her doctor asks her to cough when she has a full bladder.

Diagnostic measures to determine the cause of the incontinence

A woman presenting with a complaint of urinary incontinence requires careful examination. The social inconvenience caused by the incontinence should be evaluated. The woman should be asked if she is taking any medications, as some drugs (for example tricyclics, prazosin and lithium) may cause symptoms of urinary incontinence. General medical conditions, such as parkinsonism, multiple sclerosis and diabetic neuropathy, must be looked for and excluded, as should local bladder causes, such as bladder stone or pressure on the bladder from a myoma. The physical examination should include assessment of the perineal reflexes of segments S1–S4, and the anal sphincter tone should be tested. A specimen of midstream urine should be obtained and sent to a laboratory to exclude the possibility of bladder infections.

To try to identify the main (or the only cause) of the incontinence, tests should be arranged.

Pad test

The woman is asked to place a weighed pad (with a waterproof backing) over her vulva. Then she drinks 500 mL of sodium-free liquid over a 15-minute period. For the next 30 minutes she performs a range of activities, such as climbing a flight of stairs, walking, standing up from sitting, and washing her hands under running water. The pad is then removed and weighed again, any weight difference being urinary loss.

Urinary diary

If urge incontinence is suspected, the woman is asked to record her daily fluid intake and output each time she drinks or passes urine.

Urodynamic studies

Because the history gives a poor discrimination between the two main types of incontinence, urodynamic studies are used to provide a definitive diagnosis. This is especially important if a woman has had previous surgery for urinary incontinence. Urge incontinence and urethral sphincter incontinence can coexist, and urodynamic studies allow an assessment of which is dominant and hence whether treatment should be primarily medical or surgical. Inappropriate surgery which obstructs urinary outflow will cause even greater detrusor instability, hence the importance of reaching the right diagnosis before embarking on any form of surgery.

Urodynamic studies measure the change in intravesical and intraurethral pressure as fluid is instilled into the bladder. In urge incontinence the intravesical pressure rises early and the capacity of the bladder is diminished;

in urethral sphincter incontinence the bladder capacity is usually normal and the pressure does not rise until just before capacity is reached.

Treatment

Urge incontinence/overactive bladder syndrome

Several strategies are recommended but the success rate is variable. Behavioural therapy and pelvic floor exercises are helpful. The aim of treatment is to help the woman to increase the time between episodes of micturition, no matter how difficult she finds it. The objective is to retrain her bladder to contain more urine before detrusor activity is stimulated. Considerable support and help, preferably from a trained person, is needed.

Drugs may also be helpful. As detrusor activity is under cholinergic control, anticholinergic drugs are chosen e.g. oxybutynin (2.5–5.0 mg three times a day) or tolterodine 1–2 mg twice a day. Both have been shown to be more effective than non-drug treatments, A number of women cannot take oxybutynin because of the anticholinergic effects of dry mouth, dry skin, blurred vision or constipation. These women may find relief if they take imipramine 10 mg twice a day plus 25 mg nocte. Bladder retraining programmes for urge incontinence have a success rate of 80–90%. Adrenergic agents, such as phenylpropanolamine, are more effective than placebo, but the definitive treatment is still being sought.

Urethral sphincter incontinence

Unless the incontinence is severe, the choice of medical or surgical treatment should be offered to the patient. Obese women should try to reduce their weight, as this has been found to relieve incontinence in some cases. A chronic cough should also be treated. Postmenopausal women need additional treatment, especially if they have recurrent urinary tract symptoms. These symptoms occur because of atrophy of the urethral mucosa. The women should be treated for 2–3 months with an oestrogen vaginal pessary, ovoid or cream, as well as antibiotics if indicated. Pelvic floor exercises should be initiated (Box 39.1). The exercises must be continued for several months. An alternative, which many women may find more convenient, is the use of vaginal cones. Weighted vaginal cones (in sets of five weighing 20–90 g) are purchased. The woman inserts the lightest cone into her vagina. It is kept in by contraction of the levator ani muscle. She progresses from the lightest cone to the heaviest.

These measures effectively relieve urinary sphincter incontinence in up to 60% of affected women. If they fail, or the woman chooses surgery, several surgical approaches are possible. Most gynaecologists prefer an operation that elevates the bladder neck so that it lies within the abdominal pressure zone (Fig. 39.2) and provides support under

---

Box 39.1 Pelvic floor exercises

These exercises help a woman strengthen the muscles which act as a sling to keep the bladder, the genital organs and the rectum in their correct position. She should try to do the exercises at least once a day, for the rest of her life.

At first the exercises may be a little tiring but with perseverance she will find them easy to do. The pelvic floor exercises only take about 2 minutes of each day and relieve urinary problems.

The exercises are easy to learn. No one can detect that a woman is doing them so they may be done in company, when watching TV, while travelling on a bus or in a car while stopped at the 'stop' lights, at work, etc.

The exercises have three components:

1. When she is sitting down the woman should contract the pelvic floor muscles, as if trying to lift the genital organs from the seat. The contraction should be held for a slowly counted 5 seconds. After each contraction relax. Repeat the exercise 10 times.
2. The woman should stand up and contract the pelvic floor muscles as if she were trying to stop the flow of urine midstream, or if she were tightening her vagina. Hold the contraction for 5 seconds, then relax. Repeat the exercise 10 times.
3. Finally do a fast version of the exercise, contracting and relaxing every second, 20 times.

Women can check their progress if they wish and can make sure that they are contracting the right muscles by inserting a finger into the vagina and feeling the strength of the contraction.

If the exercises are followed as described, after a week or two she will be pleased with the improvement of the grip.

---

the urethrovesical junction. One example is shown in Figure 39.3. Another option is tension-free vaginal tape (TVT), which can be inserted under regional or local anaesthesia as a same-day procedure. The operations have similar success rates of over 90% in the immediate post-operative years, but long-term studies show that 6 years after the operation only 75% of women are continent and 15–20% have detrusor instability. Uterovaginal prolapse is increased in some treated women. Whether this is due to the operation or to a general weakness of the uterovaginal supports, which also caused the incontinence, is not known.

Women who are frail or who do not want surgery may be helped by using a bladder-neck support prosthesis. The device has two prongs, which elevate the urethrovaginal junction to its normal anatomic position (Fig. 39.4) without compressing the urethra. The device is removed at intervals for cleaning or if the woman has sexual intercourse. The appropriate size of prosthesis must be fitted by a doctor. A success rate of more than 80% is claimed.

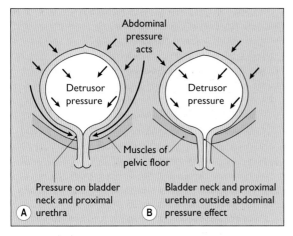

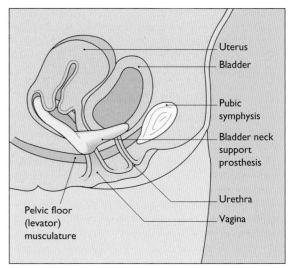

Fig. 39.4 A bladder neck support prosthesis.

Fig. 39.2 The effect of the position of the bladder neck on stress incontinence. In (A) the urethrovesical junction occupies a normal position. An increase in abdominal pressure acts equally on the detrusor pressure and on the bladder neck pressure, with the result that the pressure gradient is maintained and a positive 'closure' pressure is present. In (B) the urethrovesical junction lies outside the effects of abdominal pressure as the junction is below the pelvic floor. An increase in abdominal pressure is transmitted only to the detrusor pressure, which exceeds momentarily the intraurethral pressure. The positive closure pressure is lost and the patient passes a small amount of urine.

URINARY TRACT INFECTION

The short urethra and its intimate relationship with the vagina increases the chance that a woman will develop urinary tract infection. When the woman becomes sexually active, penile thrusting may move bacteria that have colonized the lower urethra upwards to infect the bladder. This may lead to symptomatic infection or to asymptomatic bacteriuria (>100 000 organisms per mL of urine), which affects 3–8% of sexually active women. Provided that the woman empties her bladder regularly the condition is without consequence, but should urinary stasis occur, as in pregnancy, the bacteria may grow in the urine, causing clinical acute infection. Initially, the infection is confined to the bladder, causing cystitis, but may spread either along the ureter or via the lymphatics to infect the kidney, causing pyelonephritis.

Clinical aspects

The symptoms of lower urinary tract infection (UTI) are frequency of micturition and dysuria; if the kidneys are involved, the woman will be febrile and may have rigors and loin pain.

Investigations

The woman should be asked if she has had previous attacks of UTI and whether she has an irritating vaginal discharge which, if present, should be investigated. Her recent sexual activity should be explored and a urethral discharge looked for. A midstream specimen of urine should be obtained and sent for examination and culture.

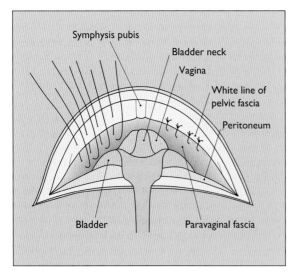

Fig. 39.3 Modified colposuspension (retropubic approach). Sutures are placed between the paravaginal fascia and the ileopectineal ligaments. These sutures elevate the bladder neck. The sutures on the right have been tied; those on the left are ready to be tied. During exertion the intra-abdominal pressure rises and presses the urethra against the symphysis pubis, thus controlling the incontinence.

Treatment

Antibiotics are prescribed. The antibiotic chosen depends on local conditions. Norfloxacin 800 mg in a single dose, or Augmentin, is currently recommended. If the patient has pyelonephritis aggressive treatment is needed. Parenteral cefalexin 1 g, followed by 500 mg 6-hourly, is appropriate therapy.

THE URETHRAL SYNDROME

In this syndrome the woman complains of dysuria, frequency and pain, which usually start 12–36 hours after sexual intercourse. The symptoms last for 1–4 days and recur when sexual intercourse is resumed, although not every time. If the symptoms are severe and recur frequently they can cause a considerable disruption to the relationship, and often sexual frustration.

Investigation includes taking a careful history and examination. Vaginal swabs should be taken, as some women with the syndrome are found to have vaginitis. A midstream specimen of urine is also taken. This either fails to show any bacterial growth, or shows a concentration of bacteria of less than 100 organisms per mL. Some women are cured if they drink 500 mL of water before intercourse, and empty the bladder completely 20–30 minutes after having sex. If this simple measure fails to cure the condition, pelvic floor exercises in combination with antibiotics may be tried.

URETHRAL PROBLEMS

Urethral prolapse

In the acute form, the entire circumference of the urethra suddenly everts and becomes engorged, as the venous return is impeded (Fig. 39.5A). The woman, who is usually elderly, complains of pain, dysuria and frequency. The immediate treatment is to reduce the prolapse and insert a catheter. Surgery may be offered later.

In the chronic form, atrophy of the urethral tissues may permit the external urinary meatus to gape and allow the posterior urethral wall to prolapse (Fig. 39.5B). The prolapse appears as a small red swelling and is painless. If it becomes infected, it becomes larger and painful. Treatment consists of applying an antiseptic ointment and an oestrogen cream. If the symptoms persist, surgery should be suggested.

Urethral caruncle

This is a pedunculated polyp arising from the posterior margin of the urinary meatus (Fig. 39.5C). It is vascular, dull red and tender. The patient complains of pain, frequency and dysuria. Treatment consists of excising the caruncle and cauterizing its bed.

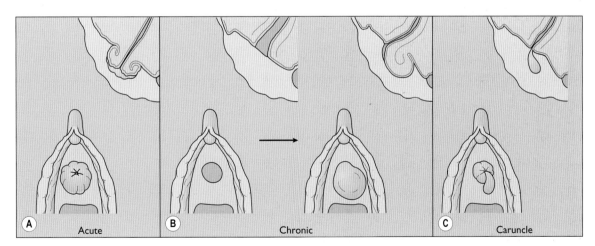

Fig. 39.5 Urethral prolapse and urethral caruncle.

Chapter | **40** |

The breast

The adult breast is of various sizes and is divided into 15–25 lobes, separated from each other by fibrous septa which radiate from the nipple. Each lobe has its own duct system, which terminates in a dilated area beneath the nipple and then opens on to the surface of the nipple as a punctate orifice. Each lobe is divided into lobules, each of which contains 10–100 acini surrounded by fatty tissue, lymphatics and blood vessels.

During the menstrual cycle, the female breast undergoes cyclical changes induced by oestradiol and progesterone. Oestradiol induces growth of the acini and, combined with progesterone in the luteal phase, causes duct development, increased vascular congestion, and fluid transudation into the breast tissues. The result is that in the late luteal phase the breasts are fuller, heavier, and may be painful.

DISORDERS OF SIZE AND SHAPE

Current fashion decrees that to be beautiful a woman's breasts should be large (but not too large), full and well supported. Many women have small breasts and some have breasts that are large and pendulous. A woman who has breasts which she perceives as too small or too large may seek medical aid. In most cases the woman is secreting normal quantities of oestrogen, so oestrogen ointments or creams will not increase breast size nor will any hormone decrease breast size.

Small breasts

The size of the breasts may appear larger if the woman has a good posture and contracts her pectoral muscles. Increase in breast size may be obtained by inserting a shaped 'form' behind the breast tissue and in front of the pectoral muscle, via an incision at the lower margin of the breast. Augmentation mammoplasty should only be undertaken by an experienced cosmetic surgeon.

Large breasts

Large, pendulous breasts not only appear unattractive (or so some women believe) but may cause shoulder pain. Treatment consists of wearing a supporting bra or undergoing a reduction mammoplasty.

BREAST DISEASES

In some women the normal cyclical enlargement of the breasts is exaggerated, with the result that the duct systems increase in size and the breasts become tender and nodular. The change may affect one segment of each breast – usually the upper, outer segment – but may involve all segments.

The condition is termed benign breast disease, which has replaced the previous diagnostic terms of mazoplasia, fibroadenosis and chronic mastitis. Benign breast disease may be localized or diffuse. Its aetiology is not known.

Localized breast disease

This type of breast disease is usually found in women aged 25–45 years and in premenopausal women, when single large cysts are found. The woman has few if any symptoms, but the discovery of the breast lump causes fear of cancer. The breast should be examined carefully, an ultrasound image made and a mammogram arranged. Once cancer has been excluded, treatment is reassurance.

Diffuse breast disease

This form is found most often in women aged 30–50. The symptoms vary from mild discomfort to severe tenderness and pain. They are worse in the luteal phase of the menstrual cycle, but may persist throughout. Palpation of the breasts reveals coarse nodular areas, as if bundles of string were in the breast.

There appears to be a considerable psychological element in the cause of breast tenderness and pain. Many of the women have or have had chronic pelvic pain and premenstrual syndrome (PMS). For this reason, it is often helpful to explore the woman's lifestyle and to talk about relationship problems. As in the management of PMS, it often helps if the woman keeps a daily diary of her symptoms, in terms of type, severity and duration, before any treatment is offered. This is because treatment is not very effective, although some women find relief by wearing a well-fitting bra day and night. There is no clear evidence that a low-fat diet or reducing caffeine intake has any effect and randomized controlled trials have failed to demonstrate any benefit from vitamin B_1 or evening primrose oil. If the tenderness and pain is severe and the above treatments have been tried, the woman may choose to try a hormonal approach. The three agents that have been shown to reduce chronic breast pain are danazol 200 mg daily, tamoxifen 10 mg daily and bromocriptine 2.5–5 mg daily. Of these the one with the least side-effects is the antioestrogen tamoxifen so that it is currently the drug of choice. In one-third of patients neither breast pain nor discomfort is relieved by any of the available treatments. If the pain is severe and debilitating, then mastectomy as a last resort can be considered.

Patients should be given a full, clear explanation of the possibility that treatment will not be successful, and the opportunity to talk with their doctor.

A recent study has found that a woman who has benign breast disease has a slightly increased risk of developing breast cancer in the premenopause. It would be wise to encourage such women to have mammograms regularly from the age of 40.

DUCT ECTASIA

The pain is localized to an area below the areola or an inner quadrant of the breast, may occur at any time during the menstrual cycle, and is increased in cold weather. Flame-shaped shadows may show on mammography. Treatment entails excising the affected wedge-shaped area.

FIBROADENOMA OF THE BREAST

Benign encapsulated tumours may arise in the breasts of women aged less than 30. Fibroadenomas are symptomless and are detected by accident or by breast self-examination. The lump is smooth and very mobile; it has been called a 'breast mouse'. Treatment consists of excision.

THE TIETZE SYNDROME

Some women complain of breast pain which is, in reality, due to an enlarged costochondral junction of one of the ribs, usually the second. The pain is localized, chronic, and not related to the premenstruum. There is no effective treatment.

BREAST CANCER

Breast cancer is the second most common cancer in women, and affects 1 woman in 8 in the USA, usually after the age of 50. Those women at greater risk of developing breast cancer are summarized in Box 40.1. Early

---

Box 40.1 Women at higher risk for breast cancer

Carriers of *BRCA1* and *BRCA2* genes
Two or more close relatives with breast or ovarian cancer
Breast cancer before age 50 years in a close relative
Family history of both breast and ovarian cancer
Male relative with breast cancer
Previous radiotherapy
Lobular carcinoma *in situ* (LCIS)
Extensive mammographic density

---

detection is the only way to control the disease, as by the time the cancer can be palpated easily, spread is likely to have occurred.

For this reason, programmes to persuade women to learn and practise breast self-examination have been developed in many countries (see p. 2). In addition, health authorities recommend that women over 35 have an annual breast examination by a doctor. This should be supplemented by mammography between the ages of 40 and 45, then annually from the age of 50 (Fig. 40.1). Two views should be taken, as this increases the detection of breast cancer and reduces recall rates. About 95% of women who have mammographic and clinical screening will have no evidence of breast cancer, 5% will require further investigation, and 1% will need biopsy to establish or exclude breast cancer. In women at high risk (Box 40.1), MRI has been shown to have a high sensitivity for detection of malignancy particularly in women younger than 40 years.

The aetiology of breast cancer has not been elucidated. A genetic factor exists, as breast cancer tends to be found in families. Three genes, *BRCA1*, *BRCA2* and a mutation of *TP53*, carry a high risk of breast cancer in younger women, although these account for only a small proportion of cases. For women with *BRCA1* mutation the life-time risk of developing breast cancer is between 55–85%, and 16–60% for ovarian cancer. For *BRCA2* the risks are similar for breast cancer but less, 11–27%, for ovarian cancer. Childbearing before the age of 30 seems to be protective.

Treatment

Early breast cancer is best treated by breast-conserving surgery and radiation therapy to the axilla. The effectiveness of adjuvant treatment using chemotherapy or tamoxifen is being studied. A meta-analysis of 145 000 women with early breast cancer has shown that those who received additional treatment following surgery had higher 5-, 10- and 15-year survival rates. For women under the age of 50 adjuvant chemotherapy for 6 months, tamoxifen for 2 years or ovarian ablation had approximately equal efficacy in prolonging survival. The treatments reduced the annual breast cancer death rate by 30%. For women over 50, tamoxifen or chemotherapy increased the survival at 10 years by 12%. Tamoxifen had fewer adverse effects.

More advanced breast carcinoma is treated by modified radical mastectomy or radiotherapy. Survival is increased in postmenopausal women under 70 who have

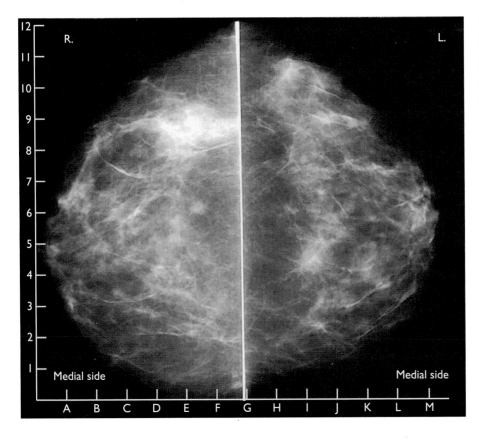

Fig. 40.1
A mammogram of a breast containing a small carcinoma at coordinates E6. A mammogram of a normal breast.

positive lymph nodes and are oestrogen receptor positive, if they are given chemotherapy (including doxorubicin, paclitaxel and cyclophosphamide) initially, followed by tamoxifen for 2–5 years. If the woman is over 70 chemotherapy may be omitted. Women who have positive nodes but are receptor negative should be prescribed chemotherapy, whereas women who have negative nodes but are receptor positive should take tamoxifen for 2–5 years.

These treatments eliminate oestrogen secretion, with the result that the patient is likely to suffer severe menopausal symptoms (hot flushes, dry vagina, bone loss), which may interfere with her social and sexual life. The use of hormone replacement therapy remains controversial. For this reason, each patient should be given sufficient information to enable her to make an informed choice.

For women with the *BRCA1–2* mutations prophylactic mastectomy may be considered although this does not totally remove the risk of developing breast cancer. Bilateral oophorectomy in the premenopausal woman reduces the risk of breast cancer by 50% and ovarian cancer by 80–95%. Selective oestrogen receptor modulators (SERMS) including tamoxifen and raloxifene decreased the risk by 50% but all have significant side-effects which need to be taken into consideration when counselling these women.

Psychosocial and physical aspects of breast cancer

Following breast-conserving surgery or a modified radical mastectomy, the majority of women have no psychiatric or sexual problems, provided a full explanation of the extent of, and problems associated with, surgery has been given by the surgeon. Breast conservation is marginally better in preserving body image and, perhaps, sexual enjoyment. About 25% of women have significant depression or anxiety.

An increasing number of women of premenopausal age are receiving chemotherapy or antioestrogen treatment after surgery, and so menopausal symptoms are causing more problems because of hot flushes and failure of vaginal lubrication. In addition, some women find difficulty in accepting the alopecia, weight changes and pallor that follow chemotherapy. The antioestrogen tamoxifen appears to cause fewer menopausal symptoms, possibly because it has mild oestrogenic effects on the vagina.

Most women, following treatment for breast cancer, are helped if they (and their partners) can talk with an experienced clinician about the problems they may develop. Questions will relate to how each partner sees the woman's body (how to find comfortable ways to have sex, and to use a water-based lubricant to avoid vaginal dryness) and what sexual enjoyment other than sexual intercourse can be experienced by the couple.

Chapter 41

Gynaecological problems in childhood and adolescence

INTERSEX

The first question a mother asks after her baby has been born is 'Is it a boy or a girl?' The answer is given after looking at the infant's genitals, but in two neonates out of 10000 the genital sex is ambiguous and the child is judged as being intersex.

Most neonates with ambiguous genitals are genetically female and have congenital adrenal hyperplasia. A few have an adrenal tumour or drug-induced virilism. In rare cases the neonate is a hermaphrodite, having a testis, an ovary and ambiguous external genitals.

Congenital adrenal hyperplasia (CAH)

This condition affects one in 10000 neonates and is due to a group of enzyme defects which prevent the synthesis of cortisone from progesterone. The lack of circulating cortisone permits the hypothalamus–pituitary to release quantities of corticotrophins, which stimulate the adrenal gland to secrete androgens, with resulting virilization of the external genitals (Fig. 41.1).

The most common enzyme defect is C21-hydroxylase deficiency (found in more than 90% of cases). In three-quarters of cases ambiguous external genitals are the only sign of the condition, but in a quarter of cases aldosterone production is lost and the patient has a salt-losing syndrome.

Any child with ambiguous genitals should be investigated for CAH, by determining the chromosomal sex and by measuring the 17-hydroxyprogesterone level (a level of more than 7 mmol/L confirming the diagnosis) and checking the serum electrolytes. Treatment should be effected urgently or death may supervene from salt loss. The infant is treated with cortisone or one of its derivatives and careful follow-up is essential, but surgical correction of the external genitals should be delayed for 3–4 years.

Other causes of intersex

Other varieties of intersexuality are not diagnosed until after puberty, when menstruation fails to start. They include gonadal dysgenesis (Turner's syndrome), testicular feminization (androgen insensitivity syndrome) and Klinefelter's syndrome (seminiferous tubular dysgenesis).

Gonadal dysgenesis

There are two varieties of this condition, pure gonadal dysgenesis and Turner's syndrome.

Pure gonadal dysgenesis

In this disorder, genital hypoplasia is detected in a girl who has normal breast development. A chromosomal analysis shows a mosaic 46, XO/XX.

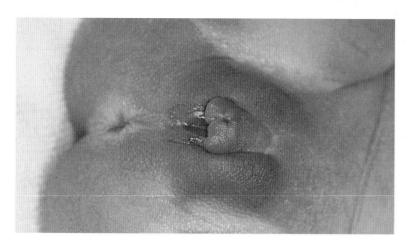

Fig. 41.1 Ambiguous external genitalia due to the adrenogenital syndrome.

Gonadal dysgenesis/Turner's syndrome

Turner's syndrome is caused by the deletion of some or all of the genes on the X chromosome. The classic Turner's syndrome karyotype is 45, X, but the majority have a mosaic pattern with a normal second cell line (e.g. 45, X/46, XX or 45, X/46, XY). The incidence is between 1/2000 and 1/5000 in liveborn infants (99% do not survive to term).

In adolescence the classic features are short stature and arrested or delayed puberty (Fig. 41.2). Only 9% with the 45, X karyotype have a complete spontaneous puberty compared with 40% of those with mosaicism. Spontaneous pregnancy is rare (2%); more likely in the mosaic form, but has been reported in the 45, X variant. The standard management is to administer growth hormone and some women can achieve normal adult height. As most have arrested pubertal development, hormone replacement therapy is carefully introduced to complete feminization over 2–3 years. These women need careful supportive counselling, especially to deal with the sexuality and infertility issues.

Testicular feminization

Physically, the person is female with female external characteristics, including good breast development (Fig. 41.3) and has been reared as a girl. She and her parents are concerned when she fails to menstruate. Examination shows that she has a short vagina, which ends blindly. Her karyotype is 46, XY, as she is genetically male. The gonads are in the abdominal cavity or in a hernial sac. They synthesize testosterone, but the body tissues lack α-reductase enzyme to convert it to di-hydroxytestosterone, and receptor cells in genital tract tissues and skin may be missing. As the testes may become malignant they should be removed and hormonal replacement treatment given.

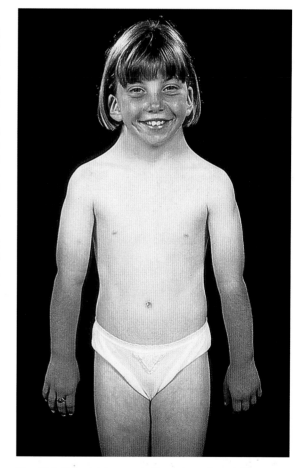

Fig. 41.2 Gonadal dysgenesis (Turner's syndrome). The patient is of short stature and has a 'webbed' neck. Pelvic examination showed a vagina and a rudimentary uterus, but palpable gonads.

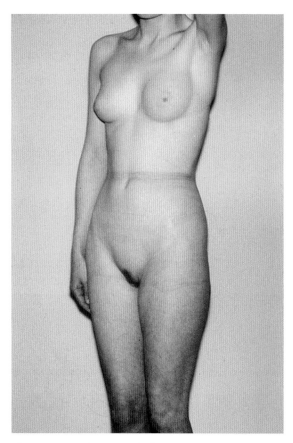

Fig. 41.3 Incomplete testicular feminization.

Klinefelter's syndrome

The person is a tall, phenotypical male whose puberty is delayed and who has a small penis and testes. The chromosome count is 47, XXY or 46, XY/XXY. The person may have a low libido. The young man needs sympathetic support, counselling and encouragement to become more assertive. Testosterone implants may improve his libido.

THE 'GENITAL CRISIS'

In a few female infants, because of tissue sensitivity, maternal oestrogen thickens the vaginal and uterine epithelium. After birth, the oestrogen is withdrawn and the child has a small withdrawal bleed per vaginam, the so-called 'genital crisis'. Similarly, a few female infants may secrete a small amount of watery milk. The parents require assurance.

FUSION OF THE LABIA MINORA

The labia may be seen to be adherent at the neonatal examination, or this may occur when the girl is a toddler. The treatment is to separate the labia with the fingers and for the mother to apply an oestrogen cream to the separated labia for 2–3 weeks to encourage epithelialization.

VULVOVAGINITIS IN PREPUBERTAL CHILDREN

Vulvovaginitis may occur at any age. The child is brought by the mother complaining of an inflamed, tender vulva and, perhaps, a vaginal discharge. The causes are listed in Table 41.1. The vulval area should be inspected and an anal swab taken for pin and thread worms. A swab should be taken from the vagina. If an intravaginal foreign body is suspected and cannot easily be detected the child should be referred to a gynaecologist who deals with children, for examination with a vaginoscope.

Treatment consists of:

- Treating an identified specific cause appropriately
- Encouraging general vulval cleanliness (and the avoidance of soap), followed by careful drying and the wearing of cotton pants day and night.

If the condition persists for more than 2 weeks in spite of these treatments, oestrogen cream may be applied to the vulva and vaginal introitus twice daily for 5 days.

PRECOCIOUS PUBERTY

Precocious puberty indicates that sexual maturation has occurred before the age of 9. Most cases are constitutional in origin, but ovarian or adrenal hormone-secreting tumours must be excluded. The investigations include:

- Full history and physical examination
- Bone age studies

Table 41.1 Vulvovaginitis: causes

			PERCENTAGE
1. Non-specific			60
2. Specific			
a. Bacterial *E. coli*	12	⎤	
N. gonorrhoeae	2	⎬	20
Other	6	⎦	
b. Fungal (*Candida*)			10
c. Protozoal (trichomonad)			5
d. Foreign body			5
e. Helminthic/viral			1

- Ultrasound, CT scan or MRI to exclude an ovarian or an adrenal tumour, and a brain scan.

Management is psychological and endocrine. The girl (and her parents) needs considerable psychological support as she perceives herself as different from her peers and may be teased. If the girl's bone age is advanced she will be taller initially but, as the epiphyses fuse earlier, she will ultimately be shorter than her peers. There is a paucity of high quality evidence about the benefits, particularly long term, of hormonal or drug treatment for precocious puberty.

PHYSICAL CHANGES OF PUBERTY AND EARLY ADOLESCENCE

The endocrinological changes that occur before and after puberty are detailed in Chapter 2. These changes manifest in physical changes (Table 41.2). If they do not parallel, fairly closely, the changes in their peers, some girls become anxious and seek reassurance. Others may develop an eating disorder.

By the age of 17 over 99% of adolescents will have reached menarche. Delay after this age may be constitutional or have a recent cause (Table 41.3). Investigations include:

- A full careful history
- A full physical examination, including a pelvic examination.

Table 41.2 Time of appearance of sexual characteristics in girls

AGE	CHARACTERISTICS
9–10	Growth of bony pelvis begins Fat deposition initiates beginnings of female contour Budding of the nipples
10–11	Budding of the breasts Appearance of pubic hair (androgens are responsible for pubic and axillary hair)
11–13	Growth of internal and external genitalia Glycogen content of the vagina increases; the height of the epithelium increases with change in cell type, and the pH is lowered. Occasionally a vaginal discharge is noted
12–14	Pigmentation of the nipples Growth and rounding of the breasts
13–15	Axillary hair appears Menarche occurs (mean 13 years, range 9–16) Pubic hair increases in amount Acne present in 60% of adolescents
16–18	Cessation of skeletal growth

Table 41.3 Primary amenorrhoea

	PERCENTAGE OF CASES
Gonadal dysgenesis (incl. Turner's syndrome)	45
Congenital absence of uterus or vagina	15
Low body weight (incl. anorexia nervosa and severe malnutrition)	10
Congenital adrenal virilism	5
Testicular feminization	5
Other (incl. hypothyroidism in 4%; systemic disease 4%)	15
Hypogonadotrophic hypogonadism (usually constitutional delayed menarche)	5

The history and examination may indicate special examinations, for example measurement of FSH; imaging of the skull or the pelvic organs; nuclear sex chromatin; laparoscopy. Treatment is discussed in Chapter 28.

MENSTRUAL DISTURBANCES IN ADOLESCENCE

Menstrual disturbances are discussed in Chapter 28. As mentioned, in the first 2 years after the menarche some young women experience oligomenorrhoea, whereas in others menstruation occurs at longer or shorter intervals. Unless the disorder persists, treatment consists of reassuring the young woman that it will settle.

Later in the teenage years dysfunctional uterine bleeding affects a small number of young women. Many of the invasive investigations listed for older women are inappropriate for teenagers. For example, hysteroscopy is invasive and usually not necessary. Treatment using hormones is the main modality, as endometrial ablation and hysterectomy are inappropriate. Hormonal treatment or treatment with NSAIDs, e.g. mefenamic acid, for 3–6 months usually controls the menstrual disturbance, after which reciprocity of the hypothalamopituitary–ovarian axis re-establishes itself, but in 5% of affected adolescents the dysfunctional uterine bleedings recur. If the menstrual disturbance does not resolve quickly with the suggested treatment, a screen for coagulation abnormalities is indicated.

Dysmenorrhoea affects many adolescent women and is considered on page 232.

Chapter | **42** |

The menopause

Menopause means the cessation of menstruation, but the term is commonly used to include the perimenopausal years and the 10 or more years following the cessation of menstruation. The period is more correctly called the climacteric.

From the mean age of 40 (±5) years a woman's ovaries become less receptive to the effects of follicle-stimulating hormone (FSH) and luteinizing hormone (LH), either because the number of receptor-binding sites on each follicle is decreasing or because increasing numbers of follicles are disappearing, or both. The effect is that oestrogen secretion declines and fluctuates and anovulation becomes more frequent. The fluctuations are a major factor in causing the menstrual disturbances that occur in some women in the years preceding the menopause (see Ch. 28). The negative feedback to the hypothalamus and pituitary gland is less effective, with the result that FSH levels begin to rise. The release of FSH is also increased by the falling levels of inhibin secreted by the ovarian follicles.

As the years pass, fewer follicles are left in the ovaries and the level of oestrogen begins to fall more rapidly. When this occurs, FSH levels continue to rise, as do LH levels, reaching a peak in the immediate post-menopause. The high circulating levels of gonadotrophins persist from this time on.

The remaining ovarian follicles become increasingly resistant to the higher FSH levels and oestrogen secretion is reduced still further until oligomenorrhoea, and later, amenorrhoea result. If the amenorrhoea persists for 12 months, with or without menopausal symptoms, the menopause has been reached. If the clinician is doubtful whether the menopause has occurred, it can be confirmed by measuring serum FSH on several occasions. A level of more than 40 IU/L indicates menopause (Table 42.1). The measurement of oestrogen levels is not helpful, as the levels of oestrone, oestradiol and oestriol fluctuate even after the menopause, particularly in the first 12 months. A change in the ratio of oestradiol to oestrone occurs, oestrone becoming the dominant circulating oestrogen. After the menopause, any circulating oestrogen detected is synthesized in the peripheral fat by aromatization of androstenedione, derived mainly from the adrenal cortex, with some from the ovarian stroma.

Table 42.1 Postmenopausal plasma hormone levels measured 1 year after the menopause

FSH (IU/L)	90–110
LH (IU/L)	60–70
Oestradiol (pmol/L)	30–100
Oestrone (pmol/L)	100–150
Total testosterone (nmol/L)	1–3
Free testosterone (pmol/L)	3–9
Dihydrotestosterone (pmol/L)	100–300

CHANGES IN THE GENITAL TRACT AFTER THE MENOPAUSE

The decline in circulating oestrogen after the menopause leads to atrophy of the organs of the genital tract and the breasts (Fig. 42.1). The ovaries, the Fallopian tubes and the uterus become progressively atrophic. In the uterus, the muscle fibres are converted into fibrous tissue and any fibroids present atrophy. The vaginal epithelium becomes thinner and less rugose, and intermediate cells replace superficial cells. The vaginal secretions diminish, as does the vaginal acidity, and pathogenic organisms grow more easily. The urethral mucosa may become atrophic. In some women, urinary symptoms of frequency, dysuria and incontinence result (see Ch. 39). The pelvic floor muscles lose their tone as their blood supply is reduced; relaxation of the muscles increases and uterovaginal prolapse may become evident (Ch. 38). The external genitals slowly become atrophic, and in old age the labia majora may lose their fat, revealing the labia minora.

SYMPTOMS OF THE CLIMACTERIC

The symptoms experienced by menopausal women result from the low levels of oestrogen. The two true menopausal symptoms are hot flushes and the vaginal symptoms of 'burning', dryness and dyspareunia. Not all women experience these symptoms. Studies show that about 25% of women have no symptoms and do not find the menopause disturbing in any way. Thirty-five per cent have mild or moderate symptoms and usually do not visit a doctor. The remaining 40% have severe menopausal symptoms, the severity of which is loosely related to the circulating level of oestradiol, and usually they occur if the level is less than 60 pmol/L.

The hot flushes occurring at night lead to sweating and insomnia, with fatigue the next day. Many other physical and psychological symptoms (such as aching painful joints, headaches, palpitations, dizziness, irritability, lack of concentration, anxiety and depression) are experienced, but most do not depend exclusively, or at all, on oestrogen deprivation.

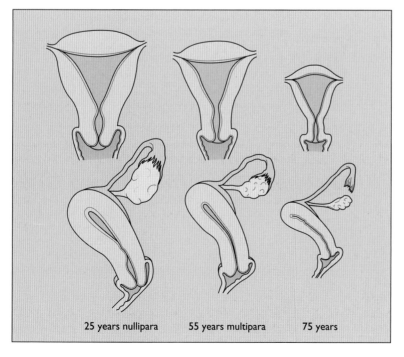

Fig. 42.1 The reduction in size of the uterus in ageing.

25 years nullipara   55 years multipara   75 years

Psychosocial factors are also involved. A woman who complains of severe premenstrual syndrome is more likely to complain of menopausal symptoms as are women who are depressed or have family conflicts.

Hot flushes

During a hot flush (hot flash in the USA) the woman experiences a feeling of heat centred on her face, which spreads to her neck and chest and may become generalized. This is associated with peripheral vasodilatation and a temporary rise in body temperature of 3°C. The cause of the flush is unknown.

Each hot flush lasts for 1–3 minutes and is often accompanied by sweating. Hot flushes may occur many times during the day and night. If they occur at night when the woman is in bed, sweating tends to be profuse and sleep is disturbed; the next day she may feel fatigued.

Hot flushes may begin in the months before the menopause but are worse after it, reaching a peak incidence 1–2 years after the menopause. The hot flushes may persist for a number of years after the menopause.

Vaginal dryness

The vaginal symptoms owing to oestrogen deprivation tend to occur later in the climacteric, if they occur at all. Vaginal dryness and 'burning' are usually reported, but some women experience marked dyspareunia, which may affect their relationship with their partner considerably. Women who have regular sexual intercourse are less likely to develop dyspareunia.

Other symptoms

Urogenital atrophy leads to urinary incontinence and recurrent urinary tract infections (see p. 311). For these conditions vaginal oestrogen therapy is recommended.

Of many other symptoms listed as being 'due' to the menopause, few are. Some menopausal women lose interest in sex, but this may be as much a function of their poor relationship as due to a hormonal deficiency. Contrary to popular belief, depression is no more common in the menopausal years than at other times. As a woman grows older her skin becomes less elastic, particularly if it is photodamaged.

LONG-TERM EFFECTS OF OESTROGEN DEFICIENCY

As well as symptoms occurring at or soon after the menopause, the long-term effects of oestrogen deficiency occur which reduce life expectancy and the quality of life. These are an increased risk of ischaemic heart disease and osteoporosis.

Ischaemic heart disease

At all ages women have a lower mortality from cardiovascular disease than do men, but in the postmenopausal years the gap closes. These observations suggested that oestrogen offers a woman some degree of protection against developing heart disease. There is no current evidence to support this conclusion and HRT does not reduce the incidence.

Osteoporosis

As women and men grow older, there is an increased tendency for their bones to become osteopenic and spinal fractures occur, leading to some symptoms of backache and a reduction in height. Other women sustain fractures of the wrist or hip from falls that would previously have been trivial. These women are likely to have osteoporosis. Postmenopausal women, deprived of oestrogen, develop osteoporosis earlier in life than men, who are protected at least until the age of 75 by circulating testosterone.

PSYCHOLOGICAL SYMPTOMS OF THE CLIMACTERIC

The perception of the menopause as threatening is culture based. In some societies women welcome it, as they are no longer able to bear children, and have greater freedom. In many western cultures, where the stress is on youth, the menopause is often perceived negatively. Relationships with a partner and children may have deteriorated, the woman may be anxious about the future, or she may feel that she is becoming less attractive.

SEXUALITY AFTER THE MENOPAUSE

Sexual desire and drive are unchanged in 60% of postmenopausal women, at least up to the age of 65–70. In 20% of postmenopausal women they are increased and in 20% reduced. The most important influence on a postmenopausal woman's sexuality is the pattern established in the reproductive years: if it was good then it will continue to be good! As men grow older, however, their sexual desire and response changes. The man may desire sex less often, it takes longer to stimulate him, and his erection is less firm and prolonged. Doctors who are consulted about a sexual problem by a postmenopausal woman may have to explain these changes. As women live longer than men, more elderly women have no partner and may seek 'permission' from a doctor if they use self-stimulatory methods to obtain sexual pleasure.

MANAGEMENT OF THE CLIMACTERIC

The management of menopausal women includes:

- Providing an explanation of the changes that are occurring
- Giving advice about nutrition and diet and answering concerns about weight
- Recommending that the woman exercises regularly
- Discussing the benefits and risks of hormone (oestrogen and progestogen) replacement treatment.

Hormone replacement treatment/ therapy (HRT)

Before prescribing HRT the doctor should carry out a general medical check, if this has not been done in the previous year. The physical examination should include an estimation of the body mass index; a breast examination, including a mammogram; a measurement of the blood pressure; and a vaginal examination, including a Pap smear.

There are compelling data which show that for a menopausal woman, small daily doses of an oestrogen, with progestogen added if she has not had a hysterectomy, will:

- Relieve the flushes and vaginal symptoms
- Induce a feeling of wellbeing
- Prevent bone loss and consequently delay the onset of osteoporosis
- Probably improve the thickness of the skin, reduce wrinkles and make the skin less dry.

HRT has not been shown to either prevent dementia including Alzheimer's or reduce the degree of dementia in established sufferers.

Contraindications to the use of HRT

A few women should not use conventional HRT (oestrogen and progestogens). These include women who have a history of a recent thromboembolism, those with acute or chronic liver disease, women who have undiagnosed uterine bleeding, and some who are diabetic, unless they are monitored carefully.

The current evidence is that the benefits of HRT are principally to relieve the symptoms of hot flushes and to prevent osteoporosis. Because of the reports of a modest increase in breast cancer in long-term users of combined oestrogen and progestogen replacement therapy, use for longer than 5 years is not recommended. This risk returns to the same level as non-users soon after cessation of therapy. Oestrogen therapy alone carries a lower risk than combined oestrogen/progesterone preparations.

Treatment choices

There are several choices of oestrogen replacement treatment. The woman may choose, for example, to take a daily oestrogen tablet, to apply an oestrogen transdermal patch every third day, or to use an oestrogenic vaginal ring, which releases very small amounts of oestrogen, to control vaginal symptoms or larger amounts to control menopausal symptoms. The advantage of this method is that the control is in the woman's hands. The dose of oestrogen is adjusted so that the symptoms are relieved. A few women, particularly those who have had a hysterectomy, choose to have an oestradiol implant every 6 months.

If the woman has not had a hysterectomy, unopposed oestrogen treatment increases the risk that she will develop an endometrial carcinoma (from 1 per 1000 women per year to 3–4 per 1000 per year). Women who have retained their uterus should be prescribed a progestogen. The combined oestrogen and progestogen should be taken each day, as 'withdrawal' bleeds occur if the progestogen is stopped.

If the woman's main problem is atrophic vaginitis, oestrogen pessaries or cream may be preferred, at least until the symptoms are relieved.

'Natural therapies' can be helpful for women with very mild symptoms but they are not effective for moderate to severe hot flushes.

Should irregular bleeding, not related to progestogen withdrawal, occur during HRT, the woman should have a transvaginal ultrasound examination of the endometrium. If the endometrium is less than 5 mm thick, endometrial adenocarcinoma is unlikely to be present. If the endometrium is 5 mm or more thick, a hysteroscopic examination of the uterine cavity and an endometrial biopsy (or a curettage) should be made.

Tibolone

Tibolone is a synthetic steroid with weak oestrogenic, progestogenic and androgenic effects. The effects on hot flushes without stimulation of endometrial cells, vaginal dryness, bone density, mood and sexual function are positive. It does carry an increased risk of developing breast cancer but this is less than for combined oestrogen/ progesterone therapies

Selective oestrogen receptor modulators (SERMs)

SERMs are compounds that mimic oestrogen in some tissues and act as an antioestrogen in others. Tamoxifen and raloxifene are used for adjuvant chemotherapy for breast cancer. One treatment regimen is to combine oestrogen, to decrease hot flushes, with a SERM that improves bone and protects against breast and endometrial cancers.

POSTMENOPAUSAL BLEEDING

Irregular vaginal bleeding may also occur in women not taking HRT. The causes are listed in Table 42.2. As 15% of women who have postmenopausal bleeding will be found

Table 42.2 Causes of postmenopausal bleeding (800 reported cases)

	PERCENTAGE
No demonstrable lesion	25
Oestrogen therapy	20
Atrophic vaginitis	15
Endometrial adenocarcinoma	15
Endometrial polyp or hyperplasia	15
Cervical carcinoma	4
Benign cervical lesions (polyps)	4
Ovarian tumour (mostly malignant)	1
Bleeding from urinary tract	1

to have a malignancy, investigations include inspection of the vagina, a Pap smear and an endometrial curettage or biopsy, even if the clinical diagnosis appears to be atrophic vaginitis or a cervical polyp. Treatment depends on the cause.

OSTEOPOROSIS

Osteoporosis is defined as a reduced bone mass per unit volume and, in clinical practice, as the relation to the degree to which bone mineral density is reduced. There are several types of osteoporosis (Box 42.1), but that which concerns women most is postmenopausal osteoporosis. The WHO has provided diagnostic criteria for the categories of osteoporosis (Fig. 42.2).

Osteoporosis is becoming a major health problem for women as they are living longer; with between 30 and 50% of women having an osteoporotic fracture if they live

---

Box 42.1 Classification of osteoporosis

Primary osteoporosis
Postmenopausal
Senile

Secondary osteoporosis
Endocrine: Cushing's syndrome, thyrotoxicosis, hypogonadism, hyperparathyroidism, anorexia nervosa, exercise-induced amenorrhoea
Drugs: corticosteroids, heparin, anticonvulsants

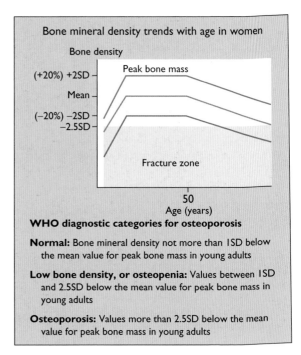

WHO diagnostic categories for osteoporosis

Normal: Bone mineral density not more than 1SD below the mean value for peak bone mass in young adults

Low bone density, or osteopenia: Values between 1SD and 2.5SD below the mean value for peak bone mass in young adults

Osteoporosis: Values more than 2.5SD below the mean value for peak bone mass in young adults

Fig. 42.2 Bone mineral density and osteoporosis.

into their 70s. Up to the age of 70, vertebral fractures leading to collapse of some vertebrae and Colles' fracture of the wrist are the most common types of fracture. After the age of 70 the frequency of hip fractures increases because older women have a greater chance of falling. In Australia, for example, over 10 000 hip fractures in a population of 16 million were reported in 1986, and the number is increasing.

The chance that a woman will develop osteoporosis depends on genetic inheritance, her peak bone mineral density (which is reached between the ages of 15 and 25), and the rate at which she loses bone. Until the age of 40 bone loss is balanced by bone formation; after this about 0.5% of the bone mass is lost annually (Fig. 42.3). Following the menopause, bone loss varies from 1 to 7% a year depending on the individual, averaging 3% a year.

This amount of bone loss continues for 10 years and then reduces to between 0.5 and 1.0% per year.

Clinical features of osteoporosis

The clinical features of vertebral body fractures, producing wedge-shaped vertebrae, are height loss, 'dowager's hump' and backache, which may be severe, and may occur suddenly after bending. However, most vertebral fractures are asymptomatic. In many cases the diagnosis of osteoporosis can be made clinically, but greater accuracy in determining the severity of the disease is obtained if a bone mineral scan is made, preferably using dual-energy X-ray absorptiometry (DEXA).

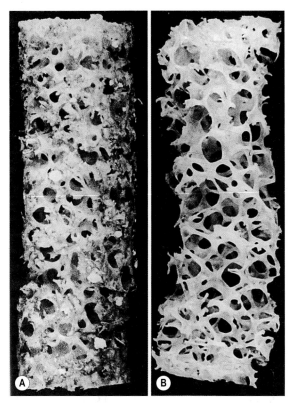

Fig. 42.3 Osteoporosis: bone from the iliac crest of a 20-year-old woman (A) compared with that of a 60-year-old woman (B).

Once osteoporosis has been established, treatment is not particularly effective. The strategy must be to prevent or delay its onset.

Prevention of osteoporosis

Adolescent and young adult women should be persuaded to take at least 800 mg of calcium a day, preferably in food. Two or three servings of milk, cheese or yoghurt will provide this amount, and the teenage woman may thus achieve her peak bone mass. Her doctor should explain that if she chooses low-fat dairy products she will not become fat, a matter of considerable concern to teenagers. Adolescent women should also take regular moderate exercise, and avoid smoking.

Young women who are amenorrhoeic for more than 6 months (for example women who have anorexia nervosa, or who are compulsive exercisers) should be prescribed an oestrogen, the contraceptive pill being a good choice.

A mature woman should take the following measures to try to prevent osteoporosis:

- Take calcium 1–1.5 g a day in food or as a supplement.
- Take regular exercise, such as walking for 30 minutes three times a week.
- Avoid smoking.

A postmenopausal woman with risk factors should also consider starting to take HRT, as oestrogen effectively prevents bone loss. If HRT is contraindicated, or she chooses not to take the hormones, an alternative is to take one of the bisphosphonates and seek specialist help. Before starting this treatment a more accurate prognosis can be obtained if her bone mineral density is measured using DEXA. Depending on the result, she should be advised whether she needs treatment or to wait and repeat the scan 2 years later (see Fig. 42.2). It is unclear whether exercise helps to reduce the rate of bone loss, but it may increase bone strength and reduce the chance of falls.

Established osteoporosis

Once clinical osteoporosis has been diagnosed, either by bone densitometry or following a fracture, treatment is more difficult. Drugs used to treat established osteoporosis act either by preventing bone resorption or by stimulating bone formation. Drugs that prevent bone resorption, such as those used in HRT (which also increases bone formation) and the bisphosphonates such as alendronate, have been shown to reduce the risk of vertebral, wrist and hip fractures in women with established osteoporosis. Calcitonin or calcitriol appears to have beneficial effects in women with corticosteroid-induced osteoporosis, Prevention remains the goal for reducing the adverse health effects of osteoporosis.

Chapter | **43** |

Anatomy of the female genital tract

THE VULVA

The labia majora are two large folds containing sebaceous and sweat glands embedded in adipose and connective tissue and covered by skin (Fig. 43.1). They form the lateral boundaries of the vulval cleft and are the homologues of the scrotum. Anteriorly, they unite in an adipose pad over the symphysis pubis to form the mons veneris. In the adult the mons is covered with hair, which terminates cephalically in a horizontal upper border. Hair also grows on the outer – but not the inner – surface of the labia majora. Posteriorly, the labia majora unite to form the posterior commissure. In childhood the labia majora contain little adipose tissue, and in older age the adipose tissue disappears. At the extremes of life, therefore, the labia majora are relatively small.

The labia minora are flat, delicate folds of skin containing connective tissue and some sebaceous glands, but no adipose tissue. On their medial aspect the keratinized epithelium of the skin changes into poorly keratinized squamous epithelium, containing many sebaceous glands. Anteriorly, the labia minora split into two parts, one passing over the clitoris to form the prepuce of the organ, the other passing beneath to form the homologue of the frenulum of the male. Posteriorly, they fuse to form the fourchette, which is always torn during parturition. In the reproductive years the labia minora are hidden by the labia majora, but in childhood and old age they appear to be more prominent as the labia majora are relatively small. The size of the labia minora varies considerably in different women, but this is of little clinical importance.

The proximal two-thirds of the internal surface of the labia minora and all the tissues internal to them are derived from the endoderm. The distal third of the internal surface of the labia minora and all of the vulva external to this is derived from the ectoderm, and the histology is that of the skin. The junction between the endodermal-derived tissues and the ectodermal-derived tissues is termed Hart's line.

The cleft between the labia minora is called the vestibule, and contains the external urethral meatus and the hymen, which lies just inside and surrounds the vaginal

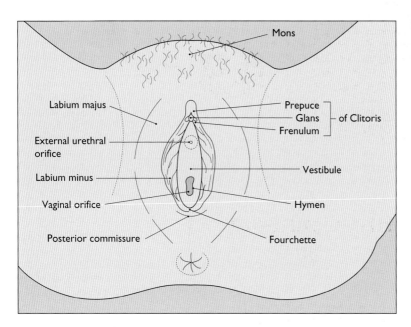

Fig. 43.1 The vulva of a virgin.

orifice. The vestibule is surmounted by the clitoris, which is the homologue of the penis, and is composed of erectile tissue. As with the penis, it becomes enlarged and stiffens during sexual excitement. The clitoris is one of the major erotic zones of the woman. Only the glans and prepuce of the clitoris are normally visible, but the corpus can be palpated along the lower surface of the symphysis pubis as a cord-like structure.

The hymen is a thin, incomplete membrane surrounding the vaginal orifice, and has one or more apertures in it that allow menstrual blood to escape. The apertures are of various shapes and sizes and the hymen varies considerably in elasticity, but is generally torn during a first coitus. An 'intact' hymen is considered a sign of virginity, but this is not reliable as in some cases coitus fails to cause a tear, and in others the hymen may be torn by digital interference. In attempting to make a decision regarding virginity, palpation to feel a circular ridge of hymenal tissue is more accurate than inspection. Although the hymen is relatively avascular, tearing at first coitus may be accompanied by a small amount of bleeding, which ceases rapidly. Childbirth causes a much greater tearing of the hymen, and after parturition only a few tags remain. These are known as carunculae myrtiformes (Fig. 43.2). Just lateral to the hymen, surrounding the vaginal orifice on each side and deep to the bulbocavernosus muscle (the sphincter vaginae), are two collections of erectile tissue – the vestibular bulbs. Embedded in the posterolateral parts of the bulbs on each side is Bartholin's gland (Fig. 43.3), which is the homologue of Cowper's gland in the male. The gland is pea-sized and not palpable unless infected. It is connected to the posterior part of the vestibule, between the hymen and

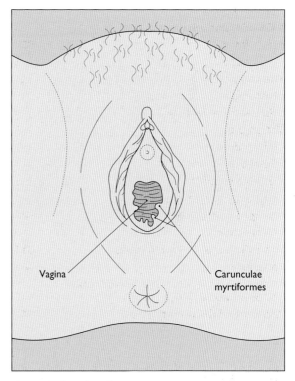

Fig. 43.2 The vulva of a parous woman.

the fourchette, by a duct some 2 cm in length. It is lined by columnar cells, which secrete a mucoid substance during sexual excitement.

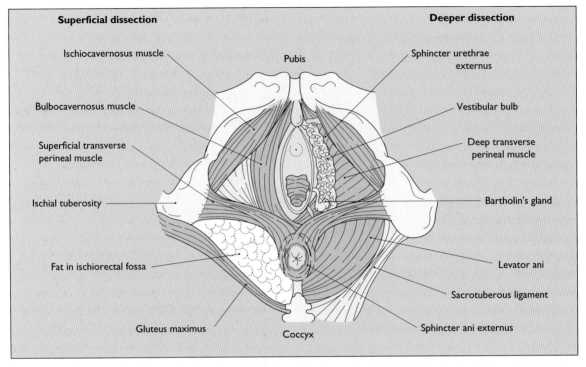

Fig. 43.3 Dissection of the perineum to show the superficial muscles, the position of Bartholin's gland and the vestibular bulb.

Vascular and nerve supply

Arteries

The external genitalia are very vascular and are supplied by branches of the internal pudendal arteries, which originate from the internal iliac arteries, and by the external pudendal arteries, deriving from the femoral arteries (Fig. 8.23).

Veins

The veins of the vulva form large venous plexuses, which become dilated during sexual excitement, and to an even greater degree during pregnancy, when varicosities are not uncommon. Most of the veins accompany the corresponding arteries, but those draining the clitoris join the vaginal and vesical venous plexuses.

Lymphatics

Lymphatic vessels form an interconnecting meshwork which extends through the labia minora, the prepuce, the fourchette and the vaginal introitus. These vessels join to form 'trunks'. The anterior trunks join with a lymphatic meshwork over the mons (which also drains the glans of the clitoris). The anterior collecting trunks pass to reach the ipsilateral and contralateral superficial femoral nodes.

The lymphatics from the labia majora also form trunks and pass to the superficial femoral nodes. There are connections between the superficial and the deep femoral nodes, which then connect with the nodes along the external iliac vessels.

The lymphatics from the clitoral shaft (which interconnect with those of the glans) pass directly to internal iliac nodes in the pelvis (Fig. 43.4). The lymphatics anastomose with those of the opposite side, and consequently bilateral or contralateral involvement is not uncommon in malignant tumours of the vulva. The vulval lymphatics also anastomose with the lymphatics of the lower third of the vagina, which drain into the external iliac nodes.

Nerve supply

The nerve supply of the vulva is described on page 83.

PELVIC FLOOR

The pelvic floor consists of the levator ani group of muscles, which arise on each side of the pelvis, (i) from the posterior surface of the pubis, (ii) from a condensation

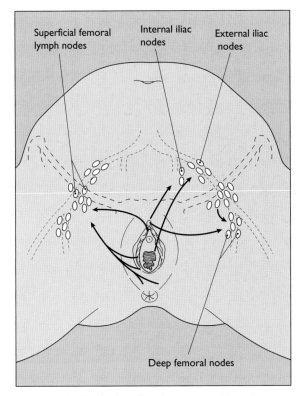

Fig. 43.4 The distribution of the lymphatics of the vulva. Extensive intercommunications exist between the lymphatics of each side.

of fascia (the white line) which covers the obturator internus muscle, and (iii) from the pelvic aspect of the ischial spine (Fig. 43.5). The muscle has several designated parts, the pubococcygeus muscle, the levator ani muscle and the coccygeus muscle (Fig. 43.6). The fibres of these muscles slope downwards and forwards and interdigitate with muscle fibres of the opposite levator ani group to form a muscular sling through which the urethra, the vagina and the rectum pass. The muscles enclosed in fascia form the pelvic diaphragm (Fig. 43.7).

Perineum

The perineum (perineal body) is the tissue that lies distal to the pelvic diaphragm. It is pyramid shaped and is bounded superiorly by the lower surface of the pelvic diaphragm; laterally by the bones and ligaments of the pelvic outlet; and below by the vulva and the anus. It can be subdivided into the urogenital triangle anteriorly and the anal triangle posteriorly by the transverse perineal muscles (Fig. 43.8). The perineum contains a number of superficial muscles, is very vascular and is filled with fatty tissue. Its importance in childbirth is that it is frequently damaged as the fetus is born.

THE VAGINA

The vagina is a fibromuscular sheath extending upwards and backwards from the vestibule, at an angle of about 85° to the horizontal, and parallel with the plane of the pelvic brim when the woman is standing erect (Fig. 43.9). The walls of the vagina, as well as being muscular, contain a well-developed venous plexus. Normally the walls are in apposition, the vagina being a potential cavity and having an H-shape in cross-section in the middle third (Fig. 43.10). In the lower third the widest diameter of the vagina is the anteroposterior, but above this the widest diameter is the transverse. Knowledge of this is important when introducing a vaginal bivalve speculum. Because of the well-developed walls, the lining epithelium tends to be lifted into ridges, or rugae, which run in a circumferential manner from two longitudinal columns running sagittally the length of the anterior and posterior vaginal walls. The formation of rugae in this manner permits the great distension without damage of which the vagina is capable. The length of the anterior vaginal wall is about 7 cm, and its upper end is invaginated by the cervix. Because of this, the posterior vaginal wall, which ends blindly, is about 2 cm longer. The vaginal vault is divided into four areas, which are related to the projecting cervix. These are the shallow anterior fornix, the capacious posterior fornix and the shallow lateral fornices (Fig 43.10). Although the vagina varies considerably in length and width, its functional size is largely determined by the tone in its muscular wall and the contractions of the surrounding muscles. These are under voluntary control. Unless the vagina has been injured or shortened at operation, anatomical variations in size do not cause difficulty or pain (dyspareunia) during coitus; most cases of dyspareunia are psychosomatic in origin.

The vagina is surrounded by several important structures. The anterior wall is in contact with the urethra, to which it is closely bound, and above this with the base of the bladder. Posteriorly, the lower third is separated from the rectum by the complex of muscles and fascia that constitutes the perineal body but, above, is in direct contact with the rectum. The upper one-quarter, including the posterior fornix, is covered by the peritoneum of the uterorectal pouch (pouch of Douglas, or cul-de-sac). The upper third of the lateral walls are in intimate contact with the pelvic connective tissue, and the fornices abut the parametrium, which contains a rich venous plexus. Lying about 1 cm above each lateral fornix are the uterine artery and the ureter (Fig. 43.11). In the middle third the lateral wall blends with the levator ani muscles, which together with the muscular vagina form one of the supports of the uterus. In the lower third the walls are related to the bulbocavernosus muscle, the bulb of the vestibule and Bartholin's glands.

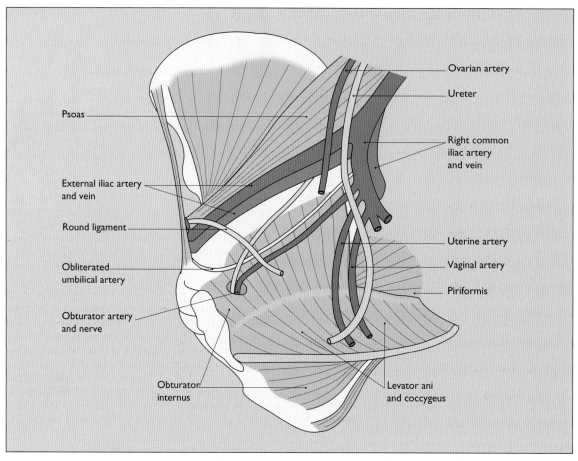

Fig. 43.5 Lateral wall of pelvis.

Fig. 43.6 The muscles that form the pelvic floor, viewed from above.

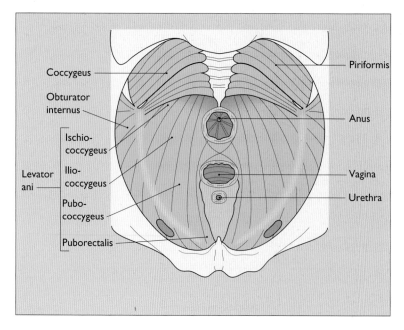

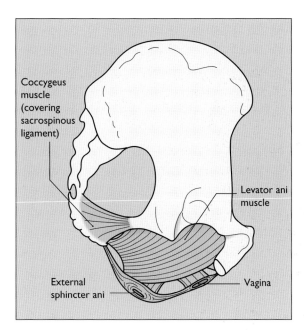

Fig. 43.7 Pelvic diaphragm – lateral view.

Histology

The vagina is lined with stratified, squamous, non-keratinized epithelium, some 10–30 cells deep, which rests upon a basement membrane and is continuous at the upper end with an identical epithelium covering the vaginal portion of the cervix. Should the epithelium be exposed to the dry external atmosphere, keratinization occurs. The cells are all derived by differentiation from the basal cells that lie upon the basement membrane. Three main cell types are described: parabasal, intermediate and superficial. The superficial cells and some intermediate cells contain glycogen. The entire epithelium shows cyclic changes during the menstrual cycle and in pregnancy, and cellular development and differentiation are controlled by the ratio of circulating oestrogens, progesterone and androgens (Fig. 43.12). The cells do not secrete mucus, but secretions seep between the cells to moisten the vagina, and the superficial cells are constantly exfoliated. The exfoliated cells release the contained glycogen, which is acted upon by Döderlein's bacilli, a normal inhabitant of the vagina, to produce lactic acid. This causes the normal acidity of the vagina and explains the relative resistance of the vagina to infection. The vaginal epithelial cells can also absorb drugs, particularly oestrogens.

The epithelium rests upon a connective tissue layer containing elastic tissue, nerves, lymphatics and blood vessels, and external to this are the thick layers of interdigitating muscle fibres, which cross in a spiral manner, the main direction being oblique rather than circular. Outside the muscle is a well-developed sheath of connective tissue, which is condensed anteriorly to form the so-called pubocervical (or vesicovaginal) fascia, and posteriorly to form the rectovaginal fascia. The condensed connective tissue fuses with, and is part of, the visceral layer of the pelvic fascia.

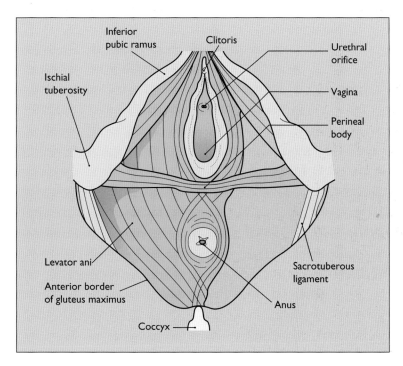

Fig. 43.8 The muscles of the female perineum. In the left half of the diagram the fat pad that fills the space has not been drawn, so as to show the lower surface of the levator ani, which forms the roof of the space.

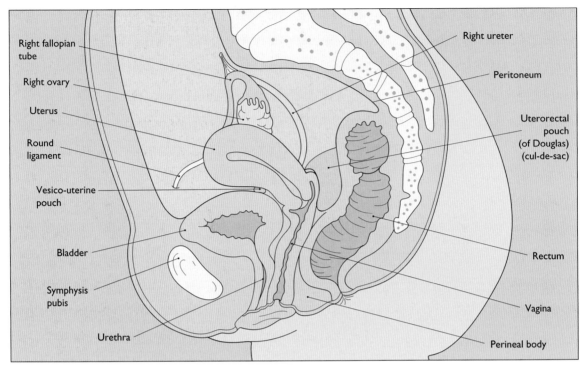

Fig. 43.9 Sagittal section of the pelvis, with the woman in the erect position.

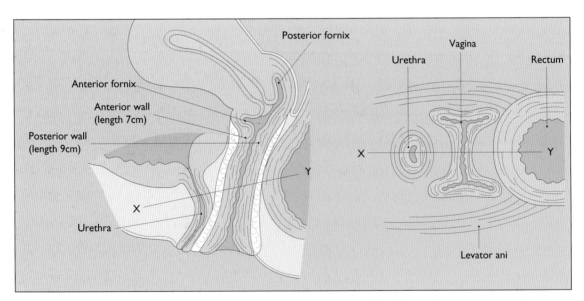

Fig. 43.10 The vagina in cross-section. Note the greater length of the posterior wall and the H-shape on a cross-section. It can be seen that the vaginal walls are normally in apposition.

Vascular connections

The arterial blood supply is from the vaginal and uterine arteries, which are branches of the internal iliac artery and which form a plexus around the vagina. A median artery arises from this plexus on the anterior and on the posterior walls. These are called azygous vaginal arteries (Fig. 43.13). The venous drainage, which goes to the internal iliac veins, is from a rich venous plexus situated on the muscular wall of the vagina, which is especially

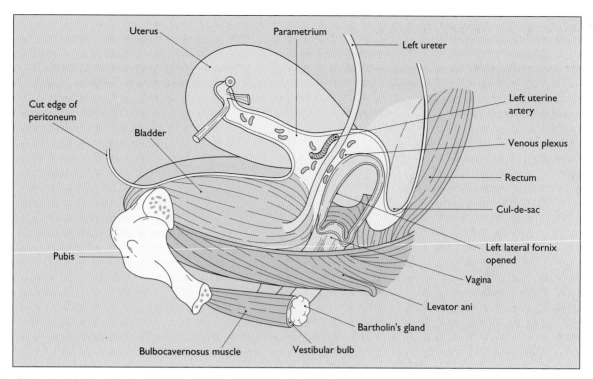

Fig. 43.11 Relationship of the parametrium to the vagina and other pelvic organs.

		Vaginal			
	Oestrogen	Epithelium	Glycogen	pH	Flora
New born	+	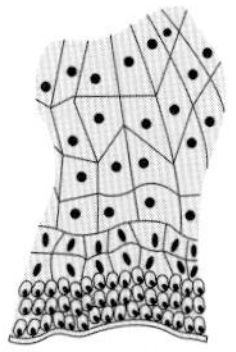	+	Acid 4–5	Sterile ↓ Doderlein's bacilli Secretion abundant
Month-old child	–	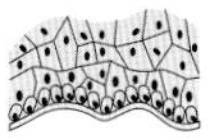	+	Alkaline >7	Sparse, coccal and varied flora. Secretion scant
Puberty	Appears	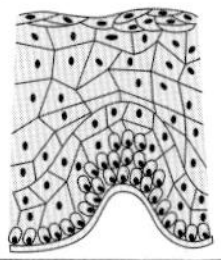	– → +	Alkaline ↓ Acid	Sparse, coccal ↓ Rich bacillary
Mature	+ +	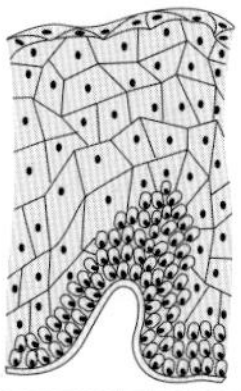	+	Acid 4–5	Doderlein's bacilli Secretion abundant
Post menopause	+ → –	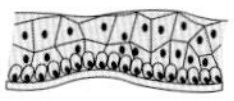	–	Neutral or alkaline 6 to >7	Varied Dependent on level of circulating oestrogen Secretion scant

Fig. 43.12 Cyclic changes in the vagina related to age.

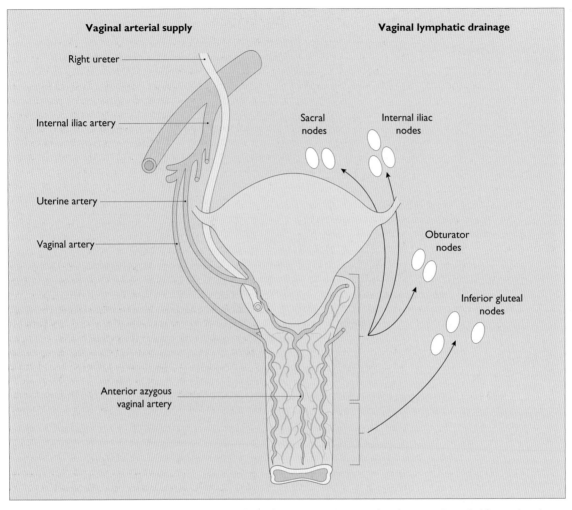

Vaginal arterial supply

Right ureter

Internal iliac artery

Uterine artery

Vaginal artery

Anterior azygous
vaginal artery

Vaginal lymphatic drainage

Sacral
nodes

Internal iliac
nodes

Obturator
nodes

Inferior gluteal
nodes

Fig. 43.13 The vaginal arterial blood supply and lymphatic drainage systems. Note that the uterus is angled forward at about 90° to the vagina, and appears foreshortened.

well developed at the lower end of the vagina and which communicates with the vesical, pudendal and haemorrhoidal venous plexuses.

The lymphatic drainage of the lower third of the vagina is to the inferior gluteal nodes, near the ischial spine. Lymphatics also link with those of the upper vagina. The lymphatic drainage from the upper two-thirds of the vagina passes to the internal iliac, the obturator and the sacral nodes.

THE UTERUS

The uterus is a thick-walled, hollow muscular organ shaped like a pear, its apex forming the cervix, which projects into the vaginal vault (Fig. 43.14). It is located in the middle of the true pelvis, lying between the bladder and the rectum. It is flattened from before backwards, and its muscular anterior and posterior walls bulge into the cavity, the walls thus being in apposition. Viewed from the front, the cavity is triangular in shape. It communicates with the peritoneal cavity via the fallopian tubes (or oviducts) above, and with the exterior via the vaginal tube below. The uterus varies in size, being largest during the reproductive years and in women who have had children. The 'average' uterus of a nulliparous woman measures about 9 cm in length, 6 cm in width at its widest part and 4 cm from before backwards, and weighs 40–60 g. The wall is 1–2 cm thick, and hence the length of the cavity measures about 7 cm. All these dimensions are increased by about 1.5 cm in women who have borne children.

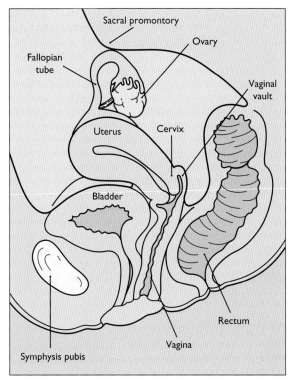

Fig. 43.14 The uterus from the side, showing the anatomical relations.

Structure

Externally the uterus is covered with peritoneum on the anterior and posterior aspects, and this forms the serosal layer. Deep to the serosal layer is the muscle layer, the myometrium, which is composed of three interdigitating layers of muscle. The outer, mainly longitudinal, layer and the inner, mainly circular, layer are poorly developed, and the bulk of the myometrium is formed from the middle layer, which is composed of obliquely interdigitating strands of muscle. Deep to the myometrium is the endometrium, which is a soft layer of variable thickness made up of tubular glands, which dip into a stroma of cells held in a fine meshwork of connective tissue. A well-developed vasculature is derived from the myometrial vessels.

The uterus is made up of a body, or corpus, an isthmus and a cervix (Fig. 43.15). The body is further divided into the area that lies above the insertion of the oviducts, and which is called the fundus. The area where the oviducts join the uterus on each side is termed the cornu. The body (including the fundus) comprises the greater portion of the organ, and is formed of thick bundles of muscle. The isthmus is a constricted annular area about 0.5 cm wide, which lies between the corpus and the cervix. The proportion of muscle begins to diminish in the isthmus, and connective tissue appears in increasing amounts. The constriction at the upper end of the isthmus is called the anatomical internal os, and the line at the lower end, where the endometrium changes into columnar cervical epithelium, is termed the histological internal os.

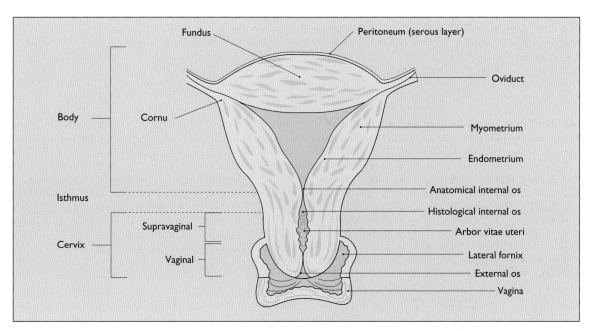

Fig. 43.15 Coronal section of the uterus, showing the cavity and the cornual areas.

On the surface of the uterus the anatomical internal os is marked by the reflection of the peritoneum, which covers the uterus, onto the superior surface of the bladder.

The cervix is fusiform or cylindrical in shape and measures about 3 cm from above downwards, half projecting into the vagina. The proportion of muscle tissue decreases rapidly in the cervix, and in its midportion only 10% of its bulk is made of muscle, the rest being connective tissue. The supravaginal portion of the cervix is surrounded by pelvic fascia, termed the parametrium, except posteriorly, where it is covered with the peritoneum of the uterorectal pouch. The vaginal portion of the cervix is cone shaped and projects into the vagina (see Fig. 43.15). It is covered with stratified squamous epithelium, which joins the columnar epithelium of the cervical canal at or near the external os. The cervical canal is spindle shaped and connects the cavity of the uterus to the vaginal cavity (see Fig. 43.15). The mucous membrane lining the canal is thrown up into anterior and posterior folds, from which circular folds radiate to give the appearance of a tree-trunk and branches. The folds are given the name arbor vitae uteri. The epithelium dips into the underlying stroma in a complicated system of clefts and crypts. The endocervical epithelium consists of columnar cells which secrete mucus, but the quality and quantity of this are under the control of the sex hormones.

Relations

The uterus normally lies bent forward at an angle of 90° to the direction of the vagina, but is freely mobile, rotating about a fulcrum at the level of the supravaginal cervix.

Anteriorly, the uterus is separated from the bladder by the vesicouterine pouch, and posteriorly is in contact with coils of bowel and the omentum. The anterior and posterior surfaces are covered with peritoneum, but its narrow lateral surfaces are in direct contact with the broad ligament and, below, with the connective tissue, venous plexuses, arteries, nerves and the ureter, which make up the substance of the parametrium. The peritoneum, which covers the anterior and posterior walls, joins at the lateral margins of the uterus to form the two leaves of the broad ligaments; and these two sheets of peritoneum remain in close proximity, except where they diverge to accommodate the round ligament (more accurately, the round muscle) and the infundibulopelvic ligament. The broad ligament extends from the lateral uterine border to the pelvic wall. Its upper border is formed by the peritoneum covering the oviduct, and below it merges anteriorly with the peritoneum of the pelvic floor, and posteriorly with the peritoneum covering the rectouterine shelf and the uterosacral ligaments (Fig. 43.16).

Uterine supports

These are discussed more fully in Chapter 38 and only a summary is presented here. The uterus is supported from below by the muscular vagina and the fibres of the levator ani muscles, which interdigitate with the middle third of the muscular vaginal sheath. An additional support of great significance is the collection of connective tissue, muscular-walled blood vessels and areolar tissue that

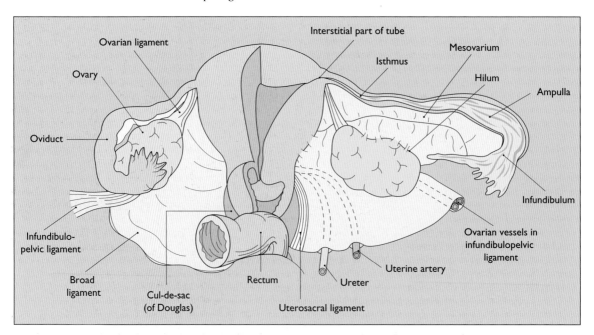

Fig. 43.16 The female pelvic organs viewed from behind. On the left the oviduct and ovary are in the position found in vivo; on the right dissection has been made.

forms a fan-shaped sheet on each side of the supravaginal cervix, and stretches from the fascia lining the pelvic wall to join the fibromuscular cervix. This fan-shaped sheet is condensed posteriorly to form the uterosacral ligaments, and medially to form the cardinal ligament, or the transverse cervical ligament (Fig. 43.17). Anteriorly, the fascia sweeps forward down the anterior wall of the vagina beneath the bladder base. This condensation is called the pubocervical fascia. Laterally, the broad ligament has a steadying effect on the uterus, and the round ligaments play a minor part in keeping the uterus in an anteverted position.

Vascular connections

The uterus is supplied by the uterine arteries, which arise from the internal iliac artery. Each vessel runs forwards and inwards in the base of the broad ligament, and crosses the ureter above it and at right-angles to it ('water under the bridge'), 1 cm lateral to the supravaginal cervix. Each gives off a descending branch which anastomoses with the ascending branches of the vaginal artery, and which supplies the lower cervix; and a circular branch to supply the upper cervix. The main trunk changes direction and passes upwards, coiled and tortuous, between the layers of the broad ligament adjacent to the lateral uterine wall, and supplies branches to the myometrium at intervals. It ends by anastomosing with the ovarian artery (Fig. 43.18). Each branch supplying the uterus divides in the outer muscular layer, to send anterior and

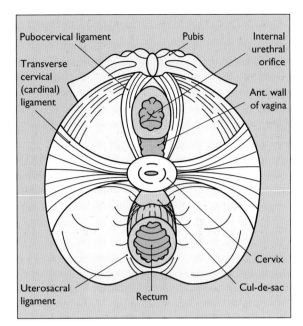

Fig. 43.17 The 'ligaments' of the cervix.

posterior branches to the myometrium, and to anastomose with those from the opposite side. These arteries give off branches at right-angles, which penetrate and supply the myometrium and, entering the endometrium, form the basal arteries.

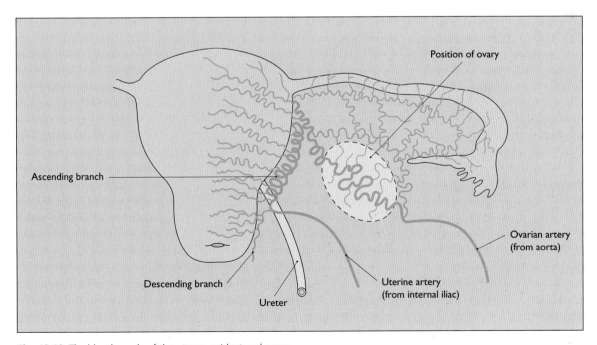

Fig. 43.18 The blood supply of the uterus, oviduct and ovary.

339

The veins of the uterus accompany the uterine artery and form pampiniform plexuses of great complexity, particularly in the parametrium, where they communicate with the veins of the bladder. The pampiniform plexus drains into the uterine vein and the ovarian vein, and has communications with the vertebral plexus of veins.

Lymphatic drainage

The lymphatic drainage of the uterus consists of three communicating networks: the deepest lies in the endometrium, the second lies in the substance of the myometrium, and the superficial network is subperitoneal. The networks form collecting trunks, which pass from the corpus between the layers of the broad ligament along with the ovarian lymphatics. These trunks then pass through the infundibulopelvic fold, and ascend, on the posterior abdominal wall, to join the nodes of the para-aortic group. A few channels pass along the round ligament to the superficial femoral nodes. The lowest two trunks communicate with the collecting trunks from the cervix, which pass through the base of the broad ligament to an inconstant node lateral to the parametrial node, to the nodes along the internal iliac arteries (the internal iliac or hypogastric nodes), and to the obturator nodes anteriorly. A few channels pass backwards along the uterosacral ligaments to the sacral nodes (Fig. 43.19).

Nerve supply

The sensory nerve fibres from the uterus, together with sensory nerve fibres from the upper vagina, pass through the 'felted' plexus of nerve ganglia that lie adjacent to the lateral aspect of the cervix on each side (the juxtacervical, or Frankenhauser's plexus). The sensory fibres then pass to the hypogastric plexus and the lumbar and thoracic chains to reach the spinal cord at T11, T12 and T13.

A few sympathetic nerve fibres derive from the lumbar sympathetic nerves. The function of these nerves seems to be limited to regulating vasodilatation. Uterine activity can continue without interruption in the absence of any nerve connection. Whether parasympathetic nerves supply the uterus has not been determined.

Motor nerves to the uterus leave the spinal cord at T6 and T7. They pass through the hypogastric plexuses and the juxtacervical plexus to reach and spread through the entire uterus. The uterus can contract without motor nerve stimulation, as occurs in labour in paraplegic women.

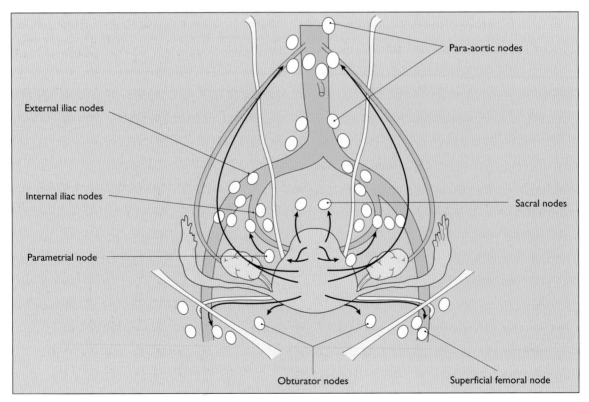

Fig. 43.19 The lymphatic drainage of the female genital organs. For clarity, the lymphatic channels have been omitted and are indicated by arrows.

THE OVIDUCTS OR FALLOPIAN TUBES

The oviducts, or Fallopian tubes, are two small muscular tubes, one on each side, which extend for about 10 cm from the uterine cornua towards the pelvic wall, forming the upper border of the broad ligaments. The outer half of each oviduct lies in contact with the ovary, curving over its superior surface to end in the abdominal ostium. Because the tube is hollow, a direct connection exists between the peritoneal cavity and the uterus. The mucous membrane lining of the tube is thrown up into folds which almost obliterate the lumen, and which are prolonged through the abdominal ostium to form the fimbriae of the tube. The oviduct can be divided into four parts. The infundibulum is the outermost portion of the tube. It includes the trumpet-shaped abdominal ostium, and lies in close proximity to the ovary. The ampulla is the longest segment of the oviduct, is normally rather tortuous, and has a relatively thin dilatable wall. The isthmus is a straight, narrow, relatively thick-walled segment, and the interstitial portion is the short, narrow portion within the uterine wall. The size of the lumen decreases from the infundibular to the interstitial portion, where it is only about 1 mm in diameter, whereas the complexity of the folds in the mucous membrane increases from the interstitial to the infundibular portions (Fig. 43.20).

The mucous membrane is lined with epithelial cells, about half of which are mucus secreting and half ciliated. The mucus secreted into the lumen is propelled towards the uterus by the action of the cilia and by peristaltic movements of the musculature of the tube. The mucus is rich in protein, and may provide nourishment for the fertilized ovum during its passage down the oviduct.

THE OVARY

The two ovaries are the homologues of the testes and are ovoid in shape. Each ovary normally lies in a shallow peritoneal fossa adjacent to the lateral pelvic wall, with its long axis in a vertical plane, but its position is influenced by movements of the uterus and broad ligament (Fig. 43.21). The ovaries have an irregular surface, are pinkish-grey in colour, and vary in size in different women and at different times of the cycle. In the infant, the ovary is a delicate, elongated structure with a smooth, glistening surface. The ovary of a neonate contains little stroma and consists mainly of primordial follicles. As infancy and childhood progress, increasing numbers of follicles degenerate and there is a progressive increase in stromal content, up to puberty. During puberty the ovary enlarges, and in the reproductive period it averages 3.5 cm in length, 2 cm in breadth and 1 cm in thickness, and weighs about 7 g. After the menopause the ovary undergoes rapid regressive changes, becoming wrinkled, white in colour and less than half the size it was in the reproductive era. Each ovary is attached to the posterior leaf of the broad ligament by a fold of peritoneum called the mesovarium, through which pass the ovarian vessels

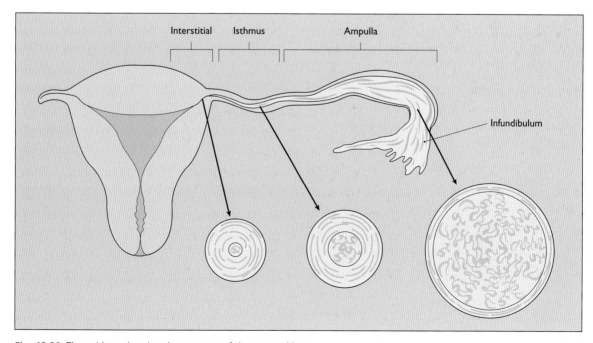

Fig. 43.20 The oviduct, showing the structure of the mucosal layer.

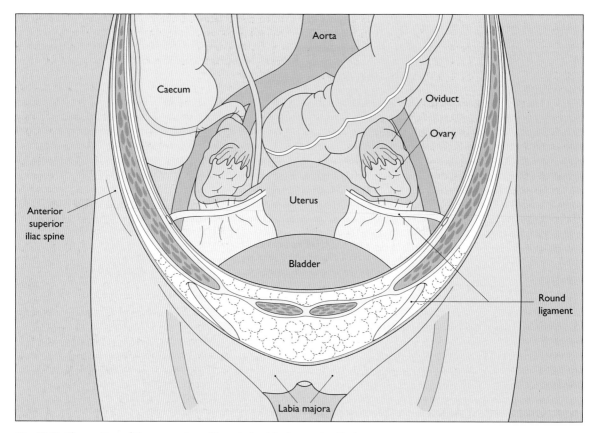

Fig. 43.21 The position of the ovary, viewed from in front in the erect patient.

and nerves (see Fig. 43.16). The peritoneum stops where the mesovarium joins the ovary, and this part of the ovary is called the hilum. The remainder of the ovarian cortex is covered by a single layer of low columnar epithelium under which is a layer of connective tissue called the tunica albuginea. This layer increases in density with increasing age.

Vascular connections and nerve supply of ovary and oviduct

The arterial, venous and lymphatic connections of both ovary and oviduct are similar, and the two organs are often referred to as the adnexae or uterine appendages.

The arterial supply is from the long, slender ovarian artery, a branch of the abdominal aorta, which arises immediately below the renal artery and crosses the inferior vena cava, the ureter and the psoas muscle on the right side, and the left psoas muscle on the left side. The vessel crosses the external iliac artery at the pelvic brim, runs between the two layers of the infundibulopelvic fold and enters the broad ligament. Within the broad ligament it runs 0.5 cm below the tube and gives off branches to the ovary via the mesovarium, and to the oviduct between the layers of the broad ligament. It ends by joining the terminal branch of

the uterine artery to form an arterial arcade. The venous drainage is into a pampiniform plexus, and then to the ovarian veins. The right ovarian vein joins the inferior vena cava, and the left ovarian vein usually enters the left renal vein.

The lymphatics of each adnexa drain to the para-aortic nodes, and there is some evidence of communicating trunks to the contralateral ovary via the subperitoneal lymphatic plexus of the fundus of the uterus.

The nerve supply of the ovary is very well developed, and arises from a sympathetic plexus which surrounds the ovarian vessels in the infundibulopelvic ligament. Its fibres derive from branches of the aortic and renal plexuses. Sensory nerves follow the arteries and are relayed in the spinal cord at the level of the tenth aortic segment. This well-developed nerve supply accounts for the extreme sensitivity of the ovary to squeezing.

ANATOMY OF THE URINARY TRACT

The urethral meatus lies in the anterior part of the vestibule, and the urethra runs upwards and backwards for 4 cm to join the bladder base at an angle. It is intimately connected with the anterior vaginal wall, and a series of small crypts open into its posterior surface in the lowest third. These are known as Skene's tubules and lie between the lateral urethral wall and the vagina. They are homologues of the male prostate, and may become the site of chronic infection.

The bladder is a muscular organ with a considerable capacity for distension. The base is relatively flat, lies parallel with the axis of the vagina, and contains the internal urinary meatus and the orifices of the ureters (Fig. 43.22). The triangular area between these three openings constitutes the trigone. The dome, or fundus, of the bladder varies in shape and position depending upon the degree of distension. It is lined by transitional epithelium, and external to this is the muscular layer. The involuntary muscle that forms the bladder can be divided into two parts, that forming the fundus, which is poorly supplied by autonomic nerves, and that forming the base (the detrusor muscle), which is richly supplied by autonomic nerves. The female urethra is a muscular tube composed of two muscle layers. It is about 4 cm long. The inner layer of muscle is longitudinal and is a direct continuation of the inner longitudinal layer of the detrusor muscle. It is embedded in dense collagen. The outer layer, which is a continuation of the outer layer of the detrusor muscle, is composed of semicircular fibres

which never form a complete ring around the urethra. They loop around the urethra, at various degrees of obliquity, turning back to reach the bladder. Collectively they form a thick muscle layer, which encircles the urethra to form a sphincter.

Elastic tissue, collagen fibres and fascial attachments are intermingled with the involuntary semicircular fibres of the urethral muscle, and with the striated voluntary fibres surrounding the mid-third of the urethra. This complex combination gives the urethra an 'inherent tone', or intraurethral pressure, which is greatest at the mid-third of its length and which is important in maintaining urinary continence.

The voluntary muscle surrounding the mid-third of the urethra is part of the levator ani muscle (the puborectalis muscle), and its contraction cuts off micturition voluntarily. It also contracts to prevent urine leakage in response to the stress of coughing, bearing down, sneezing or heavy lifting. It therefore acts as an external sphincter.

The external sphincter is under the control of the pudendal nerve, whereas the involuntary musculature is mainly under the autonomic control of the parasympathetic (cholinergic) nerves.

How does the urethra resist sudden increases in abdominal pressure? It is now known that as well as contraction of the voluntary external sphincter, the raised

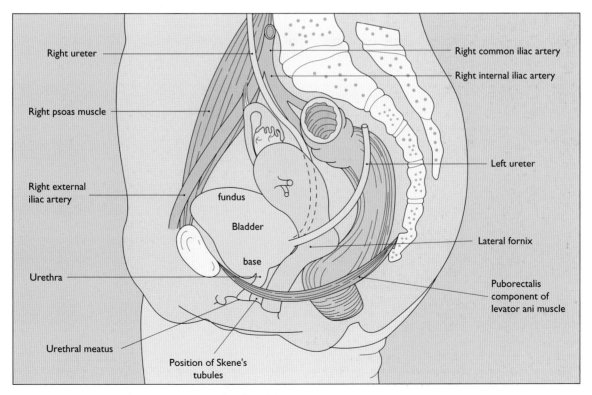

Fig. 43.22 The relations of the urinary tract within the pelvis.

abdominal pressure is transmitted not only to the bladder but also to the proximal urethra, thus increasing the intraurethral pressure as well as the intravesical pressure. This concept is important in understanding stress incontinence.

The ureters pass from the renal pelves, behind the peritoneum, lying on the psoas muscle, to enter the true pelvis anterior to the sacroiliac joint. They are separated from the joint by the ligaments of the joint, the psoas muscle and the common iliac vessels, and enter the pelvis in front of the common iliac artery at its bifurcation into the external and internal branches. Inside the true pelvis, each ureter turns downward and runs on the medial side of the internal iliac artery. In the parametrium, as it courses forward to the bladder, it is crossed by the uterine artery, and lies 1 cm lateral to the supravaginal cervix and 1 cm above the lateral fornix. It passes obliquely through the bladder wall on the posterior aspect of its base, and the ureteric orifices mark the posterior points of the trigone of the bladder (Fig. 43.23). The ureter is lined with transitional epithelium, and the main coats of its wall consist of involuntary muscle, which constantly moves as peristaltic waves pass along it. The obliquity with which the ureter enters the bladder acts as a valve preventing reflux of urine when the bladder is full.

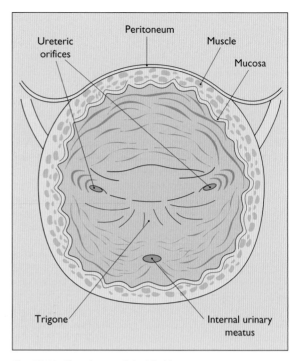

Fig. 43.23 The trigone of the bladder.

Index

Index

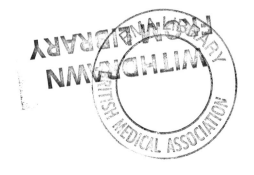